High-Yield
Brain and Behavior

High-Yield Systems
High-Yield Brain and Behavior

Barbara Fadem, PhD
Professor
Department of Psychiatry
University of Medicine and Dentistry of New Jersey
New Jersey Medical School
Newark, New Jersey

Edward A. Monaco III, MD, PhD
Resident
Department of Neurological Surgery
University of Pittsburgh Medical Center
Pittsburgh, Pennsylvania

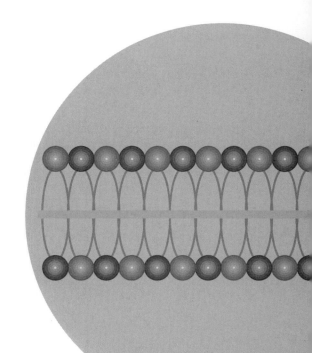

Wolters Kluwer | Lippincott Williams & Wilkins
Health
Philadelphia · Baltimore · New York · London
Buenos Aires · Hong Kong · Sydney · Tokyo

Acquisitions Editor: Crystal Taylor
Managing Editor: Kathleen Scogna
Marketing Manager: Emilie H. Moyer
Production Editor: Julie Montalbano
Designer: Holly Reid McLaughlin
Compositor: Nesbitt Graphics, Inc.
Printer: R.R. Donnelley & Sons—Willard

351 West Camden Street
Baltimore, MD 21201

530 Walnut Street
Philadelphia, PA 19106

The publisher is not responsible (as a matter of product liability, negligence, or otherwise) for any injury resulting from any material contained herein. This publication contains information relating to general principles of medical care that should not be construed as specific instructions for individual patients. Manufacturers' product information and package inserts should be reviewed for current information, including contraindications, dosages, and precautions.

Printed in the United States of America

Library of Congress Cataloging-in-Publication Data

Fadem, Barbara.
  High-yield brain and behavior / Barbara Fadem, Edward A. Monaco.
    p. ; cm. -- (High-yield systems)
  ISBN 978-0-7817-9228-8
  1. Neuropsychology--Examinations, questions, etc. 2. Neuropsychiatry--Examinations, questions, etc.
3. Neurophysiology--Examinations, questions, etc. 4. Psychophysiology--Examinations, questions, etc. I. Monaco, Edward A. II. Title. III. Series.
  [DNLM: 1. Behavior--physiology--Examination Questions. 2. Brain--physiology--Examination Questions. 3. Mental Disorders--Examination Questions. 4. Nervous System Physiology--Examination Questions. 5. Psychophysiology--methods--Examination Questions. WL 18.2 F144h 2008]
  QP360.F33 208
  612.8'2076--dc22

                                                                                2007004138

The publishers have made every effort to trace the copyright holders for borrowed material. If they have inadvertently overlooked any, they will be pleased to make the necessary arrangements at the first opportunity.

To purchase additional copies of this book, call our customer service department at **(800) 638-3030** or fax orders to **(301) 223-2320**. International customers should call **(301) 223-2300**.

Visit Lippincott Williams & Wilkins on the Internet: http://www.LWW.com. Lippincott Williams & Wilkins customer service representatives are available from 8:30 am to 6:00 pm, EST.

07 08 09 10 11
1 2 3 4 5 6 7 8 9 10

Barbara Fadem would like to dedicate this book to Jennifer Fadem Kerr, a beautiful and brilliant spark in life and beyond it.

Edward A. Monaco III would like to dedicate this book to his son, Edward IV, and his wife, Sara.

Preface

Over the past few years, American medical schools have been focused on a systems-based approach to the subject material tested in Step 1 of the United States Licensing Examination (USMLE). The High-Yield Systems series of books is aimed at providing USMLE Step 1–focused material in a systems-based manner.

This volume in the series, *High-Yield Brain and Behavior,* is a systems approach to the subjects of neuroscience and behavioral science. In medical schools, courses that cover this subject material are referred to by names such as Brain and Behavior; Mind, Brain, and Behavior; and Behavioral Neuroscience. *High-Yield Brain and Behavior.* is, to our knowledge, the first review book to address this combined course material in a USMLE-focused outline format.

The book is divided into four major sections. The first section, "Development of the Brain and Behavior," covers the maturation of the nervous system throughout life and neuropsychiatric disorders associated with different life stages. The second section, "Adult Brain and Behavior," focuses on the anatomy of the adult nervous system and the neuroanatomy and biochemistry of behavior. The third section, "Factors Influencing Patient Behavior," addresses biopsychosocial variables in behavior, such as aggression, substance abuse, and sleep as well as the doctor–patient relationship. In the fourth section neurologic and psychiatric disorders and their treatment are discussed.

Because many Step 1 questions require students to identify specific clinical problems and syndromes from brief descriptions, we have used the concept of the patient snapshot—designated by the icon at left—to provide memorable clinical portraits of patients throughout the book. The quick-access tables and diagrams also provide bites of information necessary for mastery of the important USMLE Step 1 milestone in medical education.

Acknowledgments

The authors would like to thank Kathleen Scogna and the staff at Lippincott Williams & Wilkins (LWW) for their support and assistance with this book. We are grateful also to the reviewers for their helpful suggestions and comments. We also thank Betty Sun at LWW and Dr. Ronald Dudek who conceived the High-Yield Systems series, and Dr. James Fix for the use of material from *High-Yield Neuroanatomy*.

Dr. Monaco would like to thank his partner in this endeavor, Dr. Fadem, for sharing with him her talent and insight as an author.

Contents

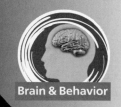
Chapter **1**

Conception Through Adolescence

I. Early Development of the Nervous System

The human nervous system consists of the central nervous system (CNS) (brain and spinal cord) and the peripheral nervous system (PNS) (sensory [afferent] neurons, motor [efferent] neurons, and autonomic neurons). The embryonic structures that give rise to the CNS and PNS are the neural tube and neural crest, respectively.

Patient Snapshot 1-1

The results of amniocentesis on a 39-year-old patient at 16 weeks' gestation reveal an elevated level of α-fetoprotein (AFP). A sonogram indicates that the female fetus has anencephaly (failure of the rostral end of the neural tube to close), resulting in total absence of the cranial vault and cerebral hemispheres. Given the severe nature of the defect and the poor prognosis for survival of the fetus, the patient and her partner elect to terminate the pregnancy.

A. Neural tube and neural crest derivatives
1. The **neural tube** develops into the CNS (Fig. 1-1).
    a. During the 3rd week of development, the ectoderm (the outermost embryonic cell layer, which gives rise to the entire nervous system) on the dorsal surface of the embryo thickens and forms the **neural plate.**
        i. A longitudinal **neural groove** develops within the neural plate.
        ii. As the groove deepens, it is bounded on each side by **neural folds.**
        iii. With further invagination, the neural folds fuse to form the **neural tube.** This fusion begins near the midpoint of the groove and extends cranially and caudally.
        iv. Neural tube closure is complete by 28 days gestation.
    b. Within the brainstem and spinal cord:
        i. The **sulcus limitans** is a longitudinal groove that serves as a landmark within the developing neural tube between ventral and dorsal structures.
        ii. The **alar plate,** the region dorsal to the sulcus limitans, becomes the sensory neurons.
        iii. The **basal plate,** the region ventral to the sulcus limitans, gives rise to the motor neurons (Fig. 1-2).
2. Cellular proliferation along the cranial end of the neural tube produces **three primary vesicles** (forebrain, midbrain, and hindbrain vesicles), which then develop

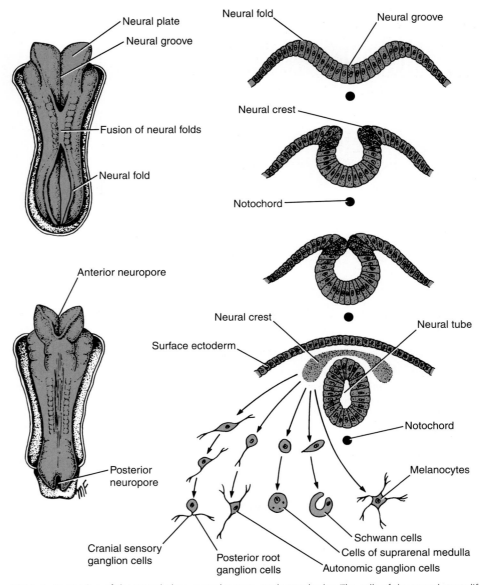

FIG 1-1. Formation of the neural plate, neural groove, and neural tube. The cells of the neural crest differentiate into posterior root ganglia cells, sensory ganglia of cranial nerves, autonomic ganglia, neurilemmal cells (Schwann cells), suprarenal medulla cells, and melanocytes. [Reprinted with permission from Snell R. Clinical Neuroanatomy, 6th ed. Baltimore, Lippincott Williams & Wilkins, 2005:499.]

        into **five secondary vesicles: telencephalon, diencephalon, mesencephalon, metencephalon,** and **myelencephalon** (Fig. 1-3; Table 1-1).

3. **α-Fetoprotein** is plasma protein found in both amniotic fluid and maternal serum. There are also high levels of AFP in fetal blood. AFP is produced by the fetal liver, gastrointestinal tract, and yolk sac. Tests to detect the AFP level can be used as indicators of the presence of a neural tube defect, such as spina bifida or anencephaly (failure of the brain to form).

    a. Typically, in the presence of an open neural tube defect, the level of AFP in the amniotic fluid and maternal serum is elevated. This is the result of leakage of AFP across the exposed open membranes of the open neural tube and then into the amniotic fluid.

    b. Conversely, AFP levels are reduced in mothers of fetuses with **Down syndrome.** Immaturity of the fetal and placental structures that synthesize AFP is believed to be the cause of this phenomenon.

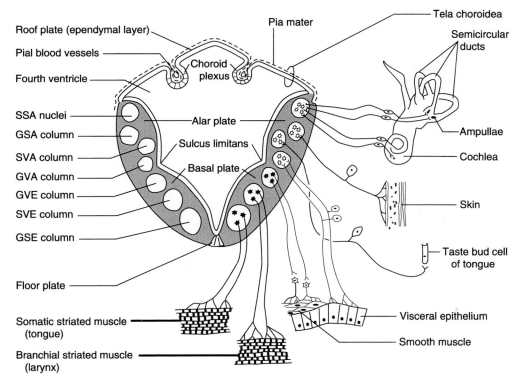

FIG 1-2. The brainstem showing the cell columns derived from the alar and basal plates. The seven cranial nerve modalities are shown. *GSA,* general somatic afferent; *GSE,* general somatic efferent; *GVA,* general visceral afferent; *GVE,* general visceral efferent; *SSA,* special somatic afferent; *SVA,* special visceral afferent; *SVE,* special visceral efferent. [Reprinted with permission from Fix J. High-Yield Neuroanatomy, 3rd ed. Baltimore, Lippincott Williams & Wilkins, 2004:25; adapted with permission from Patten BM. Human Embryology, 3rd ed. New York, McGraw Hill, 1969:298.]

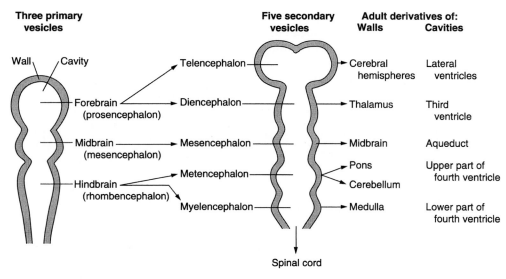

FIG 1-3. The brain vesicles indicating the adult derivatives of their walls and cavities. [Reprinted with permission from Fix J. High-Yield Neuroanatomy, 3rd ed. Baltimore, Lippincott Williams & Wilkins, 2004:25; used with permission from Moore KL. The Developing Human: Clinically Oriented Embryology, 4th ed. Philadelphia, Saunders, 1988:380.]

TABLE 1-1	THE PRIMARY DIVISIONS OF THE DEVELOPING BRAIN		
Primary Vesicle	**Primary Division**	**Subdivision (Secondary Vesicle)**	**Adult Structures**
Forebrain vesicle	Prosencephalon (forebrain)	Telencephalon	Cerebral hemispheres
			Basal ganglia
			Hippocampus
		Diencephalon	Thalamus
			Hypothalamus
			Pineal body
			Infundibulum
Midbrain vesicle	Mesencephalon (midbrain)	Mesencephalon	Tectum
			Tegmentum
			Crus cerebri
Hindbrain vesicle	Rhombencephalon (hindbrain)	Metencephalon	Pons
			Cerebellum
		Myelencephalon	Medulla oblongata

4. The **neural crest** is formed from the cells forming the lateral margin of the neural plate (Fig. 1-1).
   a. These cells are not incorporated in the neural tube and form a strip of cells that lies between the neural tube and the covering ectoderm.
   b. These cells migrate ventrolaterally and ultimately give rise to the **PNS.**
      i. The PNS consists of peripheral nerves, sensory and autonomic ganglia, and other cell groups.
      ii. The other cell groups include pseudounipolar ganglion cells of the spinal and cranial nerves, Schwann cells, multipolar autonomic ganglion cells, leptomeninges, chromaffin cells, melanocytes, odontoblasts, and the aorticopulmonary septum of the heart.

B. **Neuroanatomic changes associated with stage of life.** The brain changes dramatically throughout the life span of the human organism. Although these changes are discussed here in the context of distinct phases of life, it is important to remember that they occur throughout life.

II. Infants, Toddlers, and Preschoolers (0–6 Years)

Patient Snapshot 1-2

When a physician conducts a checkup on a 3-year-old boy and interviews the boy's mother, the physician finds that the child can ride a tricycle, can copy a circle, engages in parallel play with other children, and has about a 50-word vocabulary. The mother can understand these words, but the doctor has difficulty understanding the child's speech. The doctor concludes that while the child's motor skills and social characteristics are normal for his age, the boy is delayed in speech. By 3 years of age, the child should be speaking about 900 words and using complete sentences. His speech should also be understandable to people other than family members. Because one of the most important reasons for delayed speech in a child who is otherwise normal is a hearing problem, the physician should arrange to have the child's hearing tested as soon as possible.

In normal children, age-related attainment of motor, social, and cognitive skills is closely associated with the development of specific neurologic structures and connections (Table 1-2). The attainment of these skills also varies with factors such as the nature of the social environment and innate differences among children in responsiveness to that environment (temperament).

A. Maturation of the central nervous system. The essence of the childhood and adolescent periods is maturation of the brain to its adult state. This involves several structural changes.

1. **Myelination**
   a. The process of **myelination** is already well under way at the time of birth.
   b. The brain becomes myelinated in a stereotypic pattern, from **inferior** to **superior** and from **posterior** to **anterior.** Said another way, the brainstem and cerebellum are the **first** structures to become myelinated, later followed by the cerebral hemispheres.
   c. As myelination progresses throughout adolescence and into early adulthood, the ratio of **white matter to gray matter** increases.

2. **Increased ratio of white to gray matter volume**
   a. This is particularly striking in the **frontal** and **parietal** lobes
   b. It's positively correlated with improvement in **cognitive abilities**

3. The number of **synapses** does not remain static during development.
   a. The **addition of synapses** begins in the third trimester of pregnancy and continues through the first few years of life.
   b. The number of synapses appears to peak between 2 and 7 years of age.
   c. The subsequent decrease in **synaptic density** of many brain regions during puberty and adolescence reflects the **pruning** process, which reduces the overexuberant production of synapses created during organogenesis (Fig. 1–4).

4. **Brain weight** significantly increases during the first 5–10 years of life. It continues to increase through to the early 20s, but at a much slower pace.

B. Temperament and brain development

1. **Temperamental differences in children.** Early research showed that during infancy children tend to fall into one of three categories with respect to temperamental traits such as **activity level, reactivity to stimuli, reactions to people, mood,** and **attention span.** These temperamental traits are primarily a function of genetic and other biologic factors and remain quite stable for at least the first 25 years of life.
   a. **Easy** children are adaptable to change, show regular eating and sleeping patterns, and have a positive mood.
   b. **Difficult** children show the opposite of the traits of easy children.
   c. Although they show the traits of difficult children at first, children that are **slow to warm up** show improvement and adaptation as their experience with social contact increases.

2. Although temperament has a biologic basis, life experience can alter brain development and ultimately affect neurologic functioning.
   a. **Blocking exposure to sensory input** can alter the growth of dendrites and synapses. For example, limiting visual input in a young infant can affect development of the visual cortex and, if not corrected early, can permanently limit the child's ability to see (e.g., amblyopia).
   b. **Intellectual stimulation** can also affect brain growth. Young laboratory animals exposed to stimulating complex environments show **greater dendritic branching** and **increased synaptic density** in the neocortex than animals reared under ordinary laboratory circumstances.
   c. **Social or emotional deprivation** can also affect brain development. Neuroimaging studies indicate that children aged 7–13 years living in some

TABLE 1-2	MOTOR/PHYSICAL, SOCIAL, VERBAL/COGNITIVE DEVELOPMENT AND NEUROLOGIC ASSOCIATIONS			
	Milestones			
Age	**Motor/Physical**	**Social**	**Verbal/Cognitive**	**Neurologic Associations**
1–3 months	Lifts head when lying prone Follows objects with eyes	Is comforted by hearing a voice or being picked up Smiles in response to human face (social smile)	Shows different cries for hunger or discomfort Vocalizes in response to human attention	Connections between major brain structures are organized Rapid synaptic production Start of maturation of neuropeptide signaling systems
6 months	Turns over Reaches for objects Grasps with entire hand (raking)	Forms attachment to primary caregiver	Recognizes familiar people Repeats single sounds over and over (babbles)	Increase in size of primary motor and sensory cortices Continued synaptic production Continued maturation of neuropeptide signaling systems
8–10 months	Sits unassisted Crawls on hands and knees Pulls up to stand Transfers toys from hand to hand Picks up toys and food using pincer (thumb and forefinger) grasp	Shows stranger anxiety Plays social games (e.g., peek-a-boo)	Imitates sounds Uses gestures Responds to own name Responds to simple instructions	Spurt in synaptic density in frontal area and concurrent increase in connections to other brain regions
1.5–2 years	Stacks 3–6 blocks Climbs stairs one foot at a time Scribbles on paper Feeds self with utensil	Moves away from and then returns to mother for reassurance (rapprochement) Shows separation anxiety Shows negativity (e.g., says no)	Uses 10–250 words in one- or two-word sentences Shows object permanence Says own name Names body parts and familiar objects	Peak formation of brain association circuitry Brain 75% of adult weight Myelinization of brain continues
3–4 years	Rides tricycle Climbs stairs using alternate feet Copies circle and cross Stacks 9 blocks Uses scissors Is toilet trained Dresses independently Grooms self (e.g., brushes teeth)	Has a sense of self as male or female (gender identity) Comfortably spends part of day away from mother Plays alongside but not with another child (parallel play: ages 2–4) Engages in role playing May have imaginary companions Has curiosity about sex differences (e.g., plays doctor with other children) Has nightmares and transient phobias Has over concern	Uses about 900 words in speech Understands about 3500 words Identifies colors Speaks in complete sentences (e.g., "I can do it myself") and shows verbal self-expression Comprehends and uses prepositions (e.g., under, above)	Increased size of Broca and Wernicke areas Increased growth in interhemispheric connections in language regions Increase in synaptic density (see Fig. 1-4)

TABLE 1-2	MOTOR/PHYSICAL, SOCIAL, VERBAL/COGNITIVE DEVELOPMENT AND NEUROLOGIC ASSOCIATIONS (*CONTINUED*)			
	Milestones			
Age	Motor/Physical	Social	Verbal/Cognitive	Neurologic Associations
		about physical injury		
6–8 years	Draws a person in detail Copies square and triangle Prints letters Skips using alternate feet Ties shoelaces Rides two-wheeled bicycle	Plays cooperatively with other children Competes in games Develops an internalized moral sense of right and wrong Understand finality of death	Can think logically Can calculate simple sums Can read	Decreased neural plasticity; decreased sparing of function and limited ability to acquire language after brain damage
13–16 years	Shows motor skills near adult levels Shows development of secondary sex characteristics	Shows risk-taking behavior Develops an individual identity	Can think in an abstract "what if" fashion	Decline in number of synapses in prefrontal cortex Primary use of limbic system when assessing emotion in others
Adult	Shows adult-level motor skills Shows physical changes associated with climacterium (e.g., menopause)	Is able to develop intimate relationships with others	Shows good verbal and written self-expression Shows occupational and social productivity Shows the wisdom of age	Continuation of active corticolimbic myelination until 6th decade Primary use of the prefrontal region when assessing emotion in others

poorly managed eastern European orphanages show persistently **decreased brain metabolism** in limbic structures.

C. **Motor skills**
1. At birth, the normal infant possesses simple reflexes such as the **sucking** reflex, **startle** reflex (Moro reflex), **palmar grasp** reflex, **Babinski** reflex, and **rooting** reflex. All of these reflexes disappear during the 1st year of life (Table 1-3).
2. The **Apgar scoring system** quantifies physical functioning in newborns (Table 1-4).
3. First-time parents quickly learn that older infants and preschool children are normally active, rarely stay in one place for long, and require continual supervision.

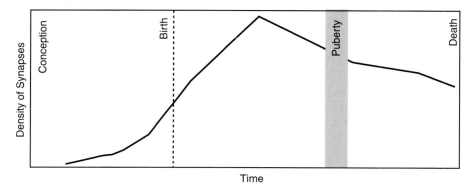

FIG 1-4. Synaptic density at different ages after conception.

TABLE 1-3	REFLEXES PRESENT AT BIRTH AND THE AGE AT WHICH THEY DISAPPEAR	
Reflex	**Description**	**Age of Disappearance**
Palmar grasp	Child's fingers grasp objects placed in palm	2 months
Rooting and sucking reflexes	Child's head turns in direction of a stroke on cheek when seeking a nipple to suck	3 months
Startle (Moro) reflex	When child is startled, his or her arms and legs extend	4 months
Babinski reflex	Dorsiflexion of largest toe when plantar surface of child's foot is stroked	12 months
Tracking reflex	Child visually follows a human face	Continues

D. Social characteristics

1. The **major social theme of the 1st year of life** is for the infant to develop a relationship with his or her primary caregiver, usually the mother. Developmental theorist Erik Erikson called this stage of life **trust vs. mistrust.**
   a. The mother–child relationship begins even before **birth.**
   b. Smiling in response to the mother (the **social smile**) occurs at 1–2 months of age and is one of the first markers of the child's social responsiveness.
   c. Crying and withdrawing in the presence of an unfamiliar person (**stranger anxiety**) **is normal** and begins at about 7 months of age.
      i. This behavior indicates that the infant has developed a specific attachment to the mother and is able to distinguish her from a stranger.
      ii. Infants exposed to many caregivers are less likely to show stranger anxiety than those exposed to few caregivers.
   d. At about 1 year, the child can maintain the mental image of an object or person without seeing it (**object permanence**).

2. The **major theme of the 2nd year of life** is to **separate from the mother** or primary caregiver, a process that is nearly complete by 3 years of age.
   a. After reaching 3 years of age, a child should be able to spend a few hours away from the mother in the care of others (e.g., in day care).
   b. A child who cannot do this after 3 years of age may be experiencing **separation anxiety disorder.**
   c. Life stress, such as moving or divorce, may result in a child's use of **regression,** a defense mechanism (see Chapter 12) in which the child temporarily behaves in a baby-like way (e.g., starts wetting the bed again).

TABLE 1-4	THE APGAR SCORING SYSTEM		
Measure	**0**	**1**	**2**
Heartbeat	Absent	Slow (<100/min)	Rapid (>100/min)
Respiration	Absent	Irregular, slow	Good, crying
Muscle tone	Flaccid, limp	Weak, inactive	Strong, active
Color of body and extremities	Both body and extremities pale or blue	Pink body, blue extremities	Pink body, pink extremities
Response to heel prick or nasal tickle	No response	Grimace	Foot withdrawal, cry, sneeze, cough

The infant is evaluated 1 min and 5 (or 10) min after birth. Each of the five measures can have a score of 0, 1, or 2 (highest score = 10). Interpretation: score > 7 = no imminent survival threat; score < 4 = imminent survival threat.

3. **Beliefs**
    a. **Fantasy and reality.** Children between 3 and 6 years of age have active imaginations. However, they can distinguish fantasy from reality (e.g., they know that **imaginary friends** are not real people), although the line between fantasy and reality may still not be sharply drawn.
    b. **Death and dying.** Preschool children do not yet understand that death is permanent.
        i.   They typically expect that a dead pet or relative will come back to life.
        ii. At about 6 years of age, children begin to understand that **death is final** and may become fearful that their parents will die and leave them.

E. **Cognitive/language skills**
    1. By 1–1.5 years of age **most children can say a few simple words** or use a few sounds that only parents can understand.
    2. The child's **vocabulary increases** rapidly after this; and by 2 years of age, the child uses about 250 words and can use two-word sentences.
    3. By 3 years of age, most children can use about 900 words and combine them into **complete sentences.** Non-family members can generally understand children of this age.
    4. Children who show delays in language should be evaluated first for **hearing problems** (Patient Snapshot 1-2).

F. **Sexual development**
    1. In the first trimester of fetal life, the androgenic secretions of the developing testes direct the differentiation of male internal and external genitalia; in the absence of these secretions during prenatal life, the **internal and external genitalia are female.**
    2. In the second trimester, **masculinization of certain brain areas** (hypothalamus, anterior commissure, corpus callosum, and thalamus) by androgenic secretions of the fetal testes occurs; and by adulthood, the brains of males and females are anatomically and functionally different (Figure 1-5).

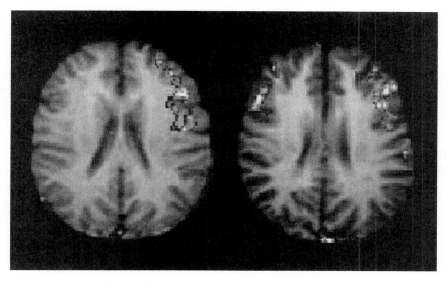

FIG 1-5. Composite functional magnetic resonance imaging (fMRI) studies of male (*left*) and female (*right*) brains showing the distribution of activation of a cognitive task—in this case, phonologic processing involving the identification of whether nonsense words (e.g., *leet* and *jeet*) rhyme. Males show unilateral activation in the left inferior frontal gyrus, whereas females show activity in both the left and the right inferior frontal gyri. [Reprinted with permission from Shaywitz BA, Shaywitz SE, Pugh KR et al. Sex differences in the functional organization of the brain for language. Nature 1995;373:607–609.]

III. School-Age Children (6–11 Years)

A. Social and interpersonal characteristics. At about 6 years of age, the child's conscience (the **superego** of Freud) and **sense of morality** begin to develop. The child can now put himself or herself in another person's place (empathy) and behave in a caring and sharing way toward others.
   1. Prefers to play with **children of the same sex;** typically avoids and is critical of those of the opposite sex
   2. Identifies with the parent of the same sex
   3. Has relationships with **adults other than parents** (teachers, group leaders)
   4. Demonstrates little interest in psychosexual issues (sexual feelings are latent and will reappear at puberty)
   5. Has internalized a **moral sense of right and wrong** (**conscience**) and understands how to follow rules
   6. Can sit still for longer periods of time and is able to engage in **complex motor tasks** (play baseball, skip rope)

B. Cognitive characteristics
   1. Learns to read and write
   2. Is **industrious** and organized (e.g., collects trading cards)
   3. Has the capacity for **logical thought** (Piaget's stage of concrete operations) and can determine that objects have more than one property (e.g., an object can be both wood and white)
   4. Understands the concepts of **conservation** and **seriation;** both of which are necessary for certain types of learning
       a. **Conservation** involves the understanding that a quantity of a substance remains the same regardless of the size of the container or shape it is in (e.g., two containers may contain the same amount of water even though one is a tall, thin tube and one is a short, wide bowl).
       b. **Seriation** involves the ability to arrange objects in order with respect to their size or other quality.
   5. Not until adolescence do some (but not all) children develop the ability for abstract reasoning (Piaget's **stage of formal operations**).

IV. Adolescence (11–20 Years)

Patient Snapshot 1-3

A worried mother calls the pediatrician after finding her 13-year-old son in the shower with another boy. The mother notes that her son is doing well in school and has a few good male friends but does not seem to be interested in girls. The physician reassures the mother that sexual practicing behavior with friends of the same or the opposite sex is normal during adolescence.

A. Developing an identity
   1. The major task of adolescence is to develop an **individual identity**—that is, a sense of who you are and where you belong in the world.
   2. To accomplish this task, teens adopt current fashions in clothing and music and **prefer to spend time with peers rather than with family.** These efforts may lead to conflict with parents.

3. If this task is not handled effectively, adolescents may experience **role confusion,** by which they do not know where they belong in the world.

4. With role confusion, adolescents may display behavioral abnormalities, such as **criminality** or an **interest in cults.**

5. Older adolescents (>16 years of age) develop **morals, ethics, self-control,** and a realistic appraisal of their own abilities; they become concerned with humanitarian issues and world problems.

B. Risk-taking behavior

1. Readiness to challenge parental rules and feelings of **omnipotence** may result in **risk-taking behavior** (failure to use condoms, driving too fast, smoking).

2. Reliance on limbic over prefrontal structures (as in adults) when making judgments may be related to this risk-taking behavior (Table 1-3).

3. Education with respect to **obvious short-term benefits** rather than references to long-term consequences of behavior are more likely to **decrease teenagers' unwanted behavior**—for example, **to encourage use of helmets while cycling,** telling a teenager that his or her face could be scarred is more helpful than telling the youngster that he or she could have long-term neurologic problems from head injury.

C. Sexual development

1. **Puberty** is marked by the development of primary and secondary sex characteristics and increased skeletal growth and occurs on average at 11–14 years of age in girls and 12–15 years of age in boys.

   a. **Alterations** in expected patterns of development (e.g., late breast development in girls, nipple enlargement in boys—usually normal but may concern the boy and his parents) may lead to psychological difficulties.

   b. **Sexual self-stimulation (masturbation)** is a normal behavior that is seen in infancy and early childhood but increases significantly with the secretion of sex hormones at puberty.

2. **Sexual expression**

   a. **Crushes** (love for an unattainable person such as a rock star) are common in young teens.

   b. Sex drives are expressed through physical activity and **masturbation** (daily masturbation is common and normal).

   c. In the United States, **first sexual intercourse** occurs on average at 16 years of age; by 19 years of age, most men and women have had sexual intercourse.

D. Homosexuality (gay or lesbian sexual orientation)

1. **Origin**

   a. **Homosexual experiences** commonly occur during adolescence. Although parents may become alarmed, such practicing is part of heterosexual as well as homosexual development.

   b. The origin of homosexuality is believed to be related to alterations in levels of **prenatal sex hormones,** resulting in anatomic changes in some hypothalamic nuclei; sex hormone levels in adult homosexual individuals are indistinguishable from those of heterosexual people of the same sex.

   c. Evidence for involvement of genetic factors includes markers on the **X chromosome** and a higher concordance rate in monozygotic than in dizygotic twins.

   d. Social factors, such as early sexual experiences with same-sex partners, are not associated with the cause of homosexuality.

   e. Homosexuality is a **normal variant of sexual expression.** Because it is not a dysfunction, no treatment is needed. People who are uncomfortable with their sexual orientation may benefit from psychological intervention to help them become more comfortable.

    2. Occurrence
        a. By most estimates, **5–10% of the population** has an exclusively homosexual sexual orientation; many more people have had at least one sexual encounter leading to arousal with a person of the same sex.
        b. There are **no significant ethnic differences** in the occurrence of homosexuality.
        c. Many people with gay and lesbian sexual orientations have experienced heterosexual sex and have had children.

E. Pregnancy
    1. More than half of all sexually active teenagers use contraceptives.
    2. Factors predisposing adolescent girls to pregnancy include **depression, poor school achievement,** and having divorced parents.
    3. Teenage pregnancy is a social problem in the United States. Although the birth rate and abortion rate in American teenagers are currently decreasing, at the start of this millennium teenagers gave birth to approximately 470,000 infants (8,500 of these infants were born to mothers <15 years of age) and had about 500,000 abortions.

V. Influence of Developmental Stage on Physician–Patient Interaction

Patient Snapshot 1-4

A 32-year-old woman and her 15-year-old daughter come to the physician's office together. The mother tells the physician that the girl has been flirting a lot with boys, which leads her to think that her daughter is having sex. She herself became pregnant at the age of 16 by a boy who later left her. The mother then asks the physician to fit her daughter for a diaphragm. During this exchange the girl sits with her arms across her chest and does not speak. The most appropriate action for the physician to take at this time is to ask the mother to leave the room and speak to the girl alone. When they are alone, the physician can ask the teenager questions about her sexuality while reassuring her that this information will not be revealed to anyone, including her mother. The physician can also provide advice about contraception to the teenager without consent or notification of her mother.

A. Interviewing children
    1. Young children (<age 12) are usually interviewed **with a parent present.**
    2. When interviewing young children, the physician should **ask direct rather than open-ended questions**—for example, "What hobbies do you have?" rather than "Tell me about yourself."
    3. To find out more about the family, ask the child to **draw a picture:** "Can you draw a picture of your family?"
    4. Ask questions in the **third person:** "Why do you think the little boy in the picture looks sad?"
    5. Get the child to **use his or her imagination:** "Let's pretend that you have two wishes, what would they be?"
    6. Gain parents' permission to speak to **teachers and other caregivers** (e.g., babysitters).

B. Interviewing adolescents
    1. Older children and adolescents (≥12) are usually interviewed **without a parent** present.

2. Adolescents worry about concerns they may find difficult to discuss with their parents (e.g., **sex** and **substance abuse**).

3. It is appropriate for the doctor to reassure the patient that information concerning sex or drugs (e.g., sexually transmitted disease, marijuana use) **will not be shared with his or her parents.**

4. The physician should **be nonjudgmental** and be able to reassure adolescents that their thoughts are normal and common among their peers.

C. Giving information to ill children and adolescents

1. It is **up to the parents to decide** if, how, and when information about a child's health will be revealed to him or her; the doctor cannot tell the child or adolescent without parental consent.

2. If the doctor needs to do a procedure on a child that will cause pain (e.g., an injection), the **doctor should tell the child what to expect** in an age-appropriate manner (e.g., a 5-year-old child would be told, "This will feel like a bug bite, but it will stop stinging after we count from one to five together.")

VI. Ethical Issues Relating to Children and Adolescents

A. Seriously ill newborns

1. When a child is born with a **serious medical condition** or is **extremely premature** (e.g., confirmed <26 weeks of gestation), the parents and the physician may have to decide whether to initiate or continue life-sustaining treatment. The major criteria used in such decisions are as follows.

   a. What is best for the child and what will the child's **quality of life** be (from the child's, not his or her parents', perspective)?

   b. If the outcome for a child cannot be predicted with any certainty, such **treatment should be initiated or continued** until such a prediction can be made.

   c. For infants confirmed to be **<26 weeks** but **>23 weeks of gestation,** parents can usually decide whether to initiate life-sustaining treatment. For infants <23 weeks of gestation or <400 g in weight, resuscitation is usually not initiated.

   d. For newborns with **anencephaly** or **confirmed trisomy 13 or 18,** life support can usually be **discontinued** even if it has already been started.

B. Treatment of minors (<18 years of age, unless emancipated)

1. Only the **parent or legal guardian** can give consent for surgical or medical treatment of a minor.

2. Parental consent is **not required** in the treatment of minors in the following instances:

   a. **Emergency** situations (e.g., when the parent or guardian cannot be located and a delay in treatment could potentially harm the child)

   b. Treatment of **sexually transmitted diseases (STDs)**

   c. Prescription of **contraceptives**

   d. Medical care during **pregnancy**

   e. Treatment of **drug and alcohol dependence**

   f. If the minor is **emancipated** because one of the following applies:

      i. The person is **married.**

      ii. The person is **self-supporting.**

      iii. The person is in the **military.**

      iv. The person is **raising a child** (even if living with his or her parents).

3. Most states require **parental notification or consent** when a minor seeks an **abortion.**

4. A **court order** can be obtained from a judge (within hours, if necessary) if a child has a life-threatening illness or accident and the **parent or guardian refuses to**

consent to an established (not an experimental) medical procedure for religious or other reasons. If there is no time to wait, the procedure should be done.

5. Testing children for **genetic disorders.** If the disorder has a pediatric onset and preventive therapy or treatment is available (e.g., cystic fibrosis), genetic testing should be offered or even required.

   a. If there are no preventive therapies or treatments for the disorder and it has a **pediatric onset** (Tay-Sachs disease), parents should have the discretion to test the child.

   b. If there are no preventive therapies or treatments for the disorder and it has an **adult onset** (Huntington disease), genetic testing usually should not be done. The child can decide whether or not to be tested when he or she is an adult.

Chapter 2

Adulthood Through Old Age

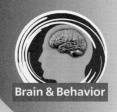

Brain & Behavior

I. Adulthood

Patient Snapshot 2-1

A 48-year-old orthopedic surgeon tells his internist that he has decided to leave his practice and open a golf pro shop. In explaining his decision he says, "I like my work, but I feel like I am getting older and that life is passing me by." The surgeon was recently diagnosed with coronary artery disease. The internist realizes that this patient is showing signs of a midlife crisis. This transitional period, often occurring in middle-aged men, not uncommonly leads to a change in profession or marital status. A midlife crisis may be precipitated by a medical illness—here, the patient's diagnosis of coronary artery disease—or an important lifestyle change. Because people who change lifestyles in middle age may be at particular risk for physical and psychological problems, such as depression and alcohol abuse, the physician should follow this patient closely with regularly scheduled visits.

A. Changes in the adult brain

1. **Myelination** clearly continues into the **5th decade** in certain regions of the brain. However, during much of adulthood (from the **2nd** to the **8th** decades), evidence suggests that the **total length** of myelinated fibers actually declines.
2. **Synaptic pruning** likely continues through adulthood but does not appear to be a major determinant of gross structure during this period.
3. **Brain weight** remains largely stable in adulthood until the age of **45–50,** at which point it begins to slowly decline. This is likely a reflection, in part, of two processes: a shift toward decreasing **white matter volume** around the age of 40 and the continued diminishment of **gray matter volume.**

B. Psychological characteristics of young adulthood (20–40 years)

1. During young adulthood, there is a **period of reappraisal** of one's life.
2. The adult's **role in society is defined,** physical development peaks, and the individual gains independence.
3. According to **Erikson,** this is the stage of **intimacy versus isolation;** if the individual does not develop the ability to sustain an intimate (e.g., **close, sexual**) **relationship with another person** by this stage of life, he or she may experience emotional isolation in the future.

C. Psychological characteristics of middle adulthood (41–64 years)

1. **Characteristics.** The person in middle adulthood possesses more **power** and **authority over others** than at earlier or later life stages.
2. **Responsibilities.** The individual either maintains a continued sense of productivity or develops a sense of emptiness (Erikson's stage of **generativity vs. stagnation**).
3. **Relationships**
   a. Many people in their middle 40s to early 50s exhibit a **midlife crisis.** This often involves a change in lifestyle, divorce, increased substance use, and/or psychiatric symptoms such as depression (see Chapter 19).

TABLE 2-1	CHARACTERISTICS OF THE STAGES OF THE SEXUAL-RESPONSE CYCLE IN MEN AND WOMEN		
Stage	**Men**	**Women**	**Both Men and Women**
Excitement	Penile erection	Clitoral erection Labial swelling Vaginal lubrication Tenting effect (rising of uterus in pelvic cavity)	Increased pulse, blood pressure, and respiration Nipple erection
Plateau	Increased size and upward movement of testes Secretion of a few drops of sperm-containing fluid	Contraction of outer third of vagina, forming orgasmic platform (enlargement of upper third of vagina)	Further increase in pulse, blood pressure, and respiration Flushing of chest and face
Orgasm	Forcible expulsion of seminal fluid	Contractions of uterus and vagina	Contractions of anal sphincter Further increase in pulse, blood pressure, and respiration
Resolution	Refractory (resting) period; length depends on age and physical condition Restimulation is not possible	Little or no refractory period	Muscle relaxation Return of sexual and cardiovascular systems to prestimulated state, over 10–15 min

Reprinted with permission from Fadem B. BRS Behavioral Science, 4th ed. Baltimore, Lippincott Williams & Wilkins, 2005:183.

    b. The midlife crisis is associated with an **awareness of one's own aging** and **death** and **severe or unexpected lifestyle changes** (e.g., death of a spouse, loss of a job, serious illness) (Patient Snapshot 2-1).

4. Sexuality. Sexuality is an important aspect of relationships in adult life. Masters and Johnson studied the **physiology of sexual response** and devised a **four-stage model** for both men and women, which consists of the excitement, plateau, orgasm, and resolution stages (Table 2-1). **Sexual dysfunctions** involve difficulty with one or more aspects of the sexual-response cycle (Table 2-2).

    a. The role of sex hormones in human sexuality

        i. Testosterone is secreted by the adrenal glands (as well as the ovaries and testes) throughout adult life and is believed to play an important role in sex drive in both men and women. **Testosterone levels are generally higher than necessary to maintain normal sexual functioning;** low testosterone levels are less likely to cause sexual dysfunction than relationship problems, unidentified illness, and stress.

        ii. Because **estrogen is only minimally involved in libido,** menopause (cessation of ovarian estrogen production) at about age 50 does not reduce the sex drive if a woman's general health is good.

    b. Sexual interest (**libido**) in men and women usually does not change significantly with increasing age.

    c. Medical treatment with **estrogens, progestins,** or **antiandrogens** (e.g., to treat prostate cancer) can decrease testosterone availability via hypothalamic feedback mechanisms, resulting in decreased sexual interest and behavior.

    d. The climacterium is the change in physiologic function that occurs during midlife.

        i. In **men,** decreases in muscle strength, endurance, and sexual performance (slower erection, diminished intensity of ejaculation, longer refractory period, and the need for more direct stimulation) occur.

        ii. Most **women** experience menopause with relatively few physical or psychological problems. Physical changes include vaginal thinning, shortening of vaginal length, and vaginal dryness. Application of moisturizing agents to the vagina can be helpful.

TABLE 2-2	CHARACTERISTICS OF THE *DIAGNOSTIC AND STATISTICAL MANUAL OF MENTAL DISORDERS,* 4TH EDITION, TEXT REVISION (DSM-IV-TR) SEXUAL DYSFUNCTIONS

Disorder	Characteristic
Hypoactive sexual desire disorder	Decreased interest in sexual activity
Sexual aversion disorder	Aversion to and avoidance of sexual activity
Female sexual arousal disorder	Inability to maintain vaginal lubrication until sex act is completed, despite adequate physical stimulation (reported in as many as 20% of women)
Male erectile disorder (commonly called impotence)	
Lifelong or primary	Has never had an erection sufficient for penetration
	Rare
Acquired or secondary	Is currently unable to maintain erections despite normal erections in past
	Most common of all male sexual disorders
Situational	Has difficulty maintaining erections in some situations, but not in others
	Common
Orgasmic disorder (male and female)	
Lifelong	Has never had an orgasm
	Reported more often in women than in men
Acquired	Is currently unable to achieve orgasm, despite adequate genital stimulation and normal orgasms in past
Premature ejaculation	Ejaculation before man would like it to occur
	Plateau phase of sexual response cycle is short or absent
	Usually accompanied by anxiety
	Second most common of all male sexual disorders
Vaginismus	Painful spasms occur in outer third of vagina, which make intercourse or pelvic examination difficult
Dyspareunia	Persistent pain occurs in association with sexual intercourse without pelvic pathology (functional dyspareunia)
	Can also be caused by pelvic pathology: pelvic inflammatory disease owing to chlamydiosis (most common) or gonorrhea (most serious)
	Occurs much more commonly in women; can occur in men

Reprinted with permission from Fadem B. BRS Behavioral Science, 4th ed. Baltimore, Lippincott Williams & Wilkins, 2005:183.

   iii. Vasomotor instability, called **hot flashes or flushes,** is a common physical problem seen in women in all countries and cultural groups and may continue for years. **Estrogen or estrogen/progesterone replacement therapy** can relieve this symptom but is used less frequently now than in the past, in part because its use is associated with increased risk of breast and uterine cancer.

II. Old Age (65+ Years)

Patient Snapshot 2-2

An 85-year-old patient tells her physician that she is concerned because she forgets the addresses and phone numbers of people she has just met and takes longer than in the past to do the Sunday crossword puzzle. She plays cards regularly with

TABLE 2-3	SOMATIC CHANGES ASSOCIATED WITH AGING	
Category	**Changes**	**Biologic and Social Outcomes**
General health	Decreased muscle mass and strength Osteoporosis	Falls and fractures (common reasons for nursing home placement) Urinary hesitancy, constipation, and incontinence
Physical function	Decreased renal and gastrointestinal function	
	Reduced bladder control	Decreased comfort during social contact, leading to social withdrawal
	Decreased pulmonary and cardiac function	Decreased energy, fatigue
Senses	Impaired vision and hearing	Declines in hearing and visual acuity, leading to social withdrawal
	Decreased responsiveness to changes in ambient temperature	Accidental burns, dehydration

friends, is well groomed, and shops and cooks for herself. The patient has a 10-year history of hypertension and coronary artery disease and no history of substance abuse. Just 1 week after her visit to the physician, the patient has a massive myocardial infarction and dies. Gross examination of the brain at autopsy reveals increased volume of the cerebral ventricles. Microscopic examination reveals cytoplasmic lipofuscin granules in the neurons and decreased myelinization but no major changes in synaptic density or neuronal number. These findings are typical of what is seen in the brain of an elderly person with no clinical signs of dementia such as this patient.

A. The aging population
1. By 2020, more than 15% of the U.S. population will be >65 years of age.
2. The **fastest-growing segment** of the population is people >85 years old.
3. With normal aging comes a **progressive decline** in aspects of **somatic** (Table 2-3) and **neurologic** (Table 2-4) functioning.

TABLE 2-4	NEUROLOGIC CHANGES ASSOCIATED WITH AGING	
Category	**Changes**	**Biological and Social Outcomes**
Neuroanatomy	Decreased brain weight Increased size of ventricles and sulci Decreased cerebral blood flow Decreased neuronal number (10–50%) Accumulation of age pigment (lipofuscin granules) in cytoplasm of neurons Breakdown of myelin sheaths Appearance of senile plaques and neurofibrillary tangles	Decreased speed of new learning (intelligence typically remains same) Decreased short-term memory Slowed response time Minor cognitive changes typically do not affect person's level of functioning or ability to live independently
Neurochemistry	Decreased availability of norepinephrine, dopamine, γ-aminobutyric acid, and acetylcholine Decreased availability of enzymes that synthesize neurotransmitters Increased availability of monoamine oxidase (breaks down neurotransmitters)	Psychiatric symptoms, such as depression and anxiety

TABLE 2-5	PSYCHOLOGICAL CHANGES ASSOCIATED WITH AGING	
Category	**Changes**	**Biological and Social Outcomes**
Self-esteem	Either a sense of ego integrity (i.e., satisfaction and pride in one's past accomplishments) or a sense of despair and worthlessness (Erikson's stage of ego integrity vs despair)	Most achieve ego integrity
Depression	More common in elderly than in general population Associated with loss of spouse, other family members, and friends; decreased social status; and decline of health Associated with memory loss and cognitive problems; thus may mimic and be misdiagnosed as Alzheimer disease (pseudodementia) (see Chapter 4)	Can be treated successfully with supportive psychotherapy in conjunction with pharmacotherapy or electroconvulsive therapy
Anxiety and fearfulness	Owing to realistic fear-inducing situations (e.g., worries about developing a physical illness or falling and breaking a bone)	Psychoactive agents may produce different effects in elderly than in younger patients (e.g., benzodiazepines can lead to falls)
Alcohol-related disorders	Present in 10–15% of geriatric population	Often not identified in elderly patients

B. Neurologic changes in old age

1. Neurologic changes include a decrease in the **number of neurons.** The extent of this loss is controversial, but the abundance of evidence indicates that, if it occurs, it is probably minimal. This is in contrast to the events that occur during **Alzheimer disease** in which there is substantial neuronal and functional loss.

2. There is also controversy about whether there are major changes in **synaptic density** in the aging brain.

3. **Brain weight** begins to rapidly decline around the **8th decade.** The changes in brain weight and size appear to reflect a **decrease** in **neuronal size** with aging. This decrease has been observed most prominently in the **frontal** and **temporal lobes.**

4. Accompanying the decreases in white and gray matter are volume increases in the **cerebral ventricles.**

5. With advancing age, there is evidence of the **breakdown** of **myelin sheaths.**

C. Psychological changes

1. With a culture **focused on youth,** adjustment to old age can be a challenge for Americans.

2. Despite the challenges, most old people have a sense of pride in their accomplishments and have achieved **ego integrity.**

3. Psychological changes associated with aging include psychiatric disorders that can mimic cognitive disorders, such as dementia (Table 2-5).

4. To gain a realistic picture of the level of functioning in elderly patients, they should be evaluated **in familiar surroundings** (e.g., their own homes).

III. Nervous System Repair and Regeneration

A. Evidence of neurogenesis in the human nervous system

1. Classically, neuroscientists have held to the dogma that the central nervous system (CNS) does not have the capacity for **repair** and **regeneration.** Even the great Ramon y Cajal said, "In adult centers the nerve paths are something fixed, ended, and immutable. Everything may die, nothing may be regenerated."

TABLE 2-6	CONSTITUTIVE NEUROGENESIS IN THE MAMMALIAN CNS		
Site	**Location of Precursors**	**Migratory Path**	**Neuronal Product**
Olfactory bulb	Subventricular zone of the lateral ventricle	Chain migration via rostral migratory stream into olfactory bulb	Majority become granule neurons, minority become periglomerular interneurons
Dentate gyrus	Subgranular zone of the dentate gyrus	Migrate short distance to granule cell layer; send dendrites to molecular layer; send axons to CA3	Hippocampal granule cells

2. Through studies of birds, rodents, nonhuman primates, and humans, it has become clear, however, that **repair** and **regeneration** of neurons (neurogenesis) **can occur** in the adult CNS.

3. There is increasing evidence for the existence of neurogenesis.

   a. Using measures of DNA replication (tritiated thymidine and bromo-deoxyuridine), investigators have demonstrated that there is **neuronal proliferation** in the adult brain.

   b. Progenitor **or precursor** cells have been found in numerous anatomic locations of the CNS that, when cultured in vitro, have the capacity for self-renewal and can be differentiated into neurons.

   c. Through the use of new molecular techniques, the **migration, differentiation**, and **integration** of precursor cells have been directly observed.

B. **Characteristics of neurogenesis**

1. One of the major obstacles in the study and understanding of neurogenesis is the observation that it occurs **constitutively** in only two locations: the **olfactory bulb** and the **dentate gyrus** of the hippocampus.

2. Table 2-6 summarizes the process of neurogenesis in these regions.

3. The reason for this limited constitutive neurogenesis is believed to be the concept of **microenvironmental permissiveness:**

   a. Several reports have shown that when **precursor** cells found in **nonneurogenic** areas are transplanted to **neurogenic** areas they can undergo differentiation into neurons.

   b. Conversely, other studies have shown that when **precursor** cells found in **neurogenic** areas are transplanted to **nonneurogenic** areas they can differentiate only into glia.

4. **Neurogenesis in the adult vs. the embryo.** Neurogenesis in the adult CNS appears to recapitulate the events of neurogenesis during the formation of the CNS.

   a. For example, neurons formed in the subventricular zone (SVZ) of the lateral ventricles are formed in **surplus** numbers.

   b. Only a fraction of the new neurons survive to maturation, a process that probably occurs by programmed cell death, or **apoptosis.**

5. Understanding the events of neurogenesis can allow physicians to someday have the tools to **repair the nervous system** after injury or neurodegenerative disease.

IV. Living and Dying

A. **Life expectancy and longevity**

1. The average life expectancy at birth in the United States is currently about **76 years;** however, this figure varies greatly by gender and race. The longest-lived group is

TABLE 2-7	LIFE EXPECTANCY (IN YEARS) AT BIRTH IN THE UNITED STATES BY SEX AND ETHNIC GROUP				
	Ethnic Group				
Sex	**African American**	**Native American**	**Hispanic American**	**White American**	**Chinese American**
Men	64.9	66.1	69.6	73.2	79.8
Women	74.1	74.4	77.1	79.6	86.1

Reprinted with permission from Institute of Medicine. Exploring the Biological Contributions to Human Health: Does Sex Matter? Washington DC, National Academy Press, 2001.

Asian Americans, particularly the Chinese, and the shortest-lived group is African Americans (Table 2-7).

2. Differences in life expectancies by gender and race have been decreasing over the past few years.

3. Factors associated with **longevity** include genetics, continued physical and occupational activity, advanced education, and social support systems (e.g., marriage).

B. Dying patients

1. In the United States, it is customary for physicians to tell all competent adult patients, including the elderly, **the complete truth** about the diagnosis and prognosis of their illness.

2. **With the patient's permission,** the physician can tell relatives this information in conjunction with or after telling the patient.

C. Stages of dying. According to Elizabeth Kübler-Ross, the process of dying involves five stages. The stages usually occur in the following order but also may be present simultaneously or occur in another order.

1. **Denial.** The patient refuses to believe that he or she is dying (e.g., "The laboratory made an error").

2. **Anger.** The patient may become angry at the physician and hospital staff ("It is your fault that I am dying. You should have checked on me weekly"). Physicians must learn not to take such comments personally (see Chapter 16).

3. **Bargaining.** The patient may try to strike a bargain with God or some higher being ("I will give half of my money to charity if I can get rid of this disease").

4. **Depression.** The patient becomes preoccupied with death and may become emotionally detached ("I feel so distant from others and so hopeless").

5. **Acceptance.** The patient is calm and accepts his or her fate ("I am putting my affairs in order").

D. Bereavement (normal grief) **versus depression** (abnormal grief). After the loss of a loved one, there is a normal grief reaction. This reaction also occurs as a result of other losses, such as loss of a body part or, for younger people, after a miscarriage or abortion. A normal grief reaction must be distinguished from depression, which is pathologic and requires immediate identification and treatment (Table 2-8).

1. Normal grief generally **subsides after 1–2 years,** although some features may continue longer. Even after they have subsided, symptoms may return on holidays or special occasions (known as the *anniversary reaction*).

2. Stressors such as bereavement can affect physical health. The **mortality rate** is high for close relatives (especially widowed men) in the 1st year of bereavement.

TABLE 2-8	CHARACTERISTICS OF BEREAVEMENT (NORMAL GRIEF) AND DEPRESSION (ABNORMAL GRIEF)
Bereavement	**Depression**
Some feelings of guilt (e.g., for not having been present at loved one's death)	Intense feelings of guilt and worthlessness (e.g., that death occurred because patient was not present)
Minor weight loss (<5 lb)	Significant weight loss (>5% of body weight)
Sadness and crying	Suicidal gesture or attempt
Difficult falling asleep	Sleeplessness, including early morning awakening
Attempts to return to work and social activities	No attempts to resume work and social activities
Moderate symptoms subside within 1 year	Moderate symptoms persist for >2 years
Treatment: support from primary-care physician, short-acting sleep agents for temporary sleep difficulties	*Treatment:* hospitalization if suicidal, antidepressants, antipsychotics, electroconvulsive therapy

Reprinted with permission from Fadem B. BRS Behavioral Science, 4th ed. Baltimore, Lippincott Williams & Wilkins, 2005:24.

V. Ethical Issues Relating to Death and Dying

A. **Legal standard of death**
1. In the United States, the legal standard of death (when a person's heart is still beating) is **irreversible cessation of all functions of the entire brain, including the brainstem.** This standard differs among states but commonly involves absence of the following
   a. Response to external events or painful stimuli
   b. Spontaneous respiration
   c. Cephalic reflexes (pupillary, corneal, pharyngeal)
   d. Electrical potentials of cerebral origin >2 mV from symmetrically placed electrodes >10 cm apart
   e. Cerebral blood flow for >30 min
2. Physicians **certify the cause of death** (e.g., natural, suicide, accident) and sign the death certificate.
3. If the patient is dead according to the legal standard, the physician is authorized to remove life support. A court order or relative's permission is not necessary.
4. The patient's **organs cannot be harvested** after death unless the patient (or parent if the patient is a minor) has signed a document (e.g., an organ donor card) or informed surrogates of his or her wish to donate.

B. **Euthanasia.** According to medical codes of ethics (e.g., those of the American Medical Association and medical specialty organizations), **euthanasia** (mercy killing) **is a criminal act and is never appropriate.**
1. **Physician-assisted suicide** is not strictly legal in most states but is not generally an indictable offense as long as the physician does not actually perform the killing (e.g., the patient injects himself or herself).
2. Under some circumstances, food, water, and medical care can be withheld from a patient who is not brain dead but whose neurologic condition is such that he or she has no reasonable prospect of recovery. While such a patient may appear to be awake (e.g., the eyes are open), the patient is not expected to ever be aware of or responsive to others or the outside world. This condition is termed a **persistent vegetative state.**
3. If a competent patient **requests cessation of artificial life support,** it is both legal and ethical for a physician to comply with this request. Such action by the physician is not considered euthanasia.

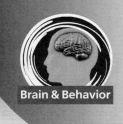

Brain & Behavior

Chapter 3

Developmental Neuropsychiatric Disorders

I. Congenital Neurologic Disorders

Patient Snapshot 3-1

An 8-year-old boy is brought to the emergency room after falling out of a tree, which he had climbed to retrieve a toy airplane. The physical examination, including a neurologic exam, is essentially normal. The X-ray examination reveals no fractures but is significant for absence of the spinous processes and posterior arches of the L4 vertebra, rendering the vertebral canal open posteriorly. Complete covering by the postvertebral muscles prevented identification of the defect on physical examination. The physician tells the parents that the child has spina bifida occulta, a condition that has been present since birth. Like this boy, children with this condition typically have normal spinal cords and spinal nerve roots and normal motor and sensory function. The parents are reassured to know that no treatment is necessary for this condition.

A. **Anatomic defects.** The most common congenital neurologic anomalies are **spina bifida, hydrocephalus,** and **anencephaly,** each occurring in about 6 per 1000 births.

1. **Neural tube defects** are a spectrum of disorders defined on the basis of their **location** (e.g., rostral versus caudal) and the **anatomy** of the defect (whether neural tissues and/or meninges are drawn into the defect [open] or not [closed]) (Table 3-1).

2. Most neural tube defects occur in isolation, but some are associated with recognizable **malformation syndromes.**

3. **Behavioral characteristics** of children with neural tube defects

a. In **isolated spina bifida,** in the absence of hydrocephalus, cognitive function is usually spared.

b. **Myelomeningocele** can be an isolated defect but is often associated with hypoplasia or agenesis of the corpus callosum, likely secondary to hydrocephalus.

   i. In **myelomeningocele with hydrocephalus,** the rostral/caudal location of the lesion is associated with neural and cognitive deficits (Fig. 3-1).

   ii. Callosal disruption results in poor transfer of information between the hemispheres. Children with myelomeningocele and callosal disruption show deficits in language comprehension. Young adults with this condition have deficiencies in reading comprehension and writing.

   iii. Lesions at T12 and above are associated with reduced cerebrum and cerebellum volumes and a higher incidence of **mental retardation.**

B. **Cerebral palsy.** Cerebral palsy (CP) is a term used to describe a group of **nonprogressive impairment syndromes** of movement and posture resulting from anomalies of the brain that arise during early development.

1. The **muscle control difficulties** that characterize CP are often accompanied by nervous system dysfunctions.

2. Other dysfunctions in CP include hearing and visual difficulties, learning disabilities, cognitive deficits, behavioral problems, and seizures.

TABLE 3-1			**OPEN AND CLOSED NEURAL TUBE DEFECTS**		
Defect	**Number per 1000 Live Births**	**Mechanism**	**Anatomy**	**Detection**[a]	**Prognosis**
Open					
Anencephaly	6	Failed closure of rostral end of neural tube	Total or partial absence of cranial vault and cerebral hemispheres	Elevated α-fetoprotein levels (serum and amniotic fluid) Low serum estriol Acetylcholinesterase activity in amniotic fluid	Uniformly lethal
Myelomeningocele	0.03–1	Defective closure of neural tube in vertebral column	Absence of posterior vertebral elements Protrusion of underlying meninges and neural structures	Elevated α-fetoprotein levels (serum and amniotic fluid)	Loss of neural function below lesion Reduced ambulation Little or no bowel/ bladder function Cranial nerve and sensory deficits Associated with Chiari malformation
Closed					
Spina bifida occulta	150–200	Absence of a spinous process and variable amounts of lamina No herniation of underlying structures	No visible exposure of meninges or neural tissue Detectable by a dimple, hair patch, or lipomatous nevus, on lumbosacral skin	CT and MRI scans at birth Often identified serendipitously (Patient Snapshot 3-1)	Usually of no clinical importance
Encephalocele	10–30	Failed closure of the neural tube at variable rostral locations, most often occipital region	Variable, skull defect often in occipital region Herniation of dysplastic brain and meninges through defect	CT and MRI scans at birth	Variable, depending on anatomic structures affected by herniation Often impaired cognitive development
Meningocele	1	Failed closure of neural tube at variable locations	Bony defect in skull or vertebral column with protrusion of meninges	CT and MRI scans at birth	Most patients are neurologically normal
Sacral agenesis	Up to 100 (in mothers with diabetes)	Variable degrees of developmental failure involving legs, lumbar, sacral, and coccygeal vertebrae and underlying spinal elements	Depends on location of lesion	CT and MRI scans at birth	Depends on location of lesion Usually distal weakness and muscle atrophy Sensory deficits Urinary symptoms

[a]In addition to fetal ultrasound and physical examination at birth.

C. **Neurocutaneous disorders.** Neurocutaneous syndromes are characterized by the presence of **neuropsychiatric abnormalities** in association with **skin manifestations.**
1. Up to 30 disorders are now characterized as neurocutaneous disorders.
2. The more common disorders are **Sturge-Weber syndrome, tuberous sclerosis,** and **neurofibromatosis** (Fig. 3-2; Table 3-2).

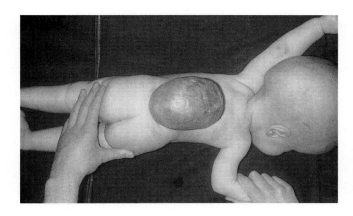

FIG 3-1. This infant has a myelomeningocele with concomitant hydro-cephalus. [Reprinted with permission from Pillitteri A. Maternal and Child Health Nursing: Care of the Childbearing and Childrearing Family, 4th ed. Philadelphia, Lippincott Williams & Wilkins, 2003.]

D. Chromosomal disorders. A number of chromosomal disorders have neurobehavioral manifestations (Table 3-3).

II. Mental Retardation

Delayed intellectual development (mental retardation) has many causes. The most common genetic causes are **Down syndrome** and **fragile X syndrome (FXS)** but there are other genetic causes of mental retardation and behavioral problems (Table 3-3).

Patient Snapshot 3-2

A 14-year-old girl with Down syndrome and an IQ of 60 is brought to the physician's office for a school physical. The parents tell the physician that the child, who was formerly friendly and outgoing, has recently seemed quiet around unfamiliar

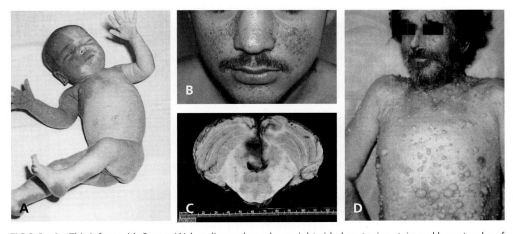

FIG 3-2. A. This infant with Sturge-Weber disease has a large right-sided port-wine stain and hypertrophy of the right upper extremity. [Reprinted with permission from O'Doherty N. Atlas of the Newborn. Philadelphia, Lippincott, 1979.] **B.** This patient with tuberous sclerosis has adenoma sebaceum (angiofibromas). Note the similarity to acne lesions. [Reprinted with permission from Goodheart HP. Goodheart's Photoguide of Common Skin Disorders, 2nd ed. Philadelphia, Lippincott Williams & Wilkins, 2003.] **C.** A horizontal section of the brain from an individual with tuberous sclerosis showing a large subependymal astrocytic nodule in the left lateral ventricle (candle drippings). [Reprinted with permission from Rubin E, Farber JL. Pathology, 4th ed. Philadelphia, Lippincott Williams & Wilkins, 2004.] **D.** This patient has multiple cutaneous neurofibromas on the face and trunk as a result of neurofibromatosis 1. [Reprinted with permission from Rubin E, Farber JL. Pathology, 3rd ed. Philadelphia, Lippincott Williams & Wilkins, 1999.]

TABLE 3-2	CUTANEOUS, NEUROLOGIC, AND NEUROPSYCHIATRIC MANIFESTATIONS OF COMMON NEUROCUTANEOUS DISORDERS		
Disorder	**Cutaneous**	**Neurologic**	**Neuropsychiatric**
Sturge-Weber syndrome	Facial angioma (port-wine stain) often in the distribution of cranial nerve V1 or V2 Leptomeningeal angioma	Progressive neurologic symptoms Seizures Focal neurologic deficits	Mental retardation (severity associated with extent of brain involvement) Behavior problems
Tuberous sclerosis	Hypopigmented ash-leaf spots on skin Angiofibromas of malar region Shagreen patches Brown fibrous forehead plaques	Cortical tubers White matter heterotopias Subependymal nodules Subependymal giant cell tumors (cause seizures and neurologic impairment, depending on extent and location)	Cognitive deficits Decreased intelligence Learning disabilities Behavior problems (e.g., autism and autistic behaviors)
Neurofibromatosis (NF) 1 and 2	Hyperpigmented macules (café au lait spots) on skin Freckling Neurofibromas Lisch nodules	Neurofibromas of spinal roots and cranial nerves Variable neurologic dysfunction (depends on site and extent; e.g., hearing loss, visual loss)	No to slight intellectual deficits Learning disabilities Visual–perceptual deficits (NF1) Attention deficit hyperactivity disorder Social difficulties

people. She is particularly shy around other teenagers. Physical examination is unremarkable. The physician explains that the teenage years can be particularly stressful for mentally retarded teens when they begin to understand that they are different and have trouble fitting in with other teenagers.

A. Down syndrome
1. Physical characteristics include a single palmar transverse crease, protruding tongue, flat facies, hypotonia, epicanthal folds, small ears, and thick neck (Fig. 3-3). These individuals have a high risk for premature aging and **Alzheimer disease**.
2. Down syndrome occurs about equally in both sexes.
3. About 95% of cases involve **trisomy of chromosome 21;** 4% involve translocation and fusion of chromosomes 21 and 13, 14, or 15; and 1% of cases are caused by mosaicism as a result of mitotic nondisjunction.

B. Fragile X syndrome (FXS)
1. FXS is associated with abnormalities in a single gene on the long arm of the X chromosome at the **Xq27 site** (the fragile site).
2. FXS occurs in both sexes but **affects males more severely.**
3. Physical characteristics include **hyperextensible joints,** large ears, elongated face, and **postpubertal enlargement of the testes.**
4. Psychological characteristics include delayed cognitive function, behavior problems such as hyperactivity and autistic behavior, and stereotypic movements such as **hand flapping.**

C. Other causes of mental retardation
1. Fetal alcohol syndrome
2. Metabolic factors affecting the mother or fetus
3. Prenatal and postnatal infection such as **rubella** and **toxoplasmosis** and maternal substance abuse
4. Many cases are of **unknown origin.**

TABLE 3-3	BEHAVIORAL MANIFESTATIONS OF CHROMOSOMAL NEUROLOGIC DISORDERS	
Chromosome	**Disorder**	**Behavioral Manifestations**
1	Dementia of the Alzheimer type (DAT)	Depression, anxiety, dementia, early onset
4	Huntington disease	Erratic behavior, psychiatric symptoms (e.g., depression), dementia
5	Sotos syndrome	Intellectual impairment, phobias, hyperphagia
7	Williams syndrome	Hypersociality, mental retardation, behavioral problems, hypotonia
8	Cohen syndrome	Autistic behavior, mental retardation, microcephaly
9	Dystonia musculorum deformans	Major depressive disorder, learning problems
	Tuberous sclerosis	Seizures, cognitive defects (Table 3-2)
11	Acute intermittent porphyria	Manic behavior, psychosis
12	Phenylketonuria	Attention deficit hyperactivity disorder (ADHD)
13	Wilson disease	Depression, personality changes, thought disorders
14	DAT	Depression, anxiety, dementia, early onset
15	Chromosome 15 inversion-duplication syndrome	Seizures, autistic behavior, hypotonia
	Prader-Willi/Angelman syndrome	Mental retardation; hypotonia; hypersocial preschooler; rage, stubbornness, rigid thinking, and self-injury in school-age and older
16	Tuberous sclerosis	Seizures, cognitive defects (Table 3-2)
17	Neurofibromatosis 1	Cognitive impairment (Table 3-2)
	Charcot-Marie-Tooth disease	Peripheral neuropathy
	Smith-Magenis syndrome	Mental retardation, impaired expressive language, stereotyped behavior, clinging and dependency, seizures
18	Tourette syndrome	Dyscontrol of language and movements
		May be mistaken for a behavior disorder
19	DAT (site of the apolipoprotein E_4 gene)	Depression, anxiety, dementia, late onset
21	Progressive myoclonic epilepsy	Cognitive regression, aphasia, mental retardation
22	Metachromatic leukodystrophy	Personality changes, psychosis, dementia
	DAT (associated with Down syndrome)	Depression, anxiety, dementia, early onset
	Neurofibromatosis 2	Hearing impairment (Table 3-2)
	DiGeorge/velocardiofacial syndrome	Psychomotor retardation, language delay, ADHD, bipolar disorder, schizophrenia, seizures
X	Fragile X syndrome	Autistic behavior
	Kallmann syndrome	No sense of smell, lack of sex drive, depression, anxiety, fatigue, insomnia
	Lesch-Nyhan syndrome	Self-mutilation and other bizarre behavior, mental retardation
	Rett syndrome	Autistic behavior, hand-wringing, breathing abnormalities

5. May also occur in conjunction with developmental disorders such as **autism** and with neurologic dysfunctions such as **seizures**

D. **Treatment.** There is no specific treatment for mental retardation. However, school systems are required by law to provide **special education** for children with special needs, such as those with mental retardation, without additional cost to parents.

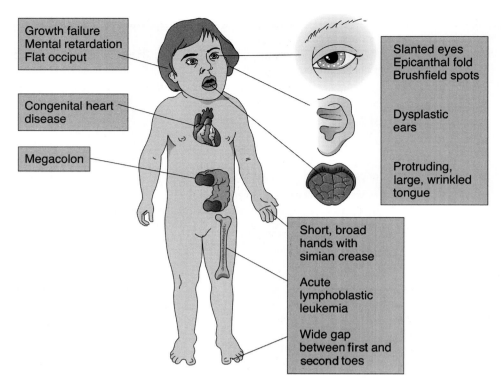

FIG 3-3. Clinical features of Down syndrome. [Reprinted with permission from Rubin E, Farber JL. Pathology, 3rd ed. Philadelphia, Lippincott Williams & Wilkins, 1999.]

E. **Prognosis**
1. School-age mentally retarded children and adolescents come to know that they are different.
2. This understanding often results in **low self-esteem,** leading to **social withdrawal** (Patient Snapshot 3-2).

III. Pervasive Developmental Disorders

The cause of the pervasive developmental disorders is **cerebral dysfunction.** Environmental and social difficulties follow from but do not cause these disorders.

Patient Snapshot 3-3

The worried parents of a 2-year-old boy take their child to the pediatrician for evaluation. They note that ever since he was an infant, their son never wanted to be held, and cried whenever he was changed or bathed. The child does not speak and does not make eye contact when spoken to. When given a toy car, the child spins one wheel over and over again. After further testing, the physician gives the child the diagnosis of autism spectrum disorder. He explains to the parents that, although there is no cure for their son's condition, behavioral therapy and educational techniques can improve the boy's ability to communicate, learn, and socialize. The doctor also recommends that the parents join a support group of other parents who have children with autism spectrum disorders.

A. Autism spectrum disorders (autistic disorder, Asperger disorder)
  1. Characteristics of autistic disorder
    a. Significant **difficulties forming social relationships** (including those with caregivers) beginning before age 3 years
    b. Significant **communication problems** (despite normal hearing); some children do not speak at all.
    c. Preference for **repetitive behavior** (e.g., spinning in place)
    d. **Self-injurious behavior** (e.g., head banging) with little evidence of pain
    e. Failure to play or to use **toys** normally
    f. Active **resistance** to alterations in the environment (e.g., getting dressed)
    g. Unusual abilities such as **savant skills** (e.g., exceptional memory or calculation skills) **are rare** but occur in some children,
  2. Asperger disorder is a mild form of autistic disorder characterized by **normal cognitive and language development** in concert with the following:
    a. Problems in social relationships (e.g., cannot gauge the emotions of others) and poor conversational skills
    b. Obsessional interests in and knowledge of **obscure subjects** that can be learned by memorization (e.g., the specifications of bicycles produced in the 1960s)
  3. Occurrence of autism spectrum disorders
    a. Seen in about 17 children per 10,000
    b. Four to five times more common in **boys**
  4. Cause. Abnormalities that give clues for the origins of autism spectrum disorders include the following:
    a. Cerebral dysfunction
      i. There is often a history of **perinatal complications.**
      ii. About 25% of children have **seizures.**
      iii. Mild problems with motor coordination such as clumsiness
      iv. **Smaller amygdala and hippocampus,** fewer Purkinje cells in the cerebellum, and less circulating oxytocin
    b. Genetic factors
      i. Higher concordance rate in monozygotic than in dizygotic twins
      ii. Chromosomes 7q, 2q, and 16p and genes on chromosome 15 have been implicated.
    c. Immunologic incompatibility between mother and fetus may be involved in some cases.
  5. Treatment
    a. Behavioral therapy to enhance social and communicative skills, decrease self-injurious behavior, and improve self-care skills
    b. Medication (e.g., antipsychotics) to control associated symptoms such as agitation and hyperactivity
    c. Supportive therapy and **counseling to parents**

B. Other pervasive developmental disorders
  1. Rett disorder
    a. Involves diminished social, verbal, and cognitive development after up to 4 years of normal functioning
    b. Occurs **only in girls** (Rett is X-linked; affected males die before birth)
    c. Characterized by stereotypical **hand-wringing movements,** ataxia, breathing problems, mental retardation, and the gradual onset of motor abnormalities
  2. Childhood disintegrative disorder
    a. Involves diminished social, verbal, cognitive, and motor development after at least 2 years of normal functioning
    b. Characterized by mental retardation

IV. Neuropsychiatric Disorders of Childhood

The **hallmark** of the neuropsychiatric disorders of childhood is maladaptive behavior resulting from underlying **abnormalities in brain function.** Children with these disorders are often misdiagnosed with behavior problems because their behavior is likely to be disruptive in school and even at home. Correct diagnosis and treatment with psychoactive medications can have a strong positive effect on academic and social functioning in these children.

A. **Attention deficit/hyperactivity disorder (ADHD)**
   1. **Characteristics**
      a. The ***Diagnostic and Statistical Manual of Mental Disorders,*** **4th edition, text revision (DSM-IV-TR)** lists three types of ADHD (Table 3-4):
         i. **Combined type**
         ii. **Predominately inattentive type**
         iii. **Predominantly hyperactive type**
      b. Evidence of ADHD must be present before age 7 and persist for at least 6 months.
      c. ADHD must occur in **at least two settings**—for example, at school and at home.
   2. The **cause** of ADHD is largely unknown.
      a. **Minor brain dysfunction** may be present but there is no compelling evidence of serious structural neurologic problems or frank mental retardation.
      b. Scientific studies **have not revealed an association** between ADHD and improper diet, excessive sugar intake, or intolerance to food additives such as artificial colors.

TABLE 3-4	DIAGNOSTIC AND STATISTICAL MANUAL OF MENTAL DISORDERS, 4TH EDITION, TEXT REVISION (DSM-IV-TR) ATTENTION DEFICIT/ HYPERACTIVITY DISORDER (ADHD) SUBTYPES
Symptoms of Hyperactivity Impulsivity (HI)	**Symptoms of Inattention**
Shows restlessness and fidgeting, squirms in seat	Makes careless mistakes owing to inattention
Shows inappropriate or excessive running and climbing	Has limited attention span
Shows excessive talking	Does not listen to direct speech
Cannot remain seated	Does not finish work or chores
Cannot play quietly	Cannot organize tasks and activities
Acts as if motor driven	Avoids sustained mental effort
Answers before questions are completed	Loses necessary objects like books or pencils
Cannot await turn	Is easily distracted
Interrupts or intrudes on conversations of others	Is forgetful
ADHD, Combined Type	
At least 6 symptoms of HI	At least 6 symptoms of inattention
ADHD, Predominately Inattentive Type	
Fewer than 6 symptoms of HI	At least 6 symptoms of inattention
ADHD, Predominately Hyperactive Type	
At least 6 symptoms of HI	Fewer than 6 symptoms of inattention

3. **Treatment** of ADHD primarily involves central nervous system (CNS) stimulants such as **methylphenidate** (Ritalin, Concerta), **dextroamphetamine sulfate** (Dexedrine), and a combination of **amphetamine and dextroamphetamine** (Adderall).

   a. CNS stimulants apparently help reduce activity level and **increase attention span,** thereby improving the child's ability to concentrate.

   b. Because stimulant drugs also **decrease appetite** (see Chapter 14), children taking them may show **inhibited growth** and failure to gain weight. These usually return to normal once the child stops taking the medication.

4. **Prognosis**

   a. Inattention and hyperactivity often result in **difficulty in school.**

   b. Because of their **problematic behavior** children with ADHD are more likely to be **physically abused** by their parents.

   c. Many children with ADHD show improvement in symptoms in adolescence, particularly decreased activity level. About 20% retain the characteristics of ADHD into adulthood.

B. **Tourette disorder**
   1. **Characteristics**

      a. Tourette disorder is a relatively rare chronic neurologic disorder that is characterized by **both involuntary motor movements and involuntary vocalizations** (motor and vocal tics).

      b. If only one type of tic is present, the diagnosis is motor tic disorder or vocal tic disorder rather than Tourette disorder.

      c. Tourette disorder usually starts with a motor tic, such as facial grimacing, that **appears between ages 7 and 8.** Vocal tics such as grunting, barking, or the involuntary use of profanity follow.

   2. **Occurrence**

      a. Tourette disorder begins **before age 18.**

      b. It is up to three times **more common in boys.**

   3. **Origin**

      a. There is a strong genetic component in Tourette disorder.

      b. There is a genetic relationship between Tourette disorder and both **ADHD** and **obsessive–compulsive disorder (OCD)** (see Chapter 20)

      c. Tourette disorder is associated with dysfunctional regulation of **dopamine** in the **caudate nucleus.**

   4. **Treatment.** Tourette disorder is treated primarily with antipsychotic agents such as risperidone (Risperdal) (see Chapter 22).

   5. **Prognosis**

      a. Children who have Tourette disorder are often perceived as **disruptive** in class and may have trouble making friends.

      b. As adults, people with Tourette disorder often have occupational and social difficulties.

V. Behavioral Disorders of Childhood

The **hallmark** of the behavioral disorders of childhood is maladaptive behavior resulting primarily from exposure to abnormal environmental situations and life stressors. Genetic and other biologic factors may also be involved but are believed to be of less importance in the cause of the behavioral disorders.

A. **Reactive attachment disorder of infancy and early childhood**

Patient Snapshot 3-4

An American couple would like to adopt a 14-month-old boy from an orphanage in Russia. They are concerned because the child has been in the institution ever since he was separated from his birth mother 4 months earlier. At the time of separation, the child showed motor and social skills normal for his age. When the couple arrives in Russia, they find that the orphanage is clean and well kept but has a high staff turnover ratio. They meet the child and find that he cannot yet walk, seems sad but does not cry, and shows little responsiveness toward them or toward anyone else. When they return to the United States and have the child evaluated, the pediatrician finds the neurologic exam unremarkable and diagnoses reactive attachment disorder of infancy, inhibited type.

1. **Overview.** Toward the end of the 1st year of life, **separation from the primary caregiver** leads to initial loud protests from normal infants (separation anxiety). With continued absence of the mother, the infant is at risk for psychiatric symptoms. The **DSM-IV-TR** term for these symptoms is **reactive attachment disorder of infancy or early childhood.**
   a. This condition has been called **failure to thrive** because it often includes poor physical growth and poor health and is potentially life-threatening.
   b. Infants may show these characteristics even when living with their mother if the **mother is physically and emotionally distant and insensitive** to their needs.
2. **Types.** There are two types of reactive attachment disorder:
   a. **Inhibited type**—child is withdrawn and unresponsive
   b. **Disinhibited type**—child approaches and attaches indiscriminately to strangers as though they were familiar to him or her
   c. The **prognosis** is better for children with the disinhibited type.
3. **Differential diagnosis.** In contrast to autism spectrum disorders in which there are neurologic abnormalities, reactive attachment disorder is seen in neurologically normal children owing to grossly pathologic socioenvironmental situations.
4. Interventions in reactive attachment disorder include:
   a. Ensuring the safety of the child, sometimes with the help of state child protective services
   b. Parental training that stresses an understanding of developmental expectations
   c. Family therapy (see Chapter 23)
   d. Early intervention school programs

B. Disruptive behavior disorders

Patient Snapshot 3-5

A worried mother reports to the physician that over the past 2 years, her 8-year-old daughter has been setting small fires at home and at school. The mother says that she recently found the child's parakeet dead on the floor with a rubber band around its neck. The child denies killing the bird and says that she sets fires because it is fun. Physical examination is unremarkable, and the child is of normal weight and height for her age. The physician's differential diagnosis includes conduct disorder. Children with conduct disorder have a poorly developed conscience and sense of morality and show behavior (e.g., setting fires) that markedly violates social norms. Torturing animals is a common manifestation of this disorder, and the brutal way the child killed the bird illustrates this characteristic.

1. **Overview.**
   a. By about age 7, most children are compliant with parental rules and show empathic feelings toward others (see Chapter 2); but some school-age children, more commonly boys, show **persistent behavior that is defiant and inappropriate** and causes problems in social relationships and school performance.

    b. Two DSM-IV-TR diagnoses for children with these characteristics are oppositional defiant disorder and conduct disorder.

2. Oppositional defiant disorder—behavior that is defiant, negative, and noncompliant but does not grossly violate social norms (e.g., argumentativeness, anger, and resentment toward authority figures)

    a. Gradual onset, usually before age 8; in girls, it more commonly begins in adolescence.

    b. A significant number of cases progress to conduct disorder.

3. Conduct disorder—behavior that **grossly violates social norms** (e.g., stealing, truancy, fire setting, animal abuse, abuse of younger children) beginning in childhood (ages 6–10) or adolescence (no symptoms before age 10)

4. Occurrence. Disruptive behavior disorders are seen in 2–16% of children <18 years but may be overdiagnosed.

5. Cause

    a. Biologic factors such as genetics and minimal brain dysfunction may be involved.

    b. Social factors that have been implicated include parental substance abuse, marital discord, mood disorders, and exposure to various types of child abuse.

6. Differential diagnosis. Depressed or anxious children and teenagers may deal with their personally unacceptable emotions by showing inappropriate, negative behavior (e.g., use of the defense mechanism acting out) (see Chapter 12) and being misdiagnosed with disruptive behavior disorders.

7. Prognosis. Most children show **remission by adulthood.** Some children show criminal behavior, antisocial personality disorder, substance abuse, and mood disorders in adulthood.

C. Separation anxiety disorder. Often called **school phobia** or **school refusal** because refusal to go to school is the major manifestation, separation anxiety disorder is characterized by an overwhelming fear of loss of a major attachment figure, particularly the mother. Because of this fear, the child avoids going to school and leaving the mother by complaining of physical symptoms such as stomach pain or headache.

1. Occurrence

    a. Separation anxiety disorder affects as many as 4% of school-age children.

    b. While the most common **age of onset is 7–8 years,** the disorder may start later. The late-onset type of separation anxiety disorder has a poorer prognosis.

2. Cause. Both social and familial factors are involved in the cause of the disorder.

    a. Stressful life events (e.g., the death of a family member)

    b. Genetic factors. Parents of children with this disorder are more likely themselves to have anxiety disorders.

3. Treatment

    a. Gradual **reintroduction of the child to school** (often accompanied by a parent) coupled with family therapy is the most effective treatment for children with this disorder.

    b. Medications such as antidepressants are useful for the associated symptoms.

4. Prognosis. Increased risk for anxiety disorders in adulthood, particularly agoraphobia.

VI. Disorders of Sexual Development

Differential exposure of the brain and body to gonadal hormones during prenatal life affects the development of gender identity, gender role, and sexual orientation (Table 3-5). Abnormalities in such exposure provide evidence for the role of these hormones in the development of masculine and feminine behavior.

TABLE 3-5	GENDER IDENTITY, GENDER ROLE, AND SEXUAL ORIENTATION		
Term	**Definition**	**Presumed Major Influence**	**Comments**
Gender identity	Sense of self as being male or female	Differential exposure to prenatal sex hormones	May or may not agree with physiologic sex or gender role (gender identity disorder)
Gender role	Expression of one's gender identity in society	Social pressure to conform to social norms	May or may not agree with physiologic sex or gender identity
Sexual orientation	Persistent and unchanging preference of people of the same sex (homosexual) or the opposite sex (heterosexual) for love and sexual expression	Differential exposure to prenatal sex hormones Genetic influences	True bisexuality is uncommon; most people have a sexual preference Homosexuality is considered a normal variant of sexual expression

Reprinted with permission from Fadem B. BRS Behavioral Science, 4th ed. Baltimore, Lippincott, Williams & Wilkins, 2005:180.

Patient Snapshot 3-6

A 17-year-old woman comes to the physician because she has never menstruated. Initial examination reveals a tall, thin female with normal external genitalia and breast development and firm, 6-cm bilateral labial masses. There are no Barr bodies in the buccal smear. The patient states that she prefers typically feminine clothes and activities and that she is attracted sexually only to men. Further evaluation of this patient reveals that this patient has androgen insensitivity syndrome.

A. **Androgen insensitivity syndrome** (AIS); formerly testicular feminization
    1. Despite an XY genotype and testes that secrete androgen, a genetic defect prevents the body cells from responding to androgen, resulting in a **female phenotype.**
    2. Testicular descent at puberty can appear as **labial or inguinal masses.**
    3. Individuals with AIS typically **identify themselves as female,** and most are heterosexual (with respect to their phenotype).

B. **Congenital virilizing adrenal hyperplasia** (CVA); formerly adrenogenital syndrome.
    1. In the presence of excessive adrenal androgen secretion prenatally, the **genitalia of a genetic female are masculinized.**
    2. Girls with CVA often show **masculinized behavior** as measured by a preference for conventionally masculine toys and a high activity level.
    3. Women with CVA are more likely to report a **lesbian sexual orientation.**

C. **Gender identity disorder** (i.e., transsexual, transgender individuals)
    1. Individuals with gender identity disorder have a pervasive psychological **feeling of being born into the body of the wrong sex,** despite a body form that is normal for their physiologic sex.
    2. This condition is also associated with **altered prenatal brain exposure to sex hormones**—for example, increased androgens in females and decreased androgens in males.
    3. In adulthood, these individuals commonly take sex hormones and **seek sex-change surgery.**

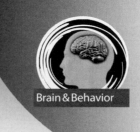

Chapter 4

Degenerative Neuropsychiatric Disorders

I. Cognitive Disorders: Delirium, Dementia, and Amnestic Disorder

Patient Snapshot 4-1

A 74-year-old man whose mental functioning was normal until 3 months ago is alert but cannot remember what to do with the phone when it rings or how to turn on the microwave. The patient, who has been hypertensive for the last 20 years, experienced a mild myocardial infarction 1 year earlier. His wife reports that, while the patient seems generally "like his old self," for the last few months he has been walking more slowly and easily loses his balance. The patient's history of cardiovascular illness, the sudden appearance of cognitive loss, and focal neurologic symptoms in the presence of well-preserved personality characteristics suggest that this patient is experiencing the onset of vascular dementia.

A. **Overview.** Because all psychiatric symptoms are mediated by the brain, it is theoretically difficult to separate organic from nonorganic disorders. Therefore, disorders **formerly called organic mental disorders** are now termed *cognitive disorders*.
   1. Cognitive disorders involve problems in **memory,** orientation, **level of consciousness,** and other intellectual functions. These difficulties are the result of abnormalities in neural chemistry, structure, or physiology **originating in the brain** or **secondary to systemic illness.**
   2. Patients with cognitive disorders may show **psychiatric symptoms** (depression, anxiety, paranoia, hallucinations, and delusions) **secondary to the cognitive problems.**
   3. The likelihood of having a cognitive disorder **increases with age.**
   4. The major cognitive disorders are **delirium, dementia,** and **amnestic disorder.** Characteristics and causes of these disorders can be found in Table 4-1.

B. **Dementia of the Alzheimer type (DAT)**
   1. **Diagnosis**
      a. DAT is the **most common type** of dementia and is diagnosed when other obvious causes for the symptoms have been eliminated.
      b. Patients show a **gradual loss of memory and intellectual abilities** that progresses to coma and **death** (usually within 8–10 years of diagnosis).
      c. For patient management and prognosis, it is important to make the distinction between **DAT** and both **pseudodementia** (depression that mimics dementia) and **normal aging** (Table 4-2).
   2. **Genetic associations** in DAT include
      a. Abnormalities of **chromosome 21** (patients with Down syndrome ultimately develop DAT)
      b. Abnormalities of **chromosomes 1 and 14** (implicated particularly in **early-onset DAT** (occurring <65 years)
      c. Possession of at least one copy of the **apolipoprotein E_4** (apoE_4) gene on **chromosome 19**
      d. Gender (higher occurrence of DAT in **women**)

35

Characteristic	Delirium	Dementia	Amnestic Disorder
TABLE 4-1		**CHARACTERISTICS AND CAUSES OF THE COGNITIVE DISORDERS**	
Hallmark	Impaired consciousness	Loss of memory and intellectual abilities	Loss of memory with few other cognitive problems
Cause	CNS disease CNS trauma CNS infection (e.g. meningitis) Systemic disease (e.g., hepatic, cardiovascular) High fever Substance abuse Substance withdrawal	DAT Vascular disease CNS disease (e.g., Huntington disease; Parkinson disease) CNS trauma CNS infection (e.g., HIV; Creutzfeldt-Jakob) Lewy body dementia Pick disease	Thiamine deficiency owing to long-term alcohol abuse, leading to destruction of mediotemporal lobe structures (mammillary bodies) Temporal lobe trauma, vascular disease, or infection (e.g., herpes simplex encephalitis)
Occurrence	More common in children and elderly Most common cause of psychiatric symptoms in medical and surgical hospital units	More common in elderly Seen in about 20% of individuals >85 years	Patients commonly have a history of alcohol abuse
Associated physical findings	Acute medical illness Autonomic dysfunction Abnormal EEG (fast wave activity or generalized slowing)	No medical illness Little autonomic dysfunction Normal EEG	
Associated psychological findings	Impaired consciousness Illusions or hallucinations (often visual and disorganized) Anxiety with psychomotor agitation Sundowning (symptoms much worse at night)	Normal consciousness No psychotic symptoms in early stages Depressed mood Little diurnal variability Confabulation (untruths told to hide memory loss), particularly in amnestic disorder	
Course	Develops quickly Fluctuating course with lucid intervals	Develops slowly Progressive downhill course	
Treatment and prognosis	Removal of the underlying medical problem will allow symptoms to resolve Increase orienting stimuli Provide a structured environment	No effective treatment, rarely reversible Pharmacotherapy and supportive therapy to treat associated psychiatric symptoms Acetylcholinesterase inhibitors or NMDA receptor antagonists (to treat DAT) Increase orienting stimuli Provide a structured environment	

CNS, central nervous system; DAT, dementia of the Alzheimer type; EEG, electroencephalogram; NMDA, N-methyl-D-aspartate. Adapted with permission from Fadem B. BRS Behavioral Science, 4th ed. Baltimore, Lippincott Williams & Wilkins, 2005:131.

TABLE 4-2		MEMORY PROBLEMS IN THE ELDERLY: COMPARISON OF CAUSES		
Condition	**Cause**	**Clinical Example**	**Major Manifestations**	**Medical Interventions**
DAT	Brain dysfunction	A 65-year-old former banker cannot remember to turn off gas jets on stove; nor can he name object in his hand (a comb)	Severe memory loss Other cognitive problems Decrease in IQ Disruption of normal life	Structured environment Acetylcholinesterase inhibitors and NMDA antagonists Ultimately, nursing home placement
Pseudodementia (depression that mimics dementia)	Depression of mood	A 65-year-old dentist cannot remember to pay her bills; she appears to be physically slowed down (psychomotor retardation) and sad	Moderate memory loss Other cognitive problems No decrease in IQ Disruption of normal life	Antidepressants ECT Psychotherapy
Normal aging	Minor changes in the normal aging brain	A 65-year-old woman forgets new phone numbers and names but functions well living on her own	Minor forgetfulness Reduction in the ability to learn new things quickly No decrease in IQ No disruption of normal life	No medical intervention Practical and emotional support from physician

DAT, dementia of the Alzheimer type; *ECT*, electroconvulsive therapy; *NMDA*, N-methyl-D-aspartate. Adapted with permission from Fadem B. BRS Behavioral Science, 4th ed. Baltimore, Lippincott Williams & Wilkins, 2005:132.

3. **Psychiatric associations**
   a. **Depression** and **anxiety** are often seen early in DAT.
   b. Patients show a **gradual lack of judgment** and inability to control impulses.
   c. Later in the illness, symptoms include **confusion** and **psychosis.**
   d. DAT has a **progressive, irreversible, downhill** course. The most effective initial interventions involve **providing a structured environment,** including practical safety measures (e.g., disconnecting the stove) and the following visual orienting cues:
      i. Labels over the doors of rooms identifying their function
      ii. Daily posting of the day of the week, date, and year
      iii. Daily written activity schedules
4. **Neurophysiologic factors**
   a. Decreased activity of acetylcholine (ACh) and reduced brain levels of **choline acetyltransferase** (the enzyme needed to synthesize ACh) are seen in DAT (see Chapter 11).
   b. Abnormal processing of amyloid precursor protein.
   c. Overstimulation of the N-methyl-D-aspartate (NMDA) receptor by **glutamate.**
5. **Gross anatomic changes** occur in DAT.
   a. **Brain ventricles** become **enlarged.**
   b. Diffuse atrophy and flattened sulci appear.
6. **Microscopic anatomic changes** occur.
   a. **Senile (amyloid) plaques** and **neurofibrillary tangles** are seen (Fig. 4-1). These changes are also seen in Down syndrome and, to a lesser extent, in normal aging.
   b. Loss of cholinergic neurons occurs in the **basal nucleus (of Meynert).**
   c. Neuronal loss and degeneration are seen in the hippocampus and cortex.
7. **Pharmacologic** interventions include the following (see also Chapter 22):
   a. **Acetylcholinesterase inhibitors**—tacrine (Cognex), donepezil (Aricept), rivastigmine (Exelon), and galantamine (Reminyl)—to temporarily **slow progression** of the disease. These agents cannot restore function already lost.
   b. **Memantine** (Namenda), an **NMDA antagonist,** was recently approved and seems to slow deterioration in patients with moderate to severe disease.

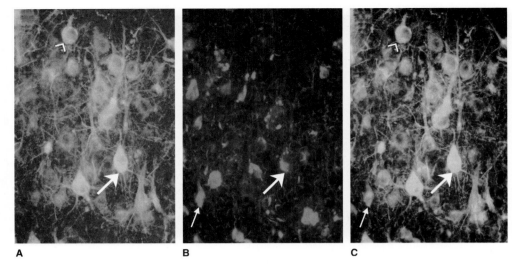

FIG 4-1. Neurons in a human brain with Alzheimer disease. Normal neurons contain neurofilaments but no neurofibrillary tangles. **A.** Brain tissue stained by a method that makes neuronal neurofilaments fluoresce, showing viable neurons. **B.** The same region of the brain as shown in part A stained to show the presence of tau within neurofibrillary tangles. **C.** Superimposition of the images in parts A and B. The neuron indicated by the *arrowhead* contains neurofilaments but no tangles and is thus healthy. The neuron indicated by the *large arrow* has neurofilaments but has also started to show accumulation of tau and thus is diseased. The neuron indicated by the *small arrow* is dead because it contains no neurofilaments. The remaining tangle is the tombstone of a neuron killed by Alzheimer disease. [Reprinted with permission from Bear MF, Connors BW, Paradiso MA. Neuroscience: Exploring the Brain, 3rd ed. Philadelphia, Lippincott Williams & Wilkins, 2006.]

    c. Psychotropic agents are used to treat associated symptoms of anxiety, depression, and psychosis.

C. Other dementias
  1. Vascular dementia (formerly multi-infarct dementia) (Fig. 4-2) (see Patient Snapshot 4-1)
    a. Multiple, small **cerebral infarctions** as a result of atherosclerosis, valvular heart disease, or arrhythmias

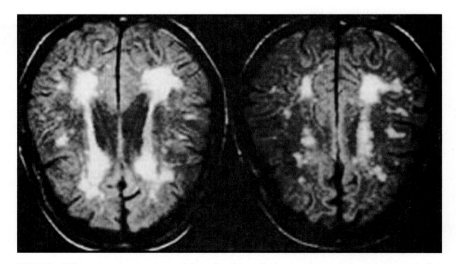

FIG 4-2. MRI proton-density transaxial studies from the brain of a patient with hypertension and vascular dementia. The hyperintensities show the extensive involvement of white matter. [Reprinted with permission from Sachdev PS, Brodaty H, Looi JC. Vascular dementia: diagnosis, management and possible prevention. Med J Aust 1999;170:81–85.]

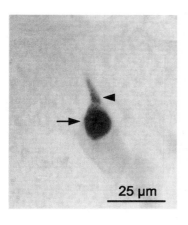

25 μm

FIG 4-3. A neuron possessing a Lewy body. *Arrow,* intraneuronal pathology in the form of a contiguous Lewy body; *arrowhead,* Lewy neurite. [Reprinted with permission from Del Tredici K, Rub U, De Vos RA, et al. Where does Parkinson disease pathology begin in the brain? J Neuropathol Exp Neurol 2002;61:413–426.]

    b. Between 30% and 40% of patients with Alzheimer disease have a **vascular component** to their symptoms.

    c. In contrast to simple DAT, vascular dementia includes the following characteristics:

        i. **Sudden** (rather than gradual) onset of cognitive dysfunction

        ii. **Stepwise** (rather than steady) loss of some function with each infarct

        iii. **Focal** neurologic symptoms (e.g., gait abnormalities)

2. **Lewy body dementia** is characterized by a gradually progressive dementia, including fluctuations in cognitive abilities, visual hallucinations, and parkinsonism.

    a. Microscopic neuroanatomic findings include spherical, eosinophilic cytoplasmic inclusions (**Lewy bodies**), which appear as round deposits of degenerating nerve cell material in brainstem and cerebral cortical tissue (Fig. 4-3).

    b. As in Alzheimer disease, Lewy body dementia is characterized by **multiple neuritic plaques,** although relatively few neurofibrillary tangles are seen.

    c. Patients often present with **positive psychotic symptoms** (e.g., hallucinations and delusions), although they typically have adverse responses to the antipsychotic medications used to treat those symptoms.

3. **Dementia owing to HIV infection**

    a. Causes

        i. **Direct infection** of the brain, causing cortical atrophy, inflammation, and demyelination

        ii. Cerebral **lymphoma**

        iii. Opportunistic **brain infections**

    b. **Death** typically occurs in one half to three quarters of patients with HIV dementia **within 6 months.**

4. **Frontotemporal dementia** (e.g., **Pick disease**) typically first presents with behavioral changes rather than with cognitive changes, as in DAT.

    a. These changes include **stereotyped/repetitive** behavior, **deterioration of personal hygiene, hyperactivity,** and **hypersexual** behavior.

    b. **Mood changes, emotional blunting,** and **apathy** also occur.

5. Other causes of dementia include brain tumor or metastasis to brain, head trauma, multiple sclerosis, and Parkinson and Huntington disease.

II. Parkinson Disease

Parkinson disease (PD) is the second most common movement disorder, behind essential tremor, and affects 1% of the population >50 years of age.

TABLE 4-3	SELECTED GENETIC MUTATIONS ASSOCIATED WITH PARKINSON DISEASE			
Locus	Gene	Chromosomal Location	Inheritance	Comments
PARK1 and PARK4	α-synuclein (SNCA); codes for the protein α-synuclein)	4q21	Autosomal dominant	PARK4 may be caused by triplication of SNCA
PARK2	Mutations in the protein parkin	6q25-q27	Autosomal recessive	Common genetic cause of early-onset Parkinson disease
PARK3	N/K	2p13	Autosomal dominant	Described in only a few kindreds
PARK8	LRRK-2 (codes for the protein dardarin)	12p11.2	Autosomal dominant	Mutant LRRK2 causes protein aggregation and cell death
				May interact with parkin

Patient Snapshot 4-2

A 62-year-old woman reports to her physician that she has been having difficulty using her right arm over the past 2 months. The arm feels clumsy and shows an intermittent tremor. Both have become progressively worse, and she feels quite depressed. She also notes that she has been seeing saliva on her pillow in the mornings. The patient seems slowed down and looks sad but denies syncope, headache, visual disturbances, or vertigo. Physical examination reveals some stiffness of the neck but no significant weakness or abnormal reflexes. It seems difficult for the patient to start walking; but once started, she walks slowly and can maintain her balance with some effort. A slight tremor of her right hand at rest is noted, which disappears when the patient reaches for a pen.

A. **Diagnosis**
   1. Diagnosis of PD is largely a clinical one based primarily on the presence of four cardinal features: **resting tremor, bradykinesia, rigidity,** and **postural instability.**
   2. Another diagnostic feature of PD is that the patient responds to **levodopa** (L-dopa) replacement therapy (Sinemet and Parcopa).

B. **Genetic associations.** There are a number of genetic mutations associated with PD (Table 4-3).
C. **Psychiatric associations.** PD is associated with **depression** and dementia.
   1. At least half of patients with PD experience **depression;** 20% of these patients are diagnosed with major depressive disorder.
   2. **Anxiety** is also often comorbid in patients with PD.
   3. Difficulties in **attention, impulse control,** and **interpreting social cues** are present to some degree in most PD patients.
   4. **Dementia** is a late development in 20–40% of PD patients.

D. **Neurophysiologic factors** (Fig. 4-4)
   1. **Depletion of dopaminergic** input to the **striatum** (caudate and putamen) is the neurochemical hallmark of PD.
   2. This depletion results in **hypoactivity of the direct, or striatonigral, pathway** and **hyperactivity of the indirect, or striatopallidal, pathway.**
      a. These changes **disinhibit** the subthalamic nucleus and **increase activity** of the globus pallidus internal segment/substantia nigra pars reticulata.
      b. The final effect is to increase inhibition on the **ventral nuclei of the thalamus** that have a role in the generation of movement, thus causing **hypokinesia.**

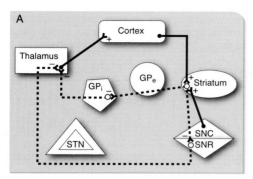 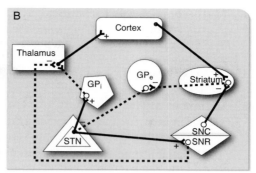

FIG 4-4. A. In a normal individual, the direct basal ganglia pathway is activated via excitatory glutamatergic input from the cortex on the striatum. Striatal output inhibits the tonically active globus pallidus pars interna (*GP$_i$*), which ultimately disinhibits thalamic output. The result is enhancement of intended movement. **B.** Activation of the indirect pathway involves decreased GABAergic output from globus pallidus pars externa (*GP$_e$*), which disinhibits the subthalamic nucleus (*STN*). Excitatory output from the subthalamic nucleus to the globus pallidus pars interna results in increased inhibition of thalamic output. The result is inhibition of unintended movement. The substantia nigra pars compacta (*SNC*) modulates the activity of both pathways. Dopaminergic output from the SNC activates the direct pathway via D$_1$ receptors in the striatum while inhibiting the indirect pathway via D$_2$ receptors. In Parkinson disease, destruction of neurons in the SNC results in decreased activation of the direct basal ganglia pathway (e.g., paucity of D$_1$ receptor activation) and decreased inhibition of the indirect pathway (e.g., paucity of D$_2$ receptor activation). The net result is decreased excitatory thalamic output and thus disordered movement. SNR: Substantia nigra pars reticulata.

    c. In other words, decreased activity of the substantia nigra pars compacta (SNC) on the direct pathway (via **decreased excitatory D$_1$ dopamine receptor** activation in the striatum) leads to decreased direct pathway activity and less movement.

    d. Decreased activity of the SNC on the indirect pathway (via **decreased inhibitory D$_2$ dopamine receptor** activation in the striatum) leads to increased indirect pathway activity and a further inhibition of movement.

E. Gross anatomic changes
    1. In PD, there is a **loss of pigmentation** in the **substantia nigra** and **locus ceruleus** (Fig. 4-5).
    2. Other brain regions affected include the **basal nucleus (of Meynert)**, the brainstem **raphe nuclei,** and the **dorsal motor nucleus of the vagus.**

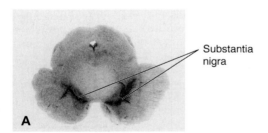

Substantia nigra

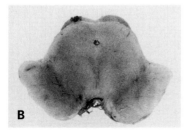

FIG 4-5. A. In a section of the midbrain of a normal subject, the darkly pigmented substantia nigra is easily seen. **B.** After destruction of the substantia nigra in Parkinson disease, the darkly pigmented region is not observed. [Reprinted with permission from Bear MF, Connors BW, Paradiso MA. Neuroscience: Exploring the Brain, 3rd ed. Philadelphia, Lippincott Williams & Wilkins, 2006:469.]

F. Microscopic anatomic changes

1. In the substantia nigra and locus ceruleus pigmented neurons are scarce, and small **extracellular deposits of melanin** (derived from necrotic neurons) are seen.
2. As in Lewy body dementia, some residual neurons may possess **Lewy bodies.**

G. Treatment of PD

1. **L-Dopa** is the most effective medication for the treatment of PD, although it becomes less effective over time (see Chapter 22).
   a. To prevent its metabolism to dopamine before crossing the blood–brain barrier and for maximal effectiveness, L-dopa is combined with a **peripheral dopamine decarboxylase inhibitor** (e.g., carbidopa).
   b. After crossing the blood–brain barrier, L-dopa is converted to dopamine and replaces that neurotransmitter in the brain.
   c. Bradykinesia, tremor, and rigidity often improve with L-dopa. Postural instability is less responsive.
   d. **Side effects** include confusion, hallucinations, psychosis, dyskinesias, dystonias, and motor fluctuations.
2. **Monoamine oxidase type B** (MAO-B) **inhibitors,** such as **selegiline** (Eldepryl), provide modest symptomatic treatment for PD by inhibiting the metabolism of dopamine.
   a. MAO-B inhibitors also may be **neuroprotective.**
   b. Selegiline should **not be taken in combination with tricyclic antidepressants or with selective serotonin reuptake inhibitors** (SSRIs) because serious adverse reactions can occur (see Chapter 22).
3. **Dopamine agonists,** such as bromocriptine (Parlodel), pergolide (Permax), pramipexole (Mirapex), and ropinirole (Requip), have the advantage of not depending on metabolic conversion or transport into the central nervous system (CNS).
4. **Catechol-*O*-methyl transferase** (COMT) **inhibitors,** such as tolcapone (Tasmar) and entacapone (Comtan), are also used for PD. These agents are L-dopa extenders that prevent central methylation of L-dopa and dopamine, thereby increasing their plasma half-lives.
5. **Anticholinergics,** such as trihexyphenidyl (Artane) and benztropine (Cogentin), are specifically useful as monotherapy in patients with tremor-dominant PD.
6. **Amantadine** has a mild anticholinergic effect and increases the release of intrinsic dopamine. It is useful for treating rigidity and bradykinesia.
7. **Surgical interventions** include thalamotomy, pallidotomy, and deep brain stimulation (see Chapter 23).
   a. **Thalamotomy** is primarily useful in the treatment of disabling tremor.
   b. Both **pallidotomy** and **deep brain stimulation** of the subthalamic nucleus reduce the excessive inhibitory output of the internal segment of the globus pallidus.

III. Huntington Disease

Huntington disease (HD) is primarily a disease of Caucasians who have northwestern European ancestry. It has an incidence rate of 1 in 20,000.

Patient Snapshot 4-3

American folk singer Woody Guthrie was born in 1912 in Oklahoma. In 1919, Guthrie's mother began to show increasingly erratic behavior, and she died in a mental hospital in 1929 without ever receiving a diagnosis. In 1940, Guthrie himself began to show erratic behavior. He stated that he "felt queer sometimes," stumbled while performing on stage, and forgot lyrics to his songs. He became increasingly angry, and his actions were increasingly bizarre. One night, he was arrested for loitering and was assumed to be under the influence of alcohol given that there was a "boozy, light-headed quality to him; his walk had become a lurch, and his speech often was decidedly slurred." Then, in rather rapid succession, he was in and out of a variety of facilities in New York City, including Bellevue Hospital (where he was diagnosed with schizophrenia) and Kings County Hospital. In 1952, he was diagnosed with Huntington disease. His physician wrote: "it has elements of schizophrenia, psychopathy and a psychoneurotic anxiety state, not to mention the mental and personality changes occurring in Huntington's chorea." Guthrie himself described his symptoms: "Face seems to twist out of shape. Can't control it. Arms dangle all around. Can't control them. Wrists feel weak and my hands wave around in odd ways. I can't stop." After years of deteriorating behavior and motor control, Woody Guthrie died in 1967.

A. **Diagnosis.** Like Parkinson disease, diagnosis of HD is primarily a clinical one. HD is characterized by the presence of chorea, cognitive decline, neurobehavioral disturbances, and a positive family history.
   1. **Chorea** consists of involuntary, continuous, abrupt, rapid, brief, unsustained, irregular movements that move from one body part to another.
   2. **Cognitive decline** is expressed as dementia, characterized by loss of recent memory and impaired judgment, concentration, and acquisition.

B. **Genetic associations**
   1. HD is an **autosomal dominant** disease of variable penetrance, caused by an unstable cytosine (C), adenine (A), and guanine (G) trinucleotide repeat expansion on **chromosome 4.**
   2. The gene for HD produces a protein with an as-yet unknown function called **huntingtin.**
   3. Repeats tend to lengthen with each successive generation, causing earlier onset. This phenomenon is called **anticipation.** There is a strong inverse correlation between the length of expansion and the age at onset.
   4. Normal individuals possess 30 or fewer **CAG repeats.** HD patients possess >36 CAG repeats.
   5. The CAG repeat is more unstable and tends to be longer when inherited paternally.

C. **Psychiatric associations**
   1. **Behavioral disturbances** are commonly present and often precede motor system involvement in HD (Patient Snapshot 4-3).
   2. These disturbances include **personality changes,** apathy, **social withdrawal, depression, agitation,** and **psychosis,** which are often first misdiagnosed as psychiatric disorders.

D. **Neurophysiologic factors** (Fig. 4-6)
   1. Loss of enkephalinergic spiny neurons of the **striatum** lessens the inhibitory influence on the external segment of the **globus pallidus.**
   2. The external segment of the globus pallidus then **increases its inhibition of the subthalamic nucleus** (STN).
   3. This decreases the facilitatory influence of the STN on the internal segment of the globus pallidus to **decrease inhibition of the motor thalamus.**
   4. Thalamocortical activity is increased as a result, and **hyperkinesis** occurs.
   5. In other words, the primary effect is to reverse the effects of striatal activity on the **indirect pathway;** therefore, disinhibiting the activity of thalamocortical projections to the motor cortex and causing hyperkinetic movements.

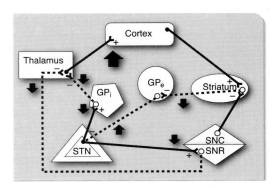

FIG 4-6. Dysregulated basal ganglia signaling in Huntington disease. Reduction in the number of striatal encephalalgic neurons decreases inhibition of the globus pallidus pars externa (*GP$_e$*), resulting in increased inhibition of the subthalamic nucleus (*STN*). Reduced excitatory signaling from the subthalamic nucleus decreases downstream GABAergic inhibitory output of the globus pallidus pars interna (*GP$_i$*) to the thalamus. The result is increased thalamic output and hyperkinesis, or chorea. SNR: Substantia nigra pars reticulata; SNC: Substantia nigra pars compacta.

E. Gross anatomic changes
   1. Prominent **atrophy** of the **caudate, putamen,** and **cerebral cortex** (primarily of the frontal and temporal regions)
   2. Imaging studies often show **enlargement of the lateral ventricles** secondary to atrophy of the caudate (Fig. 4-7).

F. Microscopic anatomic changes
   1. The **neuronal populations** (particularly small neurons) of the caudate and putamen are greatly depleted. Cortical neurons are similarly, but less severely, depleted.
   2. Moderate **astrocytic gliosis** (i.e., a **reactive proliferation of astrocytes as a consequence of neuronal destruction**) is present in affected regions.
   3. **Aggregates of huntingtin** have been detected in neurons of affected regions.

G. Therapeutic interventions
   1. There are no therapeutic interventions currently available to prevent neuronal loss in HD. Mementine, an NMDA recepta antagonist, is being tested for this use (see Table 22-1).

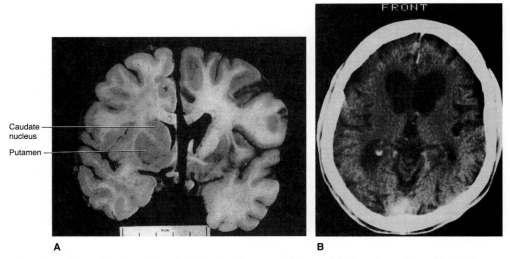

FIG 4-7. A. Coronal sections through the brain of a normal individual (*left*) and a patient with Huntington disease (*right*). Note the profound absence of basal ganglia structures in the brain of the Huntington disease patient. [Reprinted with permission from Bear MF, Connors BW, Paradiso MA. Neuroscience: Exploring the Brain, 3rd ed. Philadelphia, Lippincott Williams & Wilkins, 2006:469.] **B.** An axial CT study of the brain of a patient with advanced Huntington disease demonstrating cerebral and caudate atrophy as well as ventricular enlargement. [Reprinted with permission from Cambell WW, ed. DeJong's The Neurological Examination, 6th ed. Philadelphia, Lippincott Williams & Wilkins, 2005:419.]

   2. Treatment for HD is **symptomatic.**

   a. Dopamine antagonists are moderately effective in the treatment of chorea. Atypical antipsychotics, like clozapine and risperidone, are also useful.

   b. Conventional **antidepressant therapy** is useful for depression, but close monitoring is required to detect the production of mania or suicidal tendencies.

   c. Psychotic symptoms are treated with **atypical antipsychotics** (see Chapter 22).

IV. Amyotrophic Lateral Sclerosis

Amyotrophic lateral sclerosis (ALS) is a progressive degenerative disorder of both upper and lower motor neurons. Most people who develop ALS are between the ages of 40 and 70; the average age at diagnosis is 55 years. The disorder is more common in men, and most patients are caucasian.

Patient Snapshot 4-4

A 72-year-old man complains to his physician of a 6-month history of progressive fatigue and leg cramps. He has also noticed twitching of the muscles on his chest (fasciculations) and difficulty lifting his left foot when he walks (foot drop). He reports that on a few occasions he choked on food while swallowing. Cognitive function appears normal, and the patient denies difficulty with bowel or bladder function. Physical examination shows bilateral diffuse muscle wasting in both upper and lower extremities with prominent fasciculations in all muscle groups. Muscle tone is increased, and tendon reflexes are hyperactive in all four extremities. The patient shows a positive Babinski sign but sensory examination and coordination are normal. Electromyography shows denervation and fasciculations. The diagnosis is amyotrophic lateral sclerosis.

A. Diagnosis

   1. Diagnosis of ALS is also primarily a clinical one. Patients with ALS have **both upper and lower motor neuron symptoms.** Motor neurons controlling eye movements and sphincter function are usually spared (Table 4-4).

   2. There is typically no **evidence of sensory loss,** dementia, or cerebellar or extrapyramidal dysfunction.

   3. Electromyography (EMG) is the most useful diagnostic study and may demonstrate evidence of widespread **denervation and fasciculations.**

   4. Muscle biopsy shows **neurogenic atrophy.**

B. Genetic associations. There are both sporadic and familial forms of ALS.

   1. Familial ALS (FALS) is clinically indistinguishable from the sporadic form of ALS.

TABLE 4-4	UPPER AND LOWER MOTOR NEURON SYMPTOMS IN AMYOTROPHIC LATERAL SCLEROSIS	
Upper Motor Neuron Symptoms		**Lower Motor Neuron Symptoms**
Muscular weakness		Flaccidity
Spasticity		Atrophy
Babinski sign		Fasciculations
Hyperreflexia		Hyporeflexia

2. FALS is an **autosomal dominant** trait.
3. The most commonly implicated gene in FALS is located on **chromosome 21q** and codes for **superoxide dismutase 1** (SOD1).

C. Psychiatric associations

1. No specific psychiatric symptoms are associated with ALS.
2. However, patients with ALS must deal emotionally with the prognosis of a **chronic downhill course** ending in a few years with death.

D. Neurophysiologic factors

1. There is currently **no molecular marker** for ALS. However, mutations in the SOD1 gene may be seen.
2. Isoforms of the neurite outgrowth inhibitor protein **nogo** may show altered expression.
3. Denervation of muscles results in a **loss of the trophic** relationship thus triggering atrophy.

E. Gross anatomic changes (Fig. 4-8)

1. In ALS there is **degeneration of corticospinal, or upper, motor neurons** and observable **alterations of the lateral pyramidal pathways of the spinal cord.**
2. **Ventral roots become grossly atrophied** secondary to loss of anterior horn, or lower, motor neurons.
3. Affected **muscles are shrunken and pale.**

F. Microscopic anatomic changes

1. **Loss of large motor neurons** of the anterior horns of the lumbar cord, the cervical enlargements of the spinal cord, and the hypoglossal nucleus. This process is accompanied by **mild gliosis** (production of a dense fibrous network of neuroglia).
2. Neurofilaments aggregate in axons, forming inclusions known as **spheroids.**
3. **Loss of myelinated fibers** in the **lateral corticospinal tracts** of the spinal cord

G. Therapeutic interventions

1. No treatment is available that halts the motor neuron loss of ALS.
2. One hypothesis for the cause of ALS is that motor neurons are injured by **glutamate.**

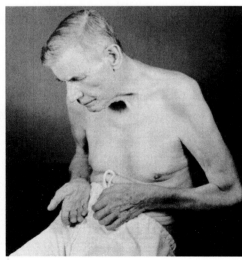

FIG 4-8. A patient with amyotrophic lateral sclerosis. Note the advanced atrophy of the muscles of the hands and shoulders. [Reprinted with permission from Cambell WW, ed. DeJong's The Neurological Examination, 6th ed. Philadelphia, Lippincott Williams & Wilkins, 2005:402.]

    a. **Riluzole** was approved by the U.S. Food and Drug Administration (FDA) because it produces a modest lengthening in survival time (e.g., 18 months vs. 15 months for placebo) in patients with ALS.

    b. Although the mechanism of riluzole's action is unknown, its pharmacologic properties include an **inhibitory** effect on glutamate release. Thus agents such as mementine may also prove useful for ALS.

3. **Symptomatic and supportive care** substantially assist patients with ALS.

4. End-of-life issues such as **patient requests to cease artificial life support** (see Chapter 4) are particularly salient for patients with ALS and their families.

Section II
ADULT BRAIN AND BEHAVIOR

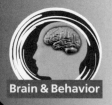

Brain & Behavior

Chapter **5**

Gross Anatomy of the Spinal Cord and Brainstem

I. Spinal Cord

The human nervous system consists of the central nervous system (CNS) and the peripheral nervous system (PNS). The CNS contains the spinal cord, the brainstem (pons, medulla, and midbrain), and the brain (cerebral hemispheres, basal ganglia, and thalamus; see Chapter 6); the PNS consists of somatosensory (afferent) neurons, motor (efferent) neurons, and autonomic neurons (see Chapter 9). Although anatomically separate, the CNS and PNS function in an interactive fashion, and both systems are involved in the expression of behavior.

Patient Snapshot 5-1

A 26-year-old medical student who has been in a multiple-vehicle accident is brought to the hospital emergency room with a suspected spinal cord injury. Physical examination reveals cutaneous hyperesthesia around the abdominal wall on the left side at the level of the umbilicus and paralysis of the left lower extremity. On the right side, the student shows partial loss of tactile skin sense of the abdomen below the umbilicus and total analgesia of the leg. X-ray examination reveals that the student has sustained an injury to the T9 vertebra, resulting in damage to the T10 segment of the spinal cord. The lack of equality in sensory and motor losses on the two sides of the body indicates that hemisection of the spinal cord has occurred. Management of this case will include consultation with specialists in physical medicine and rehabilitation to address issues concerning maximizing the patient's mobility and functioning. Spinal cord injuries such as this one commonly result in loss of bladder and bowel control as well as lack of genital sensation and erectile dysfunction. Psychological intervention can help this patient adjust to these problems as well as to manage emotional issues such as depression. Modalities such as group, cognitive, supportive, and sexual therapies will focus on helping the patient deal with difficulties caused by his increased physical dependence on others and can also help him develop means of sexual expression other than genital intercourse (see Chapter 23).

A. Gross anatomy
   1. The **spinal cord** is a continuation of the brainstem caudally and extends from the **foramen magnum** to its termination as the **conus medullaris.** In the adult, the conus is at the level of the L1 vertebra.
   2. **Basic cross-sectional anatomy of the spinal cord** (Fig. 5-1)

49

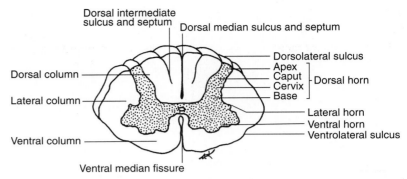

FIG 5-1. Cross section of the spinal cord with nomenclature for its sulci/fissures and regions. [Reprinted with permission from DeMyer D, ed. NMS Neuroanatomy, 2nd ed. Philadelphia, Lippincott Williams & Wilkins, 1998:110.]

    a. The **gray matter** contains neuron cell bodies and is centrally located in the cord. The **white matter** is made up of tracts containing axons and is located peripherally.

    b. The gray matter is shaped like the letter *H*, or a butterfly. In general, there are two **dorsal horns**, two **ventral horns**, two **intermediolateral horns** (**T1–L2 and S2–4**), and a **cross bar** that contains the **central canal.**

    c. The ventral horns are generally motor areas that contain, among other cell types, α-**motor neurons.** α-motor neurons exclusively innervate striated muscle by way of **motor units.** A motor unit is composed of a motor neuron, its axon, and all the muscle fibers it innervates.

3. **Tracts of the spinal cord** can be divided into ascending and descending tracts (Fig. 5-2).

    a. The **dorsal columns–medial lemniscus pathway** is an *ascending* spinal tract that is composed of the **gracile fasciculus** for the lower extremity and the **cuneate fasciculus** for the upper extremity. The sensory functions of the dorsal columns are

        i. **Touch localization**
        ii. **Form**
       iii. **Texture**
       iv. **Position sense**
       v. **Pressure**

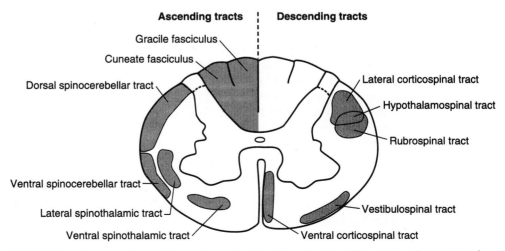

FIG 5-2. The major ascending and descending pathways of the spinal cord. [Reprinted with permission from Fix JD, ed. High-Yield Neuroanatomy, 3rd ed. Philadelphia, Lippincott Williams & Wilkins, 2005:62.]

TABLE 5-1	THE THREE MAJOR SOMATOSENSORY TRACTS OF THE SPINAL CORD		
Aspect	Dorsal Columns	Lateral Spinothalamic Tract	Ventral Spinothalamic Tract
Receptors	Pacinian and Meissner corpuscles, joint receptors, muscle spindles, Golgi tendon organs	Free nerve endings, fast- and slow-conducting pain fibers	Free nerve endings
First-order neuron	Dorsal root ganglia	Dorsal root ganglia	Dorsal root ganglion
Second-order neuron	Gracile and cuneate nuclei	Dorsal horns of the spinal cord (substantia gelatinosa)	Dorsal horns of spinal cord (substantia gelatinosa)
Third-order neuron	VPL of thalamus	VPL of thalamus	VPL of thalamus
Decussation (crossing of the midline)	Medullocervical junction	At the level of first-order neuron entry	At the level of first-order neuron entry

VPL, ventral posterolateral nucleus.

    vi. **Vibration**
   vii. **Kinesthesia**
  b. The **lateral spinothalamic tract** is a spinal tract that *ascends* in the cord along the lateral funiculus. Peripheral receptors for this tract detect
    i. **Pain**
    ii. **Temperature**
  c. The **ventral spinothalamic tract** conducts signals for light (crude) touch and pressure. This white matter tract *ascends* within the anterolateral white column. Table 5-1 summarizes the three somatosensory pathways.
  d. The **dorsal spinocerebellar tract** is an *ascending* sensory pathway that transmits proprioceptive joint information from the trunk and lower limbs to the cerebellum for the coordination of movements and maintenance of posture. This pathway involves the following:
    i. First-order sensory neurons transmit information via muscle spindles, tendon organs, and joint receptors via the dorsal root.
    ii. These axons synapse on second-order neurons of the **nucleus dorsalis** at the base of the dorsal gray column.
   iii. Second-order axons ascend within the ipsilateral dorsolateral white matter as the dorsal spinocerebellar tract.
   iv. These fibers pass through the inferior cerebellar peduncle and terminate in the cerebellar cortex.
  e. The **ventral spinocerebellar tract** is an *ascending* pathway for proprioceptive information from the trunk and upper limbs.
    i. Input comes from first-order neurons of the dorsal root ganglia possessing muscle spindles, tendon organs, and joint receptors.
    ii. These fibers synapse on second-order neurons of the **nucleus dorsalis.**
   iii. Most of the axons from second-order neurons cross the cord and ascend via the contralateral lateral white column.
   iv. Second-order axons pass through the superior cerebellar peduncle and terminate in the cerebellar cortex.
  f. The **lateral corticospinal tract** is a *descending* motor pathway that mediates **volitional motor control,** in particular the speed and agility of voluntary movements. It occupies the region of the lateral white column in the cord.
    i. Most first-order neurons (pyramidal cells) reside in layer V of the primary motor and secondary motor areas of the cerebral cortex.
    ii. Descending fibers form the **corona radiata** and pass through the **posterior limb of the internal capsule,** cerebral peduncles, and medullary pyramids, where most cross the midline (i.e., decussate). These fibers descend in the lateral white column.

   iii. The fibers that do not decussate make up the **anterior corticospinal tract** and descend in the anterior white column, only to decussate and terminate in cervical and upper thoracic cord segments.
   iv. Corticospinal fibers mostly synapse on interneurons but some synapse directly on γ-motor neurons.

   g. The **rubrospinal tract** arises from the **red nuclei** in the midbrain. Axons decussate at the level of the nuclei and *descend* through the lateral white column of the cord. Rubrospinal fibers synapse on interneurons of the anterior gray column. This tract functions to facilitate the activity of flexor muscles and inhibits the activity of extensors.

   h. The **vestibulospinal tract** participates in the maintenance of balance by facilitating the activity of extensor muscles and inhibiting the activity of flexor muscles. Axons from the lateral vestibular nucleus *descend* uncrossed in the anterior white column to synapse on interneurons of the anterior gray column.

   i. Other *descending tracts* include the following:
   i. The **tectospinal tract**—believed to regulate reflex postural movement in response to visual cues.
   ii. The **reticulospinal tract**—thought to modulate the activity of α- and γ-motor neurons.

4. The spinal cord has five levels that give off 31–32 pairs of spinal nerves (Fig. 5-3).
   a. The **cervical** level has 8 pairs of spinal nerves (C1–C8)
   b. The **thoracic** level has 12 pairs of spinal nerves (T1–T12)

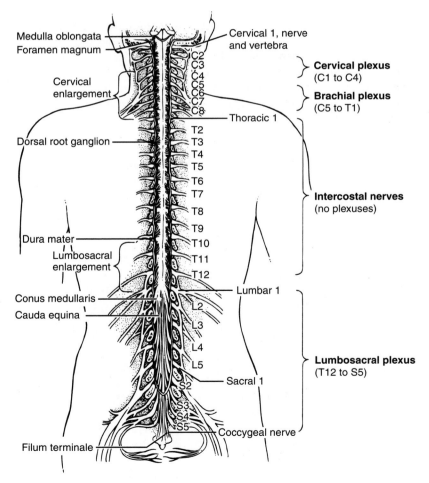

FIG 5-3. Dorsal view of the spinal cord and dorsal nerve roots in situ, after removal of the neural arches of the vertebrae. [Reprinted with permission from DeMyer D, ed. NMS Neuroanatomy, 2nd ed. Philadelphia, Lippincott Williams & Wilkins, 1998:110.]

    c. The **lumbar** level has 5 pairs of spinal nerves (L1–L5)

    d. The **sacral** level has 5 pairs of spinal nerves (S1–S5)

    e. The **coccygeal** level has 1–3 pairs of vestigial spinal nerves.

    f. The **cauda equina** is made up of the dorsal and ventral roots of the lumbosacral cord. These roots must extend downward during development to exit at their original vertebral level because the growth of the vertebral column outpaces that of the spinal cord.

        i. **Cauda equina syndrome** (CES) consists of the combination of

            (a) Urinary retention or **incontinence**

            (b) Fecal incontinence

            (c) Saddle anesthesia

            (d) Lower extremity weakness

        ii. CES is most commonly caused by a tumor, trauma, spinal infection, or lumbar disk herniation (L4–5 disk).

    g. **Spinal nerves** emerge from the vertebral column caudal to the spinal segments from which the corresponding rootlets originate. From C1 through C7, each spinal nerve emerges from the intervertebral foramen above the vertebral body of the same number. The C8 spinal nerves pass through the intervertebral foramina between the C7 and T1 vertebral bodies. Caudal to T1, spinal nerves pass through the intervertebral foramina below the corresponding vertebral level.

        i. **Intervertebral disk herniation** can occur throughout the vertebral column. It consists of herniation of the **nucleus pulposus** through the **annulus fibrosus** into the spinal canal. About 90% of cases involve herniation at the L4–5 and L5–S1 interspaces; the remaining 10% occur at the C5–6 and C6–7 interspaces.

        ii. It is important to note that the majority of lumbar disk herniations occur posterolaterally and compress the nerve root exiting from the intervertebral foramen just below. For example, posterolateral herniation of the disk between the L5 and S1 vertebral bodies puts pressure on the S1 nerve root.

            (a) Far lateral herniations stereotypically compress the nerve root exiting from the intervertebral foramen at the same level. For example, far lateral herniation of the L4–5 disk impinges on the L4 nerve root.

            (b) Central herniation can involve impingement of a number of spinal roots.

        iii. Symptoms of intervertebral disk herniation include paresthesias, anesthesia, hyporeflexia, and muscle weakness.

5. At the levels of the spinal cord that innervate the extremities, the cord is enlarged. The **cervical enlargement** extends from C5 to T1, while the **lumbosacral enlargement** extends from L3 to S2.

6. **Spinal meninges** are continuous with those of the brain.

    a. The **pia mater** is the interior-most layer and is intimately attached to the cord. It extends beyond the termination of the cord as the **filum terminale.** The pia contains the blood supply to the cord.

    b. The **arachnoid** is the intermediate layer and is named for its web-like trabeculations. The **subarachnoid space** lies between the arachnoid and the pia mater. It extends caudally to the level of the S2 vertebra and is dilated between the L1 and the S1 vertebral levels, the **lumbar cistern.**

        i. A **lumbar tap** is performed to sample the cerebrospinal fluid (CSF) contained in this subarachnoid space. It is performed by inserting a needle in the midline, between vertebrae L3 and L4 or L4 and L5.

        ii. **Spinal anesthesia** is achieved by infusing anesthetic into the lumbar cistern.

    c. The **dura mater** is the tough, fibrous external protective layer. It is not fused to the vertebral periosteum. The **subdural space** is a potential space between

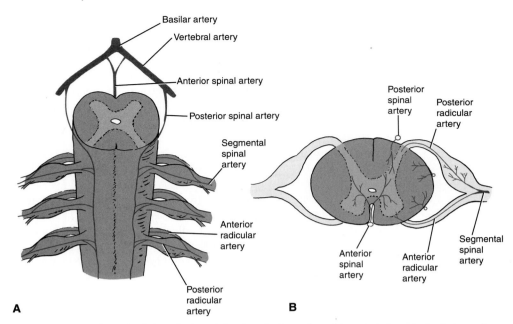

FIG 5-4. A. Arterial supply of the spinal cord showing the formation of two posterior spinal arteries and one anterior spinal artery. **B.** Transverse section of the spinal cord showing segmental spinal arteries and the radicular arteries. [Reprinted with permission from Snell RS, ed. Clinical Neuroanatomy, 6th ed. Philadelphia, Lippincott Williams & Wilkins, 2006:477.]

the dura mater and the arachnoid that does not contain CSF. The **epidural space** lies between the dura mater and the vertebral periosteum and is the location into which anesthetic is perfused to achieve **epidural anesthesia.**

B. **Blood supply** (Fig. 5-4)
   1. **Arterial supply** to the spinal cord is derived from two **posterior spinal arteries** and one **anterior spinal artery.**
      a. The **posterior spinal arteries** arise from either the **vertebral** or the **posterior inferior cerebellar arteries.** They descend along the cord close to where the dorsal roots enter. These arteries supply the posterior third of the cord.
      b. The **anterior spinal artery** is formed from two small arteries that arise from the vertebral arteries. It descends the cord within the anterior median fissure and supplies the anterior two thirds of the cord.
   2. **Venous drainage** of the spinal cord consists of a collection of six longitudinal venous channels. These venous channels are continuous with cerebral veins that drain the venous sinuses and empty primarily into the **internal vertebral venous plexus.**

C. **Spinal reflexes.** Spinal reflexes are stereotyped movements that are triggered by a specific stimulus and result in a specific action. They are known as spinal reflexes because they persist after complete transection of the spinal cord.
   1. The **muscle stretch reflex** (MSR) is a monosynaptic reflex that links a receptor neuron with an effector neuron and results in a muscle twitch in response to muscle stretch (Fig. 5-5). The functional sequence of this response is as follows:
      a. **Muscle spindles** serve as the receptors for the MSR. Upon stretch of the muscle spindle (usually via stretch of a tendon), it is activated and sends signals to the CNS via axons of α-myelinated **afferents.**

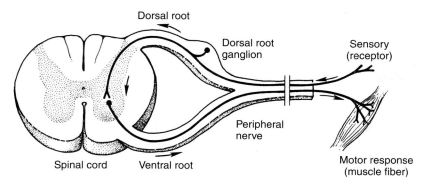

FIG 5-5. Monosynaptic reflex arc, consisting of a primary sensory neuron activating a motor neuron by a direct synapse. The motor neuron activates an effector, skeletal muscle in this case. [Reprinted with permission from DeMyer D, ed. NMS Neuroanatomy, 2nd ed. Philadelphia, Lippincott Williams & Wilkins, 1998:23.]

> **b.** The afferent axons synapse directly on α-**motor neurons** in the ventral horn.
>
> **c.** As a result, the α-motor neuron is excited, triggering an **efferent** impulse that causes muscular contraction.
>
> **d.** An example of a MSR is the **knee-jerk reflex.** Muscle stretch triggered by striking the patellar tendon causes contraction of the knee extensors and a knee jerk.

2. The **flexion and crossed-extension reflex** can serve as a protective reflex that occurs after contact with a painful stimulus. This type of reflex is mediated by polysynaptic pathways in the spinal cord (Fig. 5-6).

> **a.** The receptors that provide afferent input for this reflex are **cutaneous nociceptors,** or pain receptors.
>
> **b.** Excitatory afferent nociceptive impulses project to interneurons in the spinal cord, which project to α-motor neurons that innervate **ipsilateral** flexor muscles.

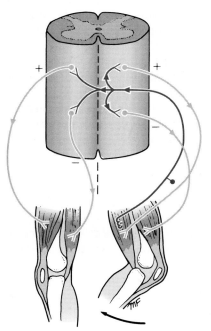

FIG 5-6. Law of reciprocal innervation and the crossed-extensor reflex. Stepping on a nail with the left foot triggers a response which results in withdrawl of that leg and activation of muscles needed to support the body by the right leg (see I.C.2.e.). [Reprinted with permission from Snell RS, ed. Clinical Neuroanatomy, 6th ed. Philadelphia, Lippincott Williams & Wilkins, 2006:162.]

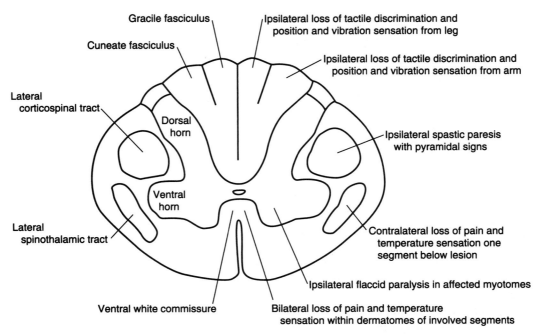

Gracile fasciculus

Cuneate fasciculus

Ipsilateral loss of tactile discrimination and position and vibration sensation from leg

Ipsilateral loss of tactile discrimination and position and vibration sensation from arm

Lateral corticospinal tract

Dorsal horn

Ipsilateral spastic paresis with pyramidal signs

Ventral horn

Lateral spinothalamic tract

Contralateral loss of pain and temperature sensation one segment below lesion

Ipsilateral flaccid paralysis in affected myotomes

Ventral white commissure

Bilateral loss of pain and temperature sensation within dermatomes of involved segments

FIG 5-7. Transverse section of the cervical spinal cord. The clinically important ascending and descending pathways are shown on the *left*. Clinical deficits that result from the interruption of these pathways are shown on the *right*. [Reprinted with permission from Fix JD, ed. High-Yield Neuroanatomy, 3rd ed. Philadelphia, Lippincott Williams & Wilkins, 2005:69.]

    c. These same impulses project to interneurons, the axons of which cross to the contralateral side of the spinal cord, that excite α-motor neurons innervating the **contralateral** extensor muscles.

    d. The result of this reflex is flexion on the side of the painful stimulus and extension on the contralateral side.

    e. An example of this reflex occurs when someone steps on a sharp object. If one steps on a nail with the left foot, flexors in the left leg are activated and the left foot is withdrawn. At the same time, extensors of the right leg are activated, serving to support the body during withdrawl (see Fig. 5-6).

D. Lesions of the spinal cord (Figs. 5-7 and 5-8)

  1. Lesions to the spinal cord can cause upper motor neuron (UMN) **signs,** lower motor neuron (LMN) **signs,** or **both.**

    a. UMN lesions result from damage to the corticospinal tract (or to the cortical neurons from which it originates) and lead to **spastic paresis** with pyramidal signs (e.g., the presence of the Babinski sign).

    b. LMN lesions result from damage to motor neurons of the spinal cord. This type of injury is observed clinically by **flaccid paralysis, areflexia, atrophy, fasciculations,** and **fibrillations. Poliomyelitis** and **Werdnig-Hoffmann disease** (a form of spinal muscular atrophy) are examples of LMN pathology (Fig. 5-8A).

    c. In **amyotrophic lateral sclerosis,** both UMNs and LMNs are affected (Fig. 5-8D). This results in a combination of UMN and LMN signs on clinical examination (and see Chapter 4).

  2. Tabes dorsalis, a condition that can be seen in patients with neurosyphilis, is the result of lesions to the **dorsal columns** (Fig. 5-8C). The result is a loss of tactile discrimination, proprioception, and vibration sense.

  3. Table 5-2 summarizes common patterns of combined motor and sensory lesions to the spinal cord.

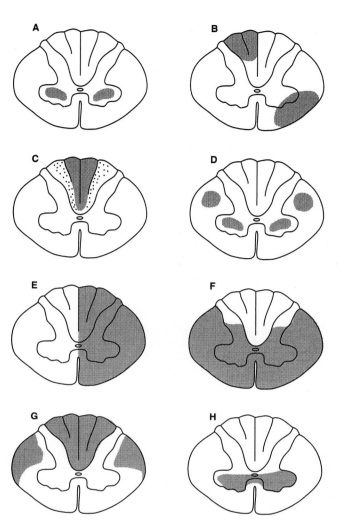

FIG 5-8. Classic lesions (hatched areas) of the spinal cord. **A.** Poliomyelitis and progressive infantile muscular atrophy (Werdnig-Hoffman disease). **B.** Multiple sclerosis. **C.** Dorsal column disease (tabes dorsalis). **D.** Amyotrophic lateral sclerosis. **E.** Hemisection of the spinal cord (Brown-Séquard syndrome). **F.** Complete ventral spinal artery occlusion. **G.** Subacute combined degeneration (vitamin B_{12} neuropathy). **H.** Syringomyelia. [Reprinted with permission from Fix JD, ed. High-Yield Neuroanatomy, 3rd ed. Philadelphia, Lippincott Williams & Wilkins, 2005:70.]

II. Brainstem

Patient Snapshot 5-2

The mother of a 9-year-old boy reports to the pediatrician that the left half of her child's face seems weak and less reactive to emotional changes than the right side. She also observes that the child's mouth seems pulled over slightly to the right, especially when he is tired. The child reports that when he eats, food gets stuck in his left cheek and the left side of his face feels weird. These symptoms began 4 months earlier and have slowly progressed. Physical examination reveals weakness of facial muscles on the left with normal strength on the right, normal facial sensation bilaterally, weakness of the lateral rectus muscle on the left, and mild weakness of the right arm and leg. After consultation, a pediatric neurologist suggests that the facial muscle and lateral rectus weakness are attributable to involvement of the left facial and abducens nuclei; the right arm and leg weakness could be the result of pontine corticospinal tract damage on the left. Preserved facial sensation indicates that the sensory nuclei of the trigeminal nerve are preserved. Imaging studies indicate that the child has a fairly well circumscribed lesion in the left pons that is consistent with an astrocytoma, a brain tumor of astrocyte origin (see Fig. 18-3).

TABLE 5-2	COMBINED MOTOR AND SENSORY LESIONS OF THE SPINAL CORD	
	Lesions	**Signs and Symptoms**
Spinal cord hemisection; Brown-Séquard syndrome (Fig. 5-8*E*)	Dorsal columns Lateral corticospinal tract Lateral spinothalamic tract Hypothalamospinal tract (T1 and above) Ventral horn	Ipsilateral loss of tactile discrimination, proprioception, and vibratory sense Ipsilateral spastic paresis and pyramidal signs below lesion Contralateral loss of pain and temperature sense one segment below lesion Ipsilateral Horner syndrome (e.g., ptosis, miosis, anhydrosis) Ipsilateral flaccid paralysis at level of lesion
Ventral spinal artery occlusion (Fig. 5-8*F*)	Lateral corticospinal tracts Lateral spinothalamic tracts Hypothalamospinal tracts (T2 and above) Ventral horns Corticospinal tracts to sacral parasympathetic centers (S2–4)	Bilateral spastic paresis and pyramidal signs below lesion Bilateral loss of pain and temperature sensation below lesion Bilateral Horner syndrome Bilateral flaccid paralysis at level of lesion Loss of voluntary bladder and bowel control
Subacute combined degeneration; B$_{12}$ neuropathy (Fig. 5-8*G*)	Dorsal columns Lateral corticospinal tracts Spinocerebellar tracts	Bilateral loss of tactile discrimination, proprioception, and vibratory sense Bilateral spastic paresis and pyramidal signs below lesions Bilateral arm and leg dystaxia
Syringomyelia; central cavitation of the cervical cord (Fig. 5-8*H*)	Ventral white commissure (decussation of lateral spinothalamic axons) Ventral horns	Bilateral loss of pain and temperature sensation Flaccid paralysis, commonly of intrinsic muscles of hands
Friedrich ataxia	Dorsal columns Lateral corticospinal tracts Spinocerebellar tracts	Bilateral loss of tactile discrimination, proprioception, and vibratory sense Bilateral spastic paresis and pyramidal signs below lesions Bilateral arm and leg dystaxia
Multiple sclerosis (Fig. 5-8*B*)	Primarily involvement of cervical cord white matter; random and asymmetric lesions	Depend on tracts affected

Because astrocytomas in children can usually be removed totally, the cure rate with surgery is about 90%.

A. **Gross anatomy.** The brainstem, extending from the pyramidal decussation to the posterior commissure, is made up of three structures (from caudal to rostral): the **medulla,** the **pons,** and the **midbrain.** Within these structures lie nuclei for cranial nerves CN III–CN XII (except for the spinal portion of CN XI) (Fig. 5-9).

1. The **medulla** is the caudal most portion of the brainstem connecting the pons with the spinal cord. The medulla contains several noteworthy structures (cranial nerves are discussed in II.B) (Fig. 5-10; Table 5-3).

2. The **pons** sits anterior to the **fourth ventricle** and the cerebellum, between the medulla and the midbrain. It has a dorsal tegmentum and a ventral base. Many of the structures of the medulla are transmitted rostrally through the pons (e.g., medial lemniscus and corticospinal tracts). It also contains several prominent structures (Fig. 5-11; Table 5-4).

3. The **midbrain** connects the pons and cerebellum to the forebrain as it passes through the opening in the tentorium cerebelli. The **cerebral aqueduct** passes

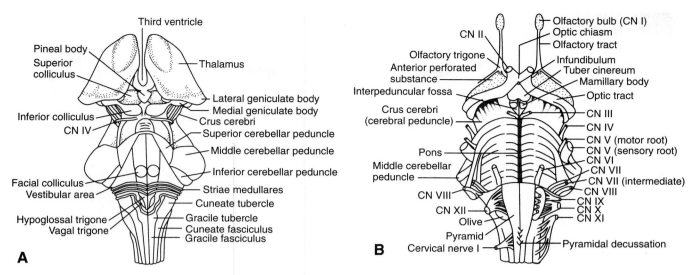

FIG 5-9. A. The dorsal surface of the brainstem. The three cerebellar peduncles have been removed to expose the rhomboid fossa. The trochlear nerve is the only nerve to exit the brainstem from the dorsal surface. The facial colliculus surmounts the genu of the facial nerve and the abducent nucleus. **B.** The ventral surface of the brainstem and the attached cranial nerves (*CN*). [Reprinted with permission from Fix JD, ed. High-Yield Neuroanatomy, 3rd ed. Philadelphia, Lippincott Williams & Wilkins, 2005:73–74.]

through the midbrain and allows for CSF flow from the third to the fourth ventricle. The cross-sectional structure of the midbrain is presented in Fig. 5-12 and Table 5-5.

B. Cranial nerves (CNs) and nuclei (Fig. 5-13)

   1. The 12 pairs of CNs can be characterized according to the modality or modalities possessed:

      a. A CN can possess **general** and/or **special** components. *Special* signifies that the nerve transmits impulses related to the special senses (vision, olfaction, gestation, audition).

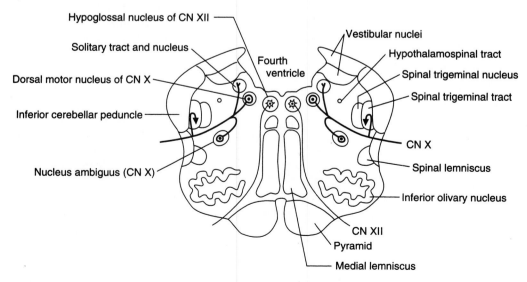

FIG 5-10. Transverse section of the medulla at the mid-olivary level. The vagus nerve (cranial nerve [*CN*] X), hypoglossal nerve (CN XII), and vestibulocochlear nerve (CN VIII) are prominent in this section. The nucleus ambiguous gives rise to special visceral efferent fibers to CN IX and XI, although only its contribution to CN X is shown. [Reprinted with permission from Fix JD, ed. High-Yield Neuroanatomy, 3rd ed. Philadelphia, Lippincott Williams & Wilkins, 2005:74.]

TABLE 5-3	MAJOR STRUCTURES IN CROSS-SECTIONAL ANATOMY OF THE MEDULLA	
Structure	**Location**	**Comment**
Pyramids	Anterior portion of medulla, separated by anterior fissure	Contain corticospinal tract fibers that originate in precentral gyrus
Decussation of pyramids	Anterior portion of medulla at base of pyramids	Where descending corticospinal tracts cross to opposite side Clinically relevant because lesions above decussation cause contralateral deficit, whereas lesions below cause ipsilateral deficit
Medial lemniscus	On each side of midline posterior to pyramids	Composed of dorsal column fibers from gracile and cuneate nuclei Conveys ascending sensory signals to thalamus
Decussation of lemnisci	Anterior to central gray matter, posterior to pyramids Just superior to decussation of pyramids	Lesions to medial lemniscal pathway result in clinically analogous deficits to pyramidal tract lesions
Nucleus ambiguus	Deep within the reticular formation	Contains large motor neurons that contribute to glossopharyngeal and vagus nerves and cranial portion of accessory nerve Its fibers innervate voluntary skeletal muscle
Inferior cerebellar peduncle	Posterolateral region of medulla	Contains primarily afferent tracts into cerebellum (e.g., dorsal spinocerebellar and olivocerebellar tracts)
Lateral spinothalamic tract	Between anterior and posterior spinocerebellar tracts on anterolateral aspects of medulla	Together with anterior spinothalamic and spinotectal tracts, makes up the spinal lemniscus
Dorsal motor nucleus of vagus nerve	Lateral to hypoglossal nuclei	Preganglionic parasympathetic fibers from this nucleus project to pulmonary, bronchial, myenteric, and submucosal plexuses

  b. A nerve can conduct **somatic** and/or **visceral** signals. Somatic nerves innervate structures embryologically associated with the body wall, whereas visceral nerves innervate embryologically splanchnic structures.

  c. A nerve can transmit impulses in the **afferent** and/or **efferent** direction. Afferent nerves are sensory nerves, and efferent nerves are motor nerves.

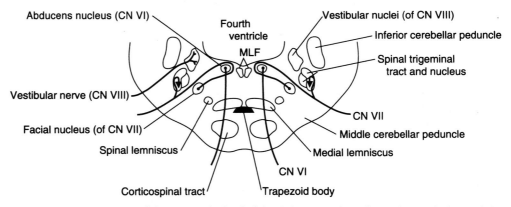

FIG 5-11. Transverse section of the pons at the level of the abducens nucleus of cranial nerve (*CN*) VI and the facial nucleus of CN VII. *MLF,* medial longitudinal fasciculus. [Reprinted with permission from Fix JD, ed. High-Yield Neuroanatomy, 3rd ed. Philadelphia, Lippincott Williams & Wilkins, 2005:75.]

TABLE 5-4	MAJOR STRUCTURES IN CROSS-SECTIONAL ANATOMY OF THE PONS	
Structure	**Location**	**Comment**
Trapezoid body	Situated along midline, anterior to medial lemnisci, posterior to pyramids	Composed of fibers from cochlear nuclei and nuclei of trapezoid body
Medial longitudinal fasciculus	Along midline at floor of fourth ventricle	Primary pathway connecting vestibular and cochlear nuclei to nuclei controlling extraocular muscles
Superior cerebellar peduncle	Posterolateral to motor nucleus of trigeminal nerve	Transmits three afferent (ventral spinocerebellar, trigeminocerebellar, and tectocerebellar tracts) and one efferent tract (dentatorubrothalamic tract)
Middle cerebellar peduncle	Along anterolateral surface of pons Lateral to superior and inferior cerebellar peduncles	Transmits afferent pontocerebellar tracts
Edinger-Westphal nucleus	Posterior to motor nucleus of oculomotor nerve	Preganglionic parasympathetic fibers from this nucleus project to postganglionic neurons of ciliary ganglion to control activity of constrictor pupillae muscle

TABLE 5-5	MAJOR STRUCTURES IN CROSS-SECTIONAL ANATOMY OF THE MIDBRAIN	
Structure	**Location**	**Comment**
Superior colliculi	Superior two eminences on dorsal surface	Large nucleus that is a center for visual reflexes
Inferior colliculi	Inferior two eminences on dorsal surface	Large nucleus that forms part of lower auditory centers
Substantia nigra	Seated between tegmentum and crus cerebri	Large motor nucleus with neurons that contain granules of melanin pigment. giving it its dark color
		Component of basal ganglia
Red nucleus	Between cerebral aqueduct and substantia nigra	Round mass of gray matter, color of which results from its abundant vascularity and an iron-containing pigment in neurons
Crus cerebri	Two anterior surface projections, separated by interpeduncular fossa	Contains important descending fiber tracts (e.g., middle three fifths is occupied by corticospinal tract)

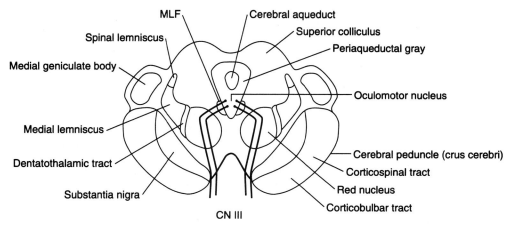

FIG 5-12. Transverse section of the midbrain at the level of the superior colliculus, oculomotor nucleus of cranial nerve (*CN*) III, and red nucleus. *MLF,* medial longitudinal fasciculus. [Reprinted with permission from Fix JD, ed. High-Yield Neuroanatomy, 3rd ed. Philadelphia, Lippincott Williams & Wilkins, 2005:76.]

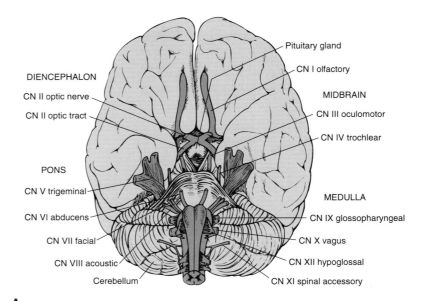

Pituitary gland
CN I olfactory

DIENCEPHALON

CN II optic nerve

CN II optic tract

MIDBRAIN

CN III oculomotor

CN IV trochlear

PONS

CN V trigeminal

CN VI abducens

CN VII facial

CN VIII acoustic

Cerebellum

MEDULLA

CN IX glossopharyngeal

CN X vagus

CN XII hypoglossal

CN XI spinal accessory

A

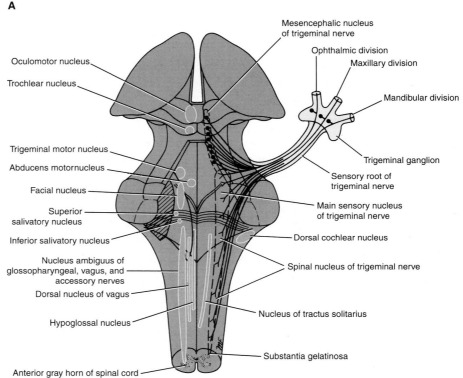

Oculomotor nucleus

Trochlear nucleus

Trigeminal motor nucleus

Abducens motornucleus

Facial nucleus

Superior salivatory nucleus

Inferior salivatory nucleus

Nucleus ambiguus of glossopharyngeal, vagus, and accessory nerves

Dorsal nucleus of vagus

Hypoglossal nucleus

Anterior gray horn of spinal cord

Mesencephalic nucleus of trigeminal nerve

Ophthalmic division

Maxillary division

Mandibular division

Trigeminal ganglion

Sensory root of trigeminal nerve

Main sensory nucleus of trigeminal nerve

Dorsal cochlear nucleus

Spinal nucleus of trigeminal nerve

Nucleus of tractus solitarius

Substantia gelatinosa

B

FIG 5-13. A. The 12 cranial nerves and brain landmarks. Note: For CN VIII, the term *acoustic nerve* is synonymous with *vestibulocochlear nerve.* [Reprinted with permission from Weber J, Kelley J. Health Assessment in Nursing, 2nd ed. Philadelphia, Lippincott Williams & Wilkins, 2003.] **B.** Position of the cranial nerve nuclei within the brainstem. *Hatched area,* position of the vestibular nuclei. [Reprinted with permission from Snell RS, ed. Clinical Neuroanatomy, 6th ed. Philadelphia, Lippincott Williams & Wilkins, 2006:194.]

    d. Therefore, there are seven functional components: general somatic efferent (**GSE**), general somatic afferent (**GSA**), general visceral efferent (**GVE**), general visceral afferent (**GVA**), special somatic afferent (**SSA**), special visceral afferent (**SVA**), and special visceral efferent (**SVE**).

   e. For easier understanding, the cranial nerves can be divided into three groups:
   i. Cranial nerves **I, II,** and **VIII** contain solely special sensory fibers (olfaction, vision, audition/vestibular function).
      (a) The nasal passages are endodermally derived; thus CN I possesses only an SVA component.
      (b) The optic (CN II) and vestibulocochlear (CN VIII) nerves possess only SSA components.
   ii. Cranial nerves **III, IV, VI,** and **XII** are essentially motor in function and innervate the striated muscles controlling the muscles of the eyes and the tongue (GSE).
      (a) Each of these cranial nerves possesses a small sensory component serving only proprioception (GSA).
      (b) The oculomotor nerve (CN III) also conveys parasympathetic fibers to the ciliary (for accommodation) and the pupilloconstrictor muscles (GVE).
   iii. The final five cranial nerves innervate structures derived from the brachial arches: **V, VII, IX, X,** and **XI.**
      (a) CN XI (accessory nerve) innervates the sternocleidomastoid and trapezius muscles and contains SVE and proprioceptive GSA components.
      (b) CN V (trigeminal nerve) innervates striated muscles for mastication (SVE) but also has a large general sensory component (facial sensation; GSA).
      (c) The facial (CN VII), glossopharyngeal (CN IX), and vagus (CN X) nerves are unique in that they possess five components: SVE, GVE, GVA, SVA, and GSA.
   f. Table 5-6 outlines the functional components of each cranial nerve.
2. All but the olfactory (CN I) and optic (CN II) nerves have cranial nerve nuclei. Figure 5-13B shows the locations of cranial nerve nuclei within the brainstem.

TABLE 5-6	FUNCTIONAL COMPONENTS OF THE CRANIAL NERVES						
Nerve	**GSE**	**SVE**	**GVE**	**GVA**	**SVA**	**GSA**	**SSA**
Sensory only							
I					+		
II							+
VIII							+
Somatomotor							
III	+		+			+[a]	
IV	+					+[a]	
VI	+					+[a]	
XII	+					+[a]	
Brachial							
V		+				+	
VII		+	+	+	+	+	
IX		+	+	+	+	+	
X		+	+	+	+	+	
XI		+				+[a]	

Adapted from DeMyer W. NMS Neuroanatomy, 2nd ed. Baltimore, Lippincott Williams & Wilkins, 1998:165.
[a]Proprioceptive GSA components only.

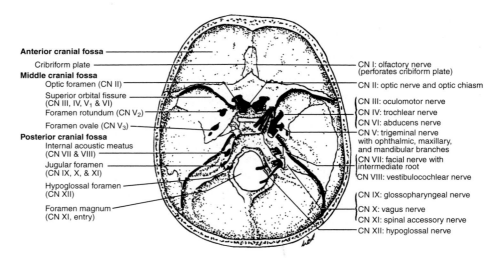

FIG 5-14. Base of the skull (calvaria removed) showing the foramina traversed by the cranial nerves. [Reprinted with permission from DeMyer D, ed. NMS Neuroanatomy, 2nd ed. Philadelphia, Lippincott Williams & Wilkins, 1998:23.]

3. Each nerve passes through a foramen in the base of the skull as it exits to its targets (Fig. 5-14).
4. Table 5-7 summarizes the 12 pairs of CNs and their nuclei, from rostral (CN I) to caudal (CN XII).
5. **Autonomic nuclei and the cranial nerves.** Four cranial nerves possess parasympathetic fibers: CN III, CN VII, CN IX, and CN X.
    a. **CN III.** Preganglionic parasympathetic fibers of the GVE component arise from the **Edinger-Westphal nucleus.** These fibers synapse on postganglionic neurons of the **ciliary ganglion.** Postganglionic fibers via the short ciliary nerves control the constrictor pupillae and ciliary muscles.
    b. **CN VII.** The facial nerve has two parasympathetic pathways:
        i. The **lacrimal pathway** begins with the preganglionic fibers of the **superior salivatory nucleus.** These fibers project to the **pterygopalatine ganglion** via the intermediate and greater petrosal nerves. Postganglionic fibers from the pterygopalatine ganglion project to the lacrimal gland of the orbit.
        ii. The **submandibular pathway** also starts with preganglionic fibers in the **superior salivatory nucleus.** The fibers project via intermediate nerve and chorda tympani to the **submandibular ganglion.** Postganglionic fibers project to the submandibular and sublingual salivary glands.
    c. **CN IX.** Preganglionic fibers from the **inferior salivatory nucleus** in the medulla project to the **otic ganglion** via the tympanic and lesser petrosal nerves. Fibers from the otic ganglion are directed at the parotid gland.
    d. **CN X.** The **dorsal motor nucleus of the vagus nerve** is the source of preganglionic parasympathetic fibers. The fibers project to the ganglia of the visceral organs by way of the vagus nerve.

C. **Reticular formation.** The **reticular formation (RF)** is a loosely arranged collection of nuclei that make up the substance of the brainstem tegmentum not otherwise occupied by cranial nerve nuclei, supplementary sensory and motor nuclei, and named long and short tracts (Fig. 5-15).
    1. **Anatomy**
        a. The RF got its name because its loose arrangement of neurons and their processes resembles a net. This is quite distinct from the usual densely packed arrangement of most CNS nuclei.

TABLE 5-7		THE CRANIAL NERVES AND NUCLEI	
Cranial Nerve	**Location of CN Nuclei**	**Path (foramina)**	**Functions**
I: olfactory	NA	Olfactory receptor cells in nasal mucosa project to olfactory bulb through cribriform plate Mitral cells of olfactory bulb project through olfactory tract and lateral olfactory stria These projections terminate in olfactory cortex and amygdala	Olfaction or smell (SVA)
II: optic	NA	Retinal ganglion cells form nerve itself and project to lateral geniculate bodies via optic canal Fibers from lateral geniculate project to primary visual cortex via visual radiations	Vision and pupillary light reflexes (afferent limb; SSA)
III: oculomotor	Rostral midbrain	GSE component arises from oculomotor nucleus of rostral midbrain It exits midbrain from interpeduncular fossa, traverses cavernous sinus, and enters orbit via superior orbital fissure GVE component derives from Edinger-Westphal nucleus, which sends preganglionic parasympathetic fibers to ciliary ganglion Postganglionic fibers from ciliary ganglion project to their targets in orbit	Control of all extraocular muscles, except lateral rectus and superior oblique Innervates levator palpebrae (GSE) Preganglionic parasympathetic fibers involved in control of constrictor pupillae muscle (miosis) and ciliary muscle (accommodation; GVE)
IV: trochlear	Caudal midbrain	Nerve arises from contralateral trochlear nucleus It decussates deep to superior medullary velum of midbrain and exits on dorsal surface of midbrain, caudal to inferior colliculus It then wraps around midbrain in subarachnoid space, passes through cavernous sinus, and enters orbit via superior orbital fissure	Innervates superior oblique muscle of eye (GSE)
V: trigeminal	Motor trigeminal nucleus (lateral midpontine tegmentum) Sensory nucleus (posterior pons lateral to motor nucleus) Spinal nucleus (continuous with sensory nucleus; extends down to second cervical segment) Mesencephalic nucleus (gray matter lateral to cerebral aqueduct; downward into pons to sensory nucleus)	Smaller motor root and larger sensory root exit anterior surface of pons and rest on temporal bone in middle cranial fossa Sensory root expands and forms trigeminal ganglion in Meckel cave, giving rise to three divisions: ophthalmic division (V_1) is purely sensory and exits cranium via superior orbital fissure, maxillary division (V_2) is purely sensory and exits cranium via foramen rotundum, mandibular division (V_3) contains sensory and motor fibers and exits through foramen ovale	Innervates muscles of mastication, tensores tympani and veli palatine, mylohyoid muscle, and anterior belly of digastric (SVE) Provides sensory innervation to face; mucous membranes of nose, mouth, and paranasal sinuses; hard palate and deep structures Also innervates dura mater of anterior and middle cranial fossa (GSA)
VI: abducens	Dorsomedial tegmentum of caudal pons	Nerve exits nucleus and passes through corticospinal tract It passes through pontine cistern and cavernous sinus and then enters orbit via superior orbital fissure	Innervates lateral rectus muscle of eye (GSE)

(continued)

TABLE 5-7		THE CRANIAL NERVES AND NUCLEI (*CONTINUED*)	
Cranial Nerve	**Location of CN Nuclei**	**Path (foramina)**	**Functions**
VII: facial	Motor nucleus (within reticular formation of lower pons) Parasympathetic nuclei (superior salivatory nuclei; lie posterolateral to motor nucleus) Sensory nucleus (upper part of nucleus of tractus solitarius, near motor nucleus)	Motor root loops posteriorly around abducens nucleus, passes beneath facial colliculus, then moves anterior to exit anterior surface of brainstem Sensory root forms from cells of geniculate ganglion and contains preganglionic parasympathetic fibers Both roots exit anterior brainstem between pons and medulla, pass laterally to CN VIII in posterior fossa, and enter internal auditory meatus and then facial canal Near medial wall of tympanic cavity, nerve forms sensory geniculate ganglion, then turns sharply backward Ultimately, motor root exits from stylomastoid foramen	Innervates ipsilateral muscles of facial expression (SVE) Parasympathetic innervation to lacrimal, submandibular, and sublingual glands (GVE) Taste from anterior two thirds of tongue (SVA) Mediates skin sensation on a small region of outer ear (GSA) Some fibers innervate soft palate and adjacent pharyngeal wall; these have no clinical significance (GVA)
VIII: vestibulocochlear	Vestibular nuclei (group of nuclei beneath floor of fourth ventricle: lateral, superior, medial, and inferior) Dorsal and ventral cochlear nuclei (on surface of anterior cerebellar peduncle in pons)	First-order vestibular sensory neurons are in vestibular ganglion, fibers of which pass through internal auditory meatus These project peripherally to hair cells in utricle and saccule, and centrally to vestibular nuclei and cerebellum First-order cochlear sensory neurons are in cochlear ganglion These project peripherally to hair cells of organ of Corti and centrally to dorsal and ventral cochlear nuclei of brainstem	Conducts signals from utricle and saccule to give information on head position (SSA) Mediates hearing (SSA)
IX: glossopharyngeal	Motor nucleus (in reticular formation of medulla; formed from superior part of nucleus ambiguus) Parasympathetic nucleus (known as inferior salivatory nucleus; in medulla) Sensory nucleus (part of nucleus of solitary tract)	Exits rostral anterolateral medulla between olive and inferior cerebellar peduncle, travels laterally in posterior fossa, exits cranium via jugular foramen Superior and inferior sensory ganglia sit along nerve near jugular foramen Nerve descends in upper neck along internal jugular vein	Innervates stylopharyngeus muscle (SVE) Parasympathetic control of parotid gland via otic ganglion (GVE) Innervates mucous membranes of posterior third of tongue, tonsil, upper pharynx, tympanic cavity, and auditory tube; also innervates carotid sinus and body (GVA) Supplies taste buds on posterior third of tongue (SVA) Sensory innervation for external ear and external auditory meatus (GSA)
X: vagus	Motor nucleus (deep in reticular formation of medulla; formed by nucleus ambiguus) Parasympathetic nucleus (beneath floor of fourth ventricle posterolateral to hypoglossal nucleus in medulla) Sensory nucleus (lower part of nucleus of tractus solitarius)	Exits rostral anterolateral medulla between olive and inferior cerebellar peduncle, travels in posterior fossa, and exits via jugular foramen Nerve descends in neck within carotid sheath after forming superior and inferior ganglia Some neck structures are innervated by branches called pharyngeal and recurrent laryngeal nerves (left of which passes under aortic arch) Right vagus enters thorax and contributes to pulmonary and esophageal plexuses, then becomes posterior trunk as it passes into abdomen via esophageal hiatus	Motor innervation to pharyngeal arch muscles of larynx, pharynx, and striated muscle of upper esophagus, uvula muscle, and levator veli palatini and palatoglossus muscles (SVE) Parasympathetic innervation to viscera of neck, thorax, and abdominal structures (to splenic flexure; GVE) Innervates mucous membranes of pharynx, larynx, esophagus, trachea, thoracic and abdominal viscera (to splenic flexure; GVA)

TABLE 5-7	THE CRANIAL NERVES AND NUCLEI (*CONTINUED*)		
Cranial Nerve	**Location of CN Nuclei**	**Path (foramina)**	**Functions**
	Cranial division of CN XI is now known as part of vagus nerve: nucleus ambiguus of medulla[a]	Left vagus contributes to same structures and becomes anterior vagal trunk as it passes through esophageal hiatus Emerges from anterior medulla between olive and inferior cerebellar peduncle, joins spinal root in posterior fossa, exits via jugular foramen, and then joins vagus nerve	Supplies taste buds in epiglottic region (SVA) Innervates infratentorial dura, external ear, external auditory meatus, and tympanic membrane GSA) Innervates intrinsic muscles of larynx (except cricothyroid; SVE)[a]
XI: spinal accessory	Spinal division: spinal nucleus in anterior gray column of first five cervical segments	Spinal division—fibers exit from spinal cord between anterior and posterior cervical nerve roots Fibers ascend through foramen magnum and then exit via jugular foramen	Spinal division: innervates sternocleidomastoid and trapezius muscles (SVE)
XII: hypoglossal	Near midline beneath floor of fourth ventricle in medulla	Exits anterior surface of medulla between pyramid and olive Exits skull by way of hypoglossal canal	Controls tongue movement (GSE)

CN, cranial nerve; *GSA*, general somatic afferent; *GSE*, general somatic efferent; *GVA*, general visceral afferent; *GVE*, general visceral efferent; *NA*, not applicable; *SSA*, special somatic afferent; *SVA*, special visceral afferent; *SVE*, special visceral efferent. Adapted from Fix JD. High Yield Neuroanatomy, 3rd ed. Philadelphia, Lippincott Williams & Wilkins, 2005:167–169.

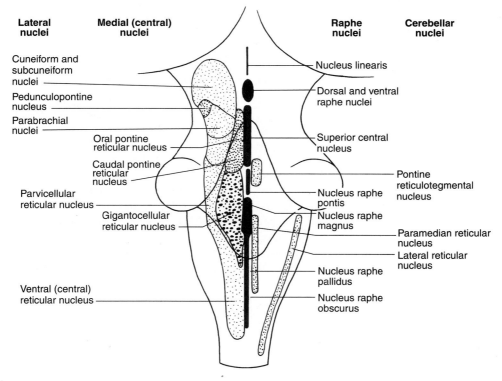

FIG 5-15. Dorsal view of the brainstem showing the location of the four groups of reticular formation nuclei. [Reprinted with permission from DeMyer D, ed. NMS Neuroanatomy, 2nd ed. Philadelphia, Lippincott Williams & Wilkins, 1998:110.]

b. The entire length of the **brainstem tegmentum,** from the medulla to the midbrain, possesses components of the RF.

c. This loose arrangement of cells is divided into three longitudinal columns: the median, medial, and lateral columns.

2. RF nuclei. The RF nuclei are classified on the basis of their location (e.g., plane or column) and the cytoarchitecture of their neurons.

    a. The **raphe nuclei** are made up of intermediate-size neurons located in the median plane of the brainstem. They extend the length of the entire median plane.

    b. The **medial (central) gigantocellular nuclei** are made up of large-size neurons. These nuclei extend through the pontomedullary tegmentum, lateral to the raphe nuclei.

    c. The **lateral parvicellular nuclei** are made up of small-celled neurons. They extend from the medullocervical junction rostrally to the midbrain and lateral to the gigantocellular nuclei.

3. Functions. The RF possesses a vast number of connections via its afferent and efferent projections. Nearly every part of the nervous system is contacted by the diffuse elements of the RF.

    a. Control of skeletal muscle

       i. Shapes the activity of α- and γ-motor neurons

      ii. Regulates muscle tone and reflex activity

     iii. In association with the vestibular system, controls the maintenance of muscle tone in antigravity muscles

     iv. Controls respiratory muscle activity

      v. Affects movement of facial-expression muscles associated with emotion

    b. Control of somatic and visceral sensations

    c. Control of the autonomic nervous system

    d. Control of the endocrine nervous system

    e. Influences the biologic clock (see also Chapter 15)

    f. The **reticular-activating system**

       i. The RF serves as a relay between multiple ascending sensory pathways and the cerebral cortex.

      ii. Relay of sensory stimuli to different parts of the cortex is believed to be responsible for determining the level of **consciousness.**

     iii. Even small **lesions** of the RF can cause profound loss of consciousness extending for a prolonged period (i.e., **coma**).

     iv. Thus the RF controls the four *A*s of sleep–wake states: **asleep, awake, alert,** and **attentive.**

D. Blood supply. Arterial blood is largely supplied to the structures of the brainstem from the posterior circulation.

1. The **medulla** is supplied by **medullary arteries,** which are small branches of the cranial portion of the vertebral arteries. The **anterior inferior cerebellar arteries (AICAs), posterior inferior cerebellar arteries (PICAs), posterior spinal,** and branches of the **basilar artery** also perfuse the medulla.

2. The **pontine arteries** are small vessels that branch from the basilar artery and enter the substance of the **pons.** The **AICAs** and **superior cerebellar artery** also participate.

3. The **midbrain** is supplied by the **posterior cerebral, superior cerebellar,** and **basilar arteries.**

Chapter 6

Gross Anatomy of the Brain and the Neuroanatomy of Behavior

I. The Brain

Patient Snapshot 6-1

A 72-year-old woman with a history of hypertension, type 2 diabetes mellitus, and hypercholesterolemia is brought to the emergency room when her son notices that she is dragging her left foot while walking. The patient, who is alert and responsive, states that the problem began suddenly 3 weeks ago. Physical examination reveals increased muscle tone in the flexors of the left arm, weakness and increased tone in the muscles of the left leg, and disturbed gait. When asked to walk, the physician observes that the patient has a problem flexing her left hip and knee such that she needs to swing her left leg in a semicircle to place her forefoot down before her heel. The patient's presentation and history suggest that she has had a stroke. Because of the weakness, the physician suspects involvement of the right precentral gyrus with concomitant destruction of upper motor neurons of the corticospinal tract. The increased muscle tone suggests loss of inhibition, resulting from involvement of extrapyramidal fibers. Management of this patient will involve reducing her cardiovascular risk factors (e.g., hypertension) to prevent future strokes as well as physical therapy and rehabilitation to address her current physical problems. Because of the proximity of the affected area to the prefrontal cortex, personality and mood changes may also occur.

A. Gross anatomy

1. The **cerebrum** is situated in the anterior and middle cranial fossae and is divided into two parts: the **diencephalon** and the **telencephalon** (Fig. 6-1).

   a. The **diencephalon** is composed of the **third ventricle** and the structures that make up its borders, including the following:

      i. The **thalamus** has been classically defined as containing 11 nuclei (Fig. 6-2). Clinically, it is thought of as a relay station for the **integration** of the sensory and motor systems.

      ii. The **subthalamus** (including the substantia nigra, the subthalamic nucleus, and portions of the red nucleus) is involved in control of muscle activity and contains relays from the tegmentum to the thalamic nuclei.

      iii. The **epithalamus** (including the habenular nucleus and the pineal gland)—the habenular nucleus is important for integration of olfactory, visceral, and somatic afferent pathways.

      iv. The **hypothalamus** (see II.B)

      v. The **optic chiasma** and **optic tract**

      vi. The **infundibulum** and **tuber cinereum**

   b. The **telencephalon** forms the **cerebral hemispheres.**

      i. The cerebral hemispheres are separated by the **longitudinal cerebral fissure,** which contains the **falx cerebri** and serves as the course of the **anterior cerebral arteries.** The surface of each cerebral hemisphere is thrown into folds or **gyri,** which are separated by **sulci;** thus increasing the surface area. Notable sulci include the **central sulcus** separating

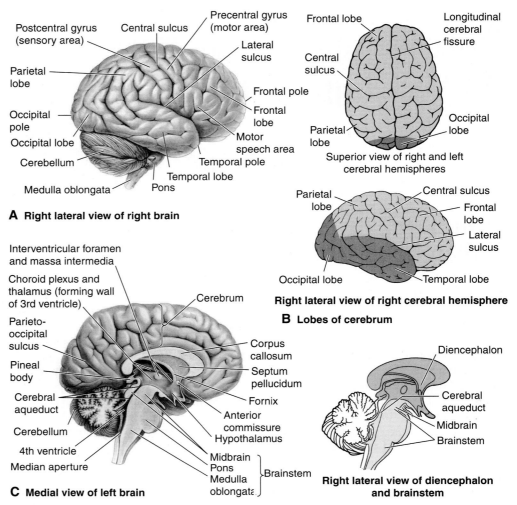

FIG 6-1. Structure of the brain. **A and B.** Observe the gyri (folds) and sulci (grooves) of the frontal, parietal, and occipital lobes. **C.** Note that the cerebral cortex also consists of gyri and sulci. The cerebral aqueduct (aqueduct of midbrain) connects the third and fourth ventricles. [Reprinted with permission from Moore KL. Clinical Oriented Anatomy, 5th ed. Baltimore, Lippincott Williams & Wilkins 2006.]

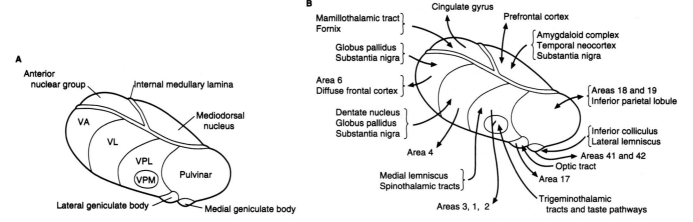

FIG 6-2. **A.** Dorsolateral aspect of the thalamus showing the major nuclei. *VA,* ventral anterior nucleus; *VL,* ventral lateral nucleus; *VPL,* ventral posterior lateral nucleus; *VPM,* ventral posterior medial nucleus. **B.** Major afferent and efferent connections. [Reprinted with permission from Fix JD. High-Yield Neuroanatomy, 3rd ed. Philadelphia, Lippincott Williams & Wilkins, 2005:117.]

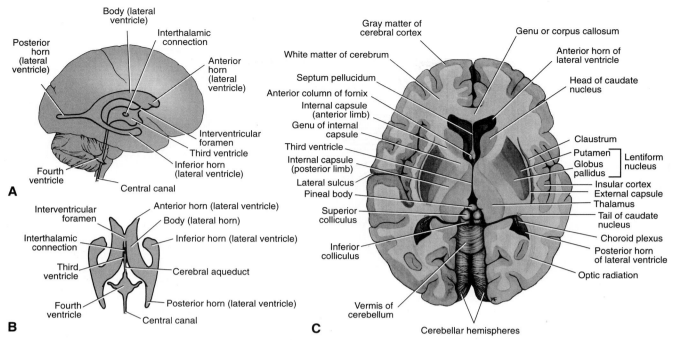

FIG 6-3. A. Lateral view of the ventricular cavities. **B.** Superior view of the ventricular cavities. **C.** Horizontal section of the cerebrum as seen from above showing the relationship among the lentiform nucleus, the caudate nucleus, the thalamus, and the internal capsule. [Reprinted with permission from Snell RS. Clinical Neuroanatomy, 6th ed. Philadelphia, Lippincott Williams & Wilkins, 2006:254–255.]

motor and sensory cortices, the **lateral sulcus,** the **parieto-occipital sulcus,** and the **calcarine sulcus.**

ii.   The surface of each cerebral hemisphere is divided into four lobes (Fig. 6-1B):

(a)   The **frontal lobe** makes up the region anterior to the central sulcus and superior to the lateral sulcus. It contains the **motor** and **premotor cortices,** the **frontal eye field, Broca speech area** (in the dominant hemisphere), and the **prefrontal cortex.**

(b)   The **parietal lobe** is bounded by the central sulcus anteriorly, the lateral sulcus inferiorly, and the parieto-occipital sulcus posteriorly. The **sensory cortex,** the **superior parietal lobule,** and the **inferior parietal lobule** are contained within the parietal lobe.

(c)   The **temporal lobe** sits inferior to the lateral sulcus and contains the **primary auditory cortex, Wernicke speech area** (in the dominant hemisphere), and **Meyer-Archambault loop.**

(d)   The **occipital lobe** makes up the remainder of the surface, seated posterior to the parieto-occipital sulcus, and contains the **visual cortex.**

iii.   **Internal structures**

(a)   The **lateral ventricles** are lined with ependyma and filled with cerebrospinal fluid (CSF). Each lateral ventricle is connected to the third ventricle via the **interventricular foramina** (of Monro) (Fig. 6-3A,B).

(b)   The **basal ganglia** are a collection of subcortical nuclei, including the **caudate nucleus,** the **putamen,** the **globus pallidus,** and the **claustrum** (Fig. 6-3C). These structures play a role in disorders of movement including Parkinson (substantia nigra) and Huntington (caudate and putamen) disorders (see Chapter 4).

(c)   Several large white matter tracts run within the cerebral hemispheres, including the **corpus callosum,** the **anterior commissure,** the **posterior commissure,** and the **fornix** (Fig. 6-4).

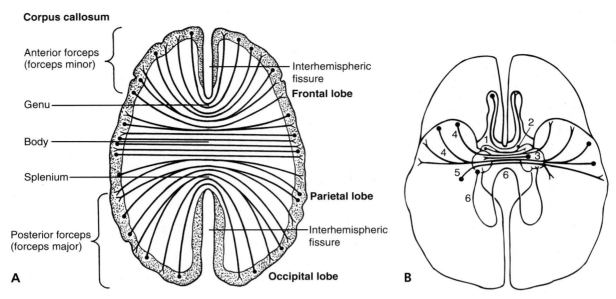

Corpus callosum

Anterior forceps (forceps minor)

Genu

Body

Splenium

Posterior forceps (forceps major)

A

Interhemispheric fissure
Frontal lobe

Parietal lobe

Interhemispheric fissure

Occipital lobe

B

FIG 6-4. A. Horizontal section through the cerebral hemispheres and corpus callosum showing the pattern of the crossing nerve fibers in the genu, body, and splenium. **B.** Ventral view of the cerebral hemispheres showing the fibers of the anterior commissure. *1,* interbulbar component; *2,* intertubercular component; *3,* interamygdaloid component; *4,* ectocortical component; *5,* interparahippocampal gyrus component; *6,* stria terminalis. [Reprinted with permission from DeMyer W. NMS Neuroanatomy, 2nd ed. Philadelphia, Lippincott Williams & Wilkins, 1998:346.]

> **(d)** Nerve fibers running from the brainstem to the cerebral cortex and back (the corticospinal tracts) form a large band named the **internal capsule** (Fig. 6-5).
>
> **2.** The **cerebellum** is a highly convoluted structure located in the posterior cranial fossa (Fig. 6-6A). It is attached to the dorsal surface of the pons via the **superior, middle,** and **inferior cerebellar peduncles.**

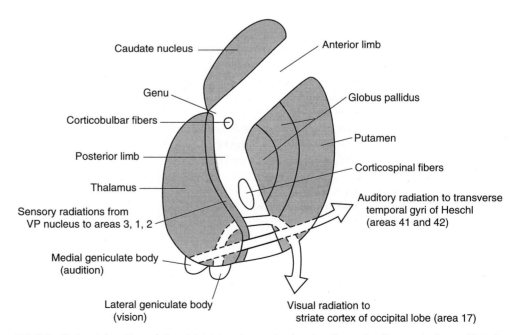

Caudate nucleus

Genu

Corticobulbar fibers

Posterior limb

Thalamus

Sensory radiations from VP nucleus to areas 3, 1, 2

Medial geniculate body (audition)

Lateral geniculate body (vision)

Anterior limb

Globus pallidus

Putamen

Corticospinal fibers

Auditory radiation to transverse temporal gyri of Heschl (areas 41 and 42)

Visual radiation to striate cortex of occipital lobe (area 17)

FIG 6-5. Horizontal section of the right internal capsule showing the major fiber projections. Clinically important tracts lie in the genu and posterior limb. Lesions of the internal capsule cause contralateral hemiparesis and contralateral hemianopia. *VP,* ventral posterior. [Reprinted with permission from Fix JD. High-Yield Neuroanatomy, 3rd ed. Philadelphia, Lippincott Williams & Wilkins, 2005:118.]

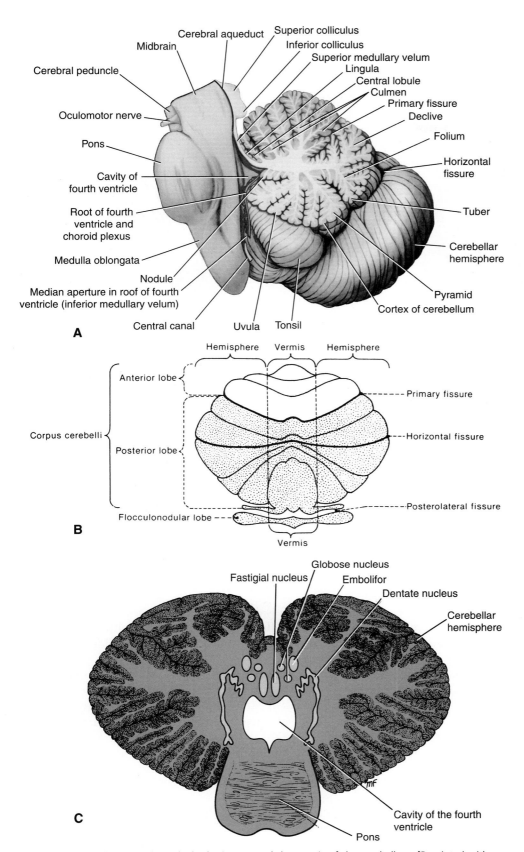

FIG 6-6. A. Sagittal section through the brainstem and the vermis of the cerebellum. [Reprinted with permission from Snell RS. Clinical Neuroanatomy, 6th ed. Philadelphia, Lippincott Williams & Wilkins, 2006:221.] **B.** Dorsal view of the cerebellum showing three sagittal subdivisions (hemisphere, vermis, and hemisphere) and three transverse subdivisions (anterior, posterior, and flocculonodular lobes). [Reprinted with permission from DeMyer W. NMS Neuroanatomy, 2nd ed. Philadelphia, Lippincott Williams & Wilkins, 1998:353.] **C.** Position of the intracerebellar nuclei. [Reprinted with permission from Snell RS. Clinical Neuroanatomy, 6th ed. Philadelphia, Lippincott Williams & Wilkins, 2006:224.]

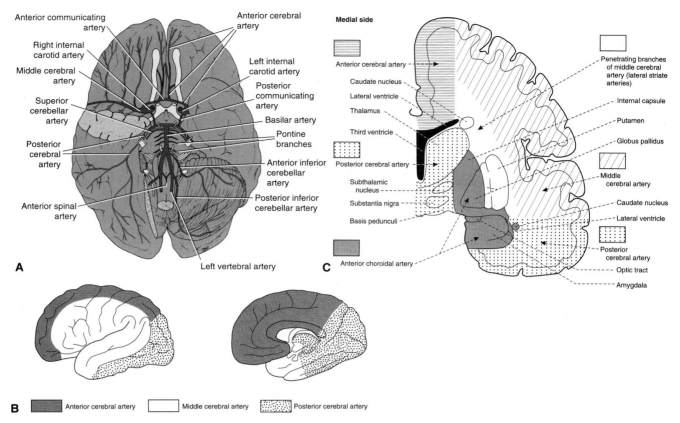

FIG 6-7. **A.** Arteries of the inferior surface of the brain. Note the formation of the circle of Willis. Part of the right temporal lobe has been removed to show the course of the middle cerebral artery. [Reprinted with permission from Snell RS. Clinical Neuroanatomy, 6th ed. Philadelphia, Lippincott Williams & Wilkins, 2006:472.] **B.** Cortical territories of the three cerebral arteries: lateral aspect (*left*) and medial and inferior aspects (*right*) of the hemisphere. [Reprinted with permission from Fix JD. High-Yield Neuroanatomy, 3rd ed. Philadelphia, Lippincott Williams & Wilkins, 2005:30.] **C.** Coronal section through the cerebral hemisphere at the level of the internal capsule and thalamus showing the major vascular territories.

a. Transversely, the cerebellum is divided into three lobes: the **anterior lobe,** the **posterior lobe,** and the **flocculonodular lobe.** Sagittally, the cerebellum is divided into **cerebellar hemispheres,** which are divided by the midline **vermis** (Fig. 6-6B).

b. Four deep nuclei are embedded within the cerebellum: the **dentate,** the **emboliform,** the **globose,** and the **fastigial nuclei** (Fig. 6-6C).

c. In general, the cerebellum has three primary functions: **maintenance of posture and balance, maintenance of muscle tone,** and **coordination of voluntary motor activity.**

B. **Blood supply**

1. The arterial blood supply to the brain is divided between the **anterior** and the **posterior circulation** (Fig. 6-7).

    a. The anterior circulation derives from the two **internal carotid arteries** and their branches:

        i. The **ophthalmic artery** branches off the internal carotid and enters the orbit via the **optic canal.** It supplies the eye, orbit, and periorbital structures.

        ii. The **posterior communicating artery** branches posteriorly to merge with the **posterior cerebral artery,** thus connecting the anterior and posterior circulations as part of the **circle of Willis.**

iii. The **anterior choroidal artery** tracks posteriorly and enters the inferior horn of the lateral ventricle to terminate at the choroid plexus. It supplies the lateral geniculate body, globus pallidus, and posterior limb of the internal capsule.

iv. The **anterior cerebral artery** is a terminal branch of the internal carotid. It runs anteriorly, enters the longitudinal fissure, and connects with its counterpart on the contralateral side via the **anterior communicating artery.** The anterior cerebral artery perfuses the medial surface of the cerebral cortex; of particular clinical importance is the leg–foot area of the motor and sensory cortices.

v. The **middle cerebral artery** is a terminal branch of the internal carotid artery. It runs laterally into the lateral sulcus and supplies the lateral convexity of the hemisphere. The following are clinically noteworthy: the Broca and Wernicke speech areas, the face and arm motor and sensory cortices, and the frontal eye fields.

b. The **posterior circulation** (e.g., vertebrobasilar system) begins with the bilateral **vertebral arteries,** themselves branches of the subclavian arteries, and terminates with branches of those arteries and of the **basilar arteries** (Fig. 6-7):

i. The **anterior spinal artery** is formed by the joining of two small inferiorly projecting branches of the vertebral arteries.

ii. The **posterior inferior cerebellar artery** (PICA) arises from the vertebral arteries and travels posteriorly between the medulla and the cerebellum to perfuse the inferior surface of the vermis, the central cerebellar nuclei, and the posterior surface of the cerebellum.

iii. The base of the pons is perfused by the **paramedian branches of the pontine arteries.**

iv. The **labyrinthine artery** follows cranial nerve (CN) VII and CN VIII into the internal acoustic meatus. It supplies the internal ear structures.

v. The **anterior inferior cerebellar artery** (AICA) arises from the basilar artery and tracks posteriorly and laterally to perfuse the anterior and inferior portions of the cerebellum.

vi. The **superior cerebellar artery** branches off the basilar artery near its termination and wraps around the cerebral peduncle. It supplies the pons, pineal gland, and superior medullary velum.

vii. The two **posterior cerebral arteries** are the terminal branches of the basilar artery. Each one joins an internal carotid artery via a **posterior communicating artery.** The posterior cerebral artery is the major blood supply to the midbrain and supplies the following structures:

(a) Thalamus

(b) Lateral and medial geniculate bodies

(c) Occipital lobe

(d) Inferior surface of the temporal lobe

c. The **circle of Willis** is an important vascular network that allows for collateral blood flow between the anterior and the posterior circulations. It is composed of the following vessels:

i. The two anterior cerebral arteries

ii. The anterior communicating artery

iii. The two posterior communicating arteries

iv. The two posterior cerebral arteries

2. The **veins of the brain** lie in the subarachnoid space and converge to drain into the **dural venous sinuses.** They are largely divided among the external and internal venous systems (Fig. 6-8):

a. The external cerebral veins are made up of the following major components: the **superior cerebral veins,** the **superficial middle cerebral vein,** the **deep middle cerebral vein,** the **anterior cerebral vein,** the **striate vein,** and the **basal vein.**

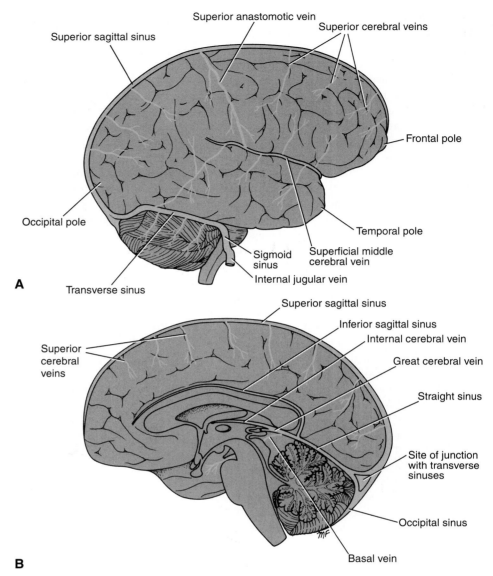

FIG 6-8. Venous drainage of the lateral (**A**) and medial (**B**) surfaces of the right cerebral hemisphere. [Reprinted with permission from Snell RS. Clinical Neuroanatomy, 6th ed. Philadelphia, Lippincott Williams & Wilkins, 2006:475.]

    b. Three major veins make up the internal venous system: the **basal vein** (of Rosenthal) and the **internal cerebral vein** join to form the **great vein** (of Galen).

    3. The **dural venous sinuses** are the primary sites of drainage for cerebral veins into the systemic venous system (Table 6-1).

C. Cerebral ventricles. The **choroid plexus** is a specialized structure that projects into the lateral, third, and fourth ventricles of the brain. It consists of infoldings of blood vessels of the pia mater, which are covered by modified ciliated ependymal cells. It secretes the CSF. Tight junctions of the choroid plexus cells form, in part, the blood–CSF barrier.

    1. The **ventricles** are lined by ependyma and contain CSF and choroid plexus. They are derived from the cavity of the neural tube.

TABLE 6-1	THE DURAL VENOUS SINUSES	
Sinus	**Location**	**Drains Into**
Superior sagittal sinus	Superior attached margin of falx cerebri	Transverse sinus, largely on right
Inferior sagittal sinus	Free margin of falx	Straight sinus
Straight sinus	Junction of falx with cerebellar tentorium	Transverse sinus, largely on left
Transverse sinus	Area of tentorium attached to occipital bone	Sigmoid sinus
Sigmoid sinus	Between transverse sinus and internal jugular vein	Jugular bulb and vein
Cavernous sinus	Parasellar area	Superior and inferior petrosal sinuses, emissary veins into superior ophthalmic vein and pterygoid plexus of veins
Superior petrosal sinus	Area of tentorium attached to petrous ridge of temporal bone	Transverse sinus
Inferior petrosal sinus	Line of the petro-occipital suture	Jugular bulb

2. The two **lateral ventricles** communicate with the third ventricle through the **interventricular foramina** (of Monro).

3. The **third ventricle** is located between the medial walls of the diencephalon. It communicates with the fourth ventricle through the cerebral aqueduct.

4. The **cerebral aqueduct** (of Sylvius) connects the third and fourth ventricles. It has no choroid plexus. Blockage of the cerebral aqueduct results in noncommunicating hydrocephalus.

5. The **fourth ventricle** communicates with the subarachnoid space through three foramina: the two lateral foramina (of Luschka) and the one medial foramen (of Magendie).

6. **Hydrocephalus** is dilation of the cerebral ventricles caused by one of the following:
   a. An abnormal increase in the formation of the fluid
   b. A blockage of the CSF pathways
   c. A decrease in the absorption of the fluid
   d. Hydrocephalus is characterized by excessive accumulation of CSF in the cerebral ventricles or subarachnoid space.
      i. **Noncommunicating hydrocephalus** results from obstruction within the ventricular system (e.g., congenital aqueductal stenosis).
      ii. **Communicating hydrocephalus** results from blockage within the subarachnoid space (e.g., adhesions after meningitis).
      iii. **Normal-pressure hydrocephalus** occurs when the CSF is not absorbed by the arachnoid villi.
         (a) It may occur secondary to posttraumatic meningeal hemorrhage.
         (b) Clinically, it is characterized by the triad of progressive dementia, ataxic gait, and urinary incontinence. (**Remember: wacky, wobbly, and wet.**)
      iv. **Hydrocephalus ex vacuo** results from loss of cells in the caudate nucleus (e.g., Huntington disease).
      v. **Pseudotumor cerebri** (benign intracranial hypertension) results from increased resistance to CSF outflow at the arachnoid villi. It occurs in obese young women and is characterized by papilledema without mass, elevated CSF pressure, and deteriorating vision. The ventricles may be slit-like on radiographic imaging.

7. **Cerebrospinal fluid** is a colorless, acellular fluid. It flows through the ventricles and into the subarachnoid space. Approximately 130 mL of CSF is contained within the ventricles and subarachnoid space. The functions of CSF are to

TABLE 6-2	CEREBROSPINAL FLUID PROFILES IN SUBARACHNOID HEMORRHAGE, BACTERIAL MENINGITIS, AND VIRAL ENCEPHALITIS			
Cerebrospinal Fluid	**Normal[a]**	**Subarachnoid Hemorrhage**	**Bacterial Meningitis**	**Viral Encephalitis**
Color	Clear	Bloody	Cloudy	Clear, cloudy
Cell count/mm^3	<5 lymphocytes	Red blood cells present	>1000 polymorphonuclear leukocytes	25–500 lymphocytes
Protein	<45 mg/dL	Normal to slightly elevated	Elevated >100 mg/dL	Slightly elevated <100 mg/dL
Glucose	~66% of blood glucose (normal blood glucose: 80–120 mg/dL)	Normal	Reduced	Normal

[a]Cell counts in infants: <10 cells/mm^3; protein in infants = 20–170 mg/dL.
Adapted in part with permission from Fix JD. High-Yield Neuroanatomy, 3rd ed. Philadelphia, Lippincott Williams & Wilkins, 2005:24.

a. Support and cushion the central nervous system, thus protecting it against concussive injury
b. Transport hormones and hormone-releasing factors
c. Remove metabolic waste products through absorption
d. The **composition of CSF** is clinically relevant (Table 6-2).

II. Neuroanatomy of Behavior

The cerebral cortex is the area of the CNS most closely associated with behavior. Behavioral alterations seen in people with **lesions** of **the frontal, temporal, parietal,** and **occipital lobes** caused by accident, disease, or surgery illustrate the major neuropsychiatric functions of these brain areas (Table 6-3). Specific aspects of neural control of language and memory, homeostatic mechanisms (including eating behavior), personality characteristics, and emotional behavior are discussed in this section.

TABLE 6-3	NEUROPSYCHIATRIC EFFECTS OF BRAIN LESIONS
Location of Lesion	**Effect of Lesion on Behavior**
Frontal lobes	Mood changes
	Difficulties with motivation, concentration, attention, orientation, and problem solving (dorsolateral lesions)
	Difficulties with judgment, inhibitions, emotions, and personality changes (orbitofrontal lesions)
	Inability to speak fluently (Broca aphasia: left-sided lesions)
Temporal lobes	Impaired memory
	Changes in aggressive behavior
	Inability to understand language (Wernicke aphasia: left-sided lesions)
Parietal lobes	Impaired processing of visual–spatial information (e.g., cannot copy a line drawing correctly: right-sided lesions)
	Impaired processing of verbal information (e.g., cannot tell right from left, do simple math, name fingers, or write; Gerstmann syndrome: left-sided lesions)
Occipital lobes	Visual hallucinations
	Blindness

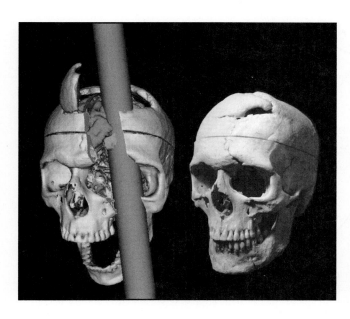

FIG 6-9. Computer-generated three-dimensional reconstructions of a thin-slice computed tomography scan of the skull of Phineas Gage and the tamping iron that caused the injury. The image on the right shows reconstruction of the injury as viewed from the outside. Ratiu et al., 2004. The tale of Phineas Gage, digitally remastered. Journal of Neurotrauma, 21(5):637-643 and Images in Clinical Medicine, New England Journal of Medicine, 351:21.

Patient Snapshot 6-2

In 1848 in a small Vermont town, the foreman of a construction gang was setting an explosive charge using a 3-lb, yard-long, 1.25-in.-wide tamping iron. The charge went off unexpectedly, blowing the iron into his head through his left cheek bone. The iron passed lateral to the optic nerve, through the anterior frontal cortex and white matter and out the top of his head (Fig. 6-9). Remarkably, the foreman survived. After his brain lesion healed, the foreman had few obvious neurologic problems but did show significant personality changes. A hardworking, responsible, personable individual before the accident, the foreman after the accident showed outbursts of anger and little concern for others. A respectful, energetic, persistent, and organized person before the accident, he began to show an inability to carry out plans and a lack of self-control. This, the well-known case of Phineas Gage, is often cited as the first evidence that the frontal cortex has significant involvement in aspects of personality and social behavior.

A. Language and memory

1. **Language** is a complex entity that can be defined as the ability to encode ideas into signals. It includes verbal and nonverbal forms of communicating and understanding. It is made up of words and grammar. **Words** are associations between sounds and meaning. **Grammar** is the system or set of rules that dictate how words are combined.

   a. The ability to develop language is believed to be **intrinsic** to humans.

   b. **Anatomy of language.** Based on numerous anatomic studies, the major regions of the brain important for speech and language have been identified (Fig. 6-10).

      i. Lesions to the **Broca area** affecting speech were first described in 1861 by neurosurgeon Paul Broca. The Broca area is located in the posterior part of the **inferior frontal gyrus** in the **dominant hemisphere** and brings about the formation of spoken words.

      ii. The **Wernicke area** was first described in 1874 by Carl Wernicke. It is located in the **dominant hemisphere** in the posterior part of the **superior temporal gyrus** and permits the understanding of written and spoken language.

      iii. The Broca and Wernicke areas are connected by a nerve fiber bundle called the **arcuate fasciculus.**

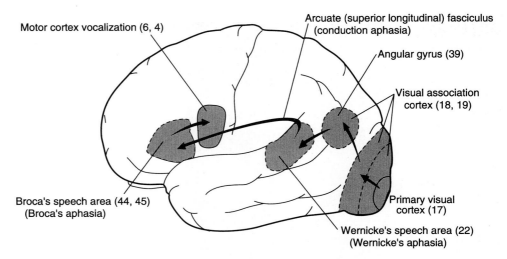

FIG 6-10. Cortical areas of the dominant hemisphere that play an important role in language production. The visual image of a word is projected from the visual cortex (Brodmann area 17) to the visual association cortices (Brodmann areas 18 and 19) and then to the angular gyrus (Brodmann area 39). Further processing occurs in the Wernicke speech area (Brodmann area 22), where the auditory form of the word is recalled. Through the arcuate fasciculus, this information reaches the Broca speech area (Brodmann areas 44 and 45), where motor speech programs control the vocalization mechanisms of the precentral gyrus. Lesions of the Broca speech area, Wernicke speech area, or the arcuate fasciculus result in dysphasia. [Reprinted with permission from Fix JD. High-Yield Neuroanatomy, 3rd ed. Philadelphia, Lippincott Williams & Wilkins, 2005:158.]

    c. **Aphasia** is defined as an acquired language disorder. Study of these disorders has been facilitated by the availability of patients with specific patterns of damage to the brain. These analyses have identified unique language deficits and their corresponding anatomic lesions (Table 6-4).

2. **Memory** is a mental ability that serves to process information so that it will be available for use at a later time.

    a. Cognitive neuroscientists classify memory into two basic categories:

        i. **Explicit** or **declarative memory** is the knowledge of **facts** (e.g., what we know about things or people or places) and what these facts mean. This type of memory must be recalled **consciously** to use it.

TABLE 6-4		THE MAJOR TYPES OF APHASIA		
Aphasia	**Site of Brain Damage**	**Speech**	**Comprehension**	**Repetition**
Broca	Left posterior frontal cortex and underlying structures	Nonfluent and effortful	Mostly preserved for single words and simple sentences	Impaired
Wernicke	Left posterior, superior, and middle temporal lobe cortices	Fluent, abundant, well articulated, and melodic	Impaired	Impaired
Conduction	Left superior temporal and supramarginal gyri	Fluent, some defects with articulation	Intact or largely retained	Impaired
Global	Very large left perisylvian lesion	Scant, nonfluent	Impaired	Impaired
Transcortical motor	Anterior or superior to Broca area	Explosive, nonfluent	Intact or largely retained	Intact or largely retained
Transcortical sensory	Posterior or inferior to Wernicke area	Scant, fluent	Impaired	Intact or largely retained

Data from DeMyer W. NMS Neuroanatomy, 2nd ed. Philadelphia, Lippincott Williams & Wilkins, 1998:362; and Bear MF, Connors BW, Paradiso MA. Neuroscience: Exploring the Brain, 3rd ed. Philadelphia, Lippincott Williams & Wilkins, 2006:622.

TABLE 6-5	SUMMARY OF MEMORY SYSTEMS	
Memory System	**Primary Anatomic Structures**	**Duration**
Episodic memory (e-xplicit/declarative)	Medial temporal lobes, anterior thalamic nuclei, fornix, mammillary bodies, prefrontal cortex	Minutes to years
Semantic memory (explicit/declarative)	Inferolateral temporal lobes	Minutes to years
Procedural memory (implicit/nondeclarative)	Basal ganglia, cerebellum, supplementary motor area	Minutes to years
Working memory (implicit/ nondeclarative)	Phonologic: prefrontal cortex, Broca area, Wernicke area	Seconds to minutes
	Spatial: prefrontal cortex, visual-association areas	

    ii. **Implicit** or **nondeclarative memory** is memory that is expressed as a change in behavior. It involves information about how to perform something (e.g., how to ride a bike) and is recalled **unconsciously.**

  b. Memory can be further subcategorized on the basis of the specific **type of material** being remembered. Anatomic structures involved in the subcategories of memory are listed in Table 6-5.

    i. The system that is used to recall **personal experiences** or **events** (e.g., what you had for breakfast yesterday) is called **episodic memory.** Episodic memory is explicit or declarative and must be recalled consciously. The anatomic domain of episodic memory was determined by studying anatomic lesions in amnestic patients.

      (a) Individuals with episodic memory dysfunction have difficulty recalling events. This dysfunction is said to follow **Ribot's law,** which states that memory of events nearest to the time of injury are the most vulnerable, whereas remote memories are relatively resistant.

      (b) Episodic memory dysfunction can result in an impairment in the ability to remember new events after injury, or **anterograde amnesia,** and an inability to retrieve recently learned information, or **retrograde amnesia.**

    ii. **Semantic memory** is another form of explicit or declarative memory. It involves the general store of conceptual and factual information (e.g., the color of a banana or the capital of Montana) that is not linked specifically to an experience. The study of patients with dysfunction of semantic memory has localized this type of memory to a region of the brain distinct from those governing episodic memory, the **inferolateral temporal lobe. Alzheimer disease** is the most common clinical disorder of semantic memory (see Chapter 4).

    iii. When one is learning behavioral or cognitive skills and algorithms that will be used in an unconscious and automatic way, one is using **procedural memory.** Because of its use in an unconscious way, procedural memory is most often implicit but can be explicit. Anatomically, it is localized to the **basal ganglia, supplementary motor area,** and **cerebellum.**

    iv. **Working memory** is quite distinct from the three types of memory just discussed. It is the shortest duration memory and involves the ability to **temporarily** maintain and manipulate information that one needs to keep in mind. Working memory involves a combination of attention, concentration, and short-term memory. It can be divided into two types:

      (a) Memory for **phonologic** information involves temporarily keeping facts and figures in mind, like keeping a phone number in your head. This type of memory is localized to the dominant hemisphere.

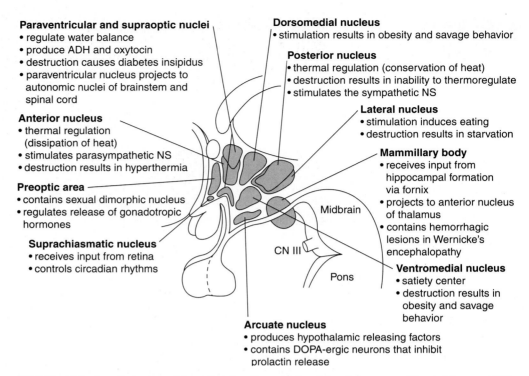

Paraventricular and supraoptic nuclei
• regulate water balance
• produce ADH and oxytocin
• destruction causes diabetes insipidus
• paraventricular nucleus projects to autonomic nuclei of brainstem and spinal cord

Anterior nucleus
• thermal regulation (dissipation of heat)
• stimulates parasympathetic NS
• destruction results in hyperthermia

Preoptic area
• contains sexual dimorphic nucleus
• regulates release of gonadotropic hormones

Suprachiasmatic nucleus
• receives input from retina
• controls circadian rhythms

Dorsomedial nucleus
• stimulation results in obesity and savage behavior

Posterior nucleus
• thermal regulation (conservation of heat)
• destruction results in inability to thermoregulate
• stimulates the sympathetic NS

Lateral nucleus
• stimulation induces eating
• destruction results in starvation

Mammillary body
• receives input from hippocampal formation via fornix
• projects to anterior nucleus of thalamus
• contains hemorrhagic lesions in Wernicke's encephalopathy

Midbrain

CN III

Pons

Ventromedial nucleus
• satiety center
• destruction results in obesity and savage behavior

Arcuate nucleus
• produces hypothalamic releasing factors
• contains DOPA-ergic neurons that inhibit prolactin release

FIG 6-11. Major hypothalamic nuclei and their functions. *ADH,* antidiuretic hormone; *CN,* cranial nerve; *DOPA,* dopamine; *NS* = nervous system. [Reprinted with permission from Fix JD. High-Yield Neuroanatomy, 3rd ed. Philadelphia, Lippincott Williams & Wilkins, 2005:132.]

(b) Memory for **spatial** information involves briefly remembering the spatial arrangement of things, such as following directions that someone has described verbally. This type of memory is localized to the nondominant hemisphere.

B. **Hypothalamic function**
1. The **hypothalamus** modulates the activity of the autonomic nervous system, the endocrine system, and the limbic system. In so doing, it governs body homeostasis. The hypothalamus also has a role in emotional behavior.
2. **Anatomy**
   a. The hypothalamus is a part of the diencephalon and extends from near the optic chiasm to the caudal border of the mammillary bodies. It is bounded by the thalamus superiorly, internal capsule laterally, optic chiasm and lamina terminalis anteriorly, and wall of the third ventricle medioposteriorly.
   b. Microscopically, the hypothalamus is divided into small collections of nerve cells called nuclei. Each has specialized functions (Fig. 6-11).
3. **Afferent and efferent connections** (Table 6-6)
4. **Hypothalamohypophyseal tract** (Fig. 6-12)
   a. The **hypothalamohypophseal tract** connects the **supraoptic** and **paraventricular nuclei** with the posterior lobe of the pituitary gland (the neurohypophysis). The axons from these nuclei release their hormonal products in the posterior pituitary, where they are absorbed into the bloodstream.
   b. **Vasopressin** (antidiuretic hormone) is the major product of the supraoptic nucleus. It serves to cause vasoconstriction and to inhibit diuresis. The antidiuretic function targets the distal convoluted tubules and collecting system of the kidney, triggering an increase in the reabsorption of water. The release of vasopressin is stimulated by an increase in osmotic pressure in the blood circulating through the supraoptic nucleus (an osmoreceptor).

Pathway	Origin	Destination
Afferent		
Medial and spinal lemnisci, tractus solitarius, reticular formation	Viscera and somatic structures	Hypothalamic nuclei
Visual fibers	Retina	Suprachiasmatic nucleus
Medial forebrain bundle	Olfactory mucous membrane	Hypothalamic nuclei
Auditory fibers	Inner ear	Hypothalamic nuclei
Corticohypothalamic fibers	Frontal lobe of cerebral cortex	Hypothalamic nuclei
Hippocampal–hypothalamic fibers; likely main output pathway of limbic system	Hippocampus	Nuclei of mammillary bodies
Amygdalohypothalamic fibers	Amygdaloid complex	Hypothalamic nuclei
Thalamohypothalamic fibers	Dorsomedial and midline nuclei of thalamus	Hypothalamic nuclei
Tegmental fibers	Tegmentum of midbrain	Hypothalamic nuclei
Efferent		
Descending fibers in reticular formation to brainstem and spinal cord	Preoptic, anterior, posterior, and lateral nuclei of hypothalamus	Craniosacral parasympathetic and thoracolumbar sympathetic outflows
Mammillothalamic tract	Nuclei of mammillary bodies	Anterior nucleus of thalamus; relayed to cingulated gyrus
Mammillotegmental tract	Nuclei of mammillary bodies	Reticular formation in tegmentum of brainstem
Multiple pathways	Hypothalamic nuclei	Limbic system

Reprinted with permission from Snell RS. Clinical Neuroanatomy, 6th ed. Philadelphia, Lippincott Williams & Wilkins, 2006:382.

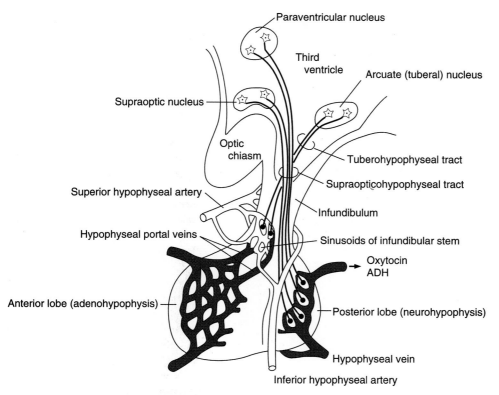

FIG 6-12. The hypophyseal portal system. The paraventricular and supraoptic nuclei produce antidiuretic hormone (*ADH*) and oxytocin and transport them through the supraopticohypophyseal tract to the capillary bed of the neurohypophysis. The arcuate nucleus of the infundibulum transports hypothalamic-stimulating hormones through the tuberohypophysial tract to the sinusoids of the infundibular stem. These sinusoids then drain into the secondary capillary plexus in the adenohypophysis. [Reprinted with permission from Fix JD. High-Yield Neuroanatomy, 3rd ed. Philadelphia, Lippincott Williams & Wilkins, 2005:133.]

    c. **Oxytocin** is the major product of the paraventricular nucleus. It is a hormone that stimulates smooth muscle contraction of the uterus and myoepithelial cells of breast epithelium. Oxytocin is strongly stimulated by breastfeeding.

    d. **Hypophyseal portal system**

        i. The **hypophyseal portal system** is a capillary-to-capillary network in the anterior lobe of the pituitary (adenohypophysis), which allows for regulation of the anterior pituitary via secretion of releasing and inhibitory hormones by hypothalamus (Fig. 6-12).

        ii. Axons from the medial zone of the hypothalamus project to the **median eminence** and **infundibulum** of the pituitary and release their hormone products into the superior end of the portal system. The portal system carries these hormones inferiorly into the anterior lobe, where they can regulate the activity of the secretory cells there.

        iii. Table 6-7 shows the hypothalamic regulation, anterior pituitary hormone, and the functions of the respective hormonal systems. An easy way to remember the hormonal products of the anterior pituitary is by the acronym FLAT PiG for FSH (follicle-stimulating hormone), LH (luteinizing hormone), ACTH (adrenocorticotropic hormone), TSH (thyroid-stimulating hormone), prolactin, and GH (growth hormone).

5. **Summary of the homeostatic functions of the hypothalamus**

    a. Modulates the activity of the **autonomic nervous system.** Activity in the **anterior hypothalamus** promotes parasympathetic stimulation; activity in the **posterior hypothalamus** is important for sympathetic output.

    b. **Endocrine** function is modulated by the effects of releasing-inhibitory proteins.

    c. **Serum osmolarity** is controlled by the release of **vasopressin. Thirst** is also modulated through this system, via the actions of the supraoptic nucleus as an osmoreceptor.

    d. **Oxytocin** is important for uterine contraction during delivery and milk release via myoepithelial cell contraction.

    e. The **anterior hypothalamus** regulates body temperature by controlling the mechanisms of heat loss. The **posterior hypothalamus** controls the mechanisms of heat production.

6. **Summary of the behavioral functions of the hypothalamus**

    a. A **hunger center** is located in the lateral region of the hypothalamus. In animal studies, damage to this region results in lack of appetite. Conversely, a

TABLE 6-7	REGULATION AND FUNCTION OF THE HORMONAL NETWORK OF THE HYPOPHYSEAL PORTAL SYSTEM	
Releasing/Inhibiting Hormone	**Anterior Pituitary Product**	**Function**
Follicle-stimulating hormone-releasing hormone, luteinizing a hormone-releasing hormone[a]	Follicle-stimulating hormone, luteinizing hormone	Females: stimulates ovarian follicle development and the production of estrogen and progesterone
		Males: regulates spermatogenesis and testosterone production
Corticotropin-releasing hormone	Adrenocorticotropic hormone	Stimulates adrenal corticosteroid and sex hormone production
Thyrotropin-releasing hormone	Thyroid-stimulating hormone	Increases thyroid hormone production
Prolactin-releasing hormone	Prolactin	Stimulates lactogenesis
Prolactin-inhibiting hormone, dopamine	Prolactin	Inhibits lactogenesis
Growth hormone-releasing hormone	Growth hormone	Promotes growth at epiphyseal centers of cartilage
Growth hormone-inhibiting hormone or somatostatin	Growth hormone (decreased production)	Reduces growth at epiphyseal centers of cartilage

[a]The presence of these hormones remains a matter of debate. Reprinted with permission from Snell RS. Clinical Neuroanatomy, 6th ed. Philadelphia, Lippincott Williams & Wilkins, 2006:385.

satiety center is located in the ventromedial region. Damage to this region on animal experimentation has been shown to lead to obesity (Fig. 6-11).

b. **Emotional behaviors** are affected by connections between the hypothalamus, the limbic system, and the prefrontal cortex.

c. **Circadian rhythms** are affected by activity of the hypothalamus (see Chapter 15).

C. Clinical correlates of prefrontal activity

1. The three major prefrontal subdivisions—the **orbitofrontal region,** the **dorsolateral convexity,** and the **medial region**—have specialized behavioral functions.

   a. The **orbitofrontal cortex** is a center for the biologic control of inhibition, emotions, and drive states. It is also part of the dopamine-driven reward circuit of the brain and is activated in addicts exposed to drug-related cues.

   b. The dorsolateral convexity influences behavior and personality and has executive responsibilities involving activities such as formulating plans, maintaining attention and concentration, and changing problem-solving strategies when needed.

   c. The **medial region** has connections to the basal ganglia and accessory cortical motor areas and is involved primarily in motor activity.

2. The emotional-behavioral functions of the frontal lobes are **lateralized.**

   a. Lesions of **the left prefrontal** area, both cortical and subcortical, may result in **depression.**

   b. Lesions of **the right prefrontal** area are more likely to produce manifestations of **elevated mood.**

   c. Functional MRI (fMRI) studies reveal that positive mood is associated with activation of the left prefrontal area and stress area with activation of the right prefrontal.

   d. **Schizophrenia and obsessive–compulsive disorder (OCD),** both of which are characterized by behavioral and affective changes (see Chapters 19 and 20), are associated with decreased bilateral prefrontal cortical activity.

D. Limbic system and emotional behavior (Fig. 6-13). The **limbic system** is a loose collection of structures, such as the hippocampus and amygdala, that modulates activity

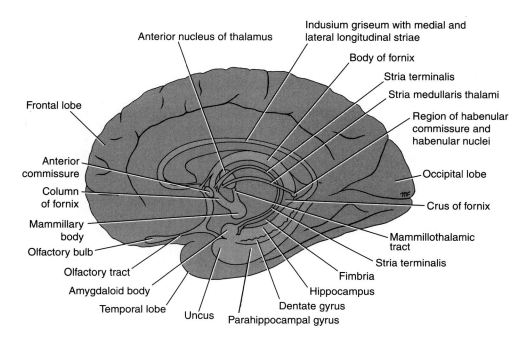

FIG 6-13. Medial aspect of the right cerebral hemisphere showing structures that form the limbic system. [Reprinted with permission from Snell RS. Clinical Neuroanatomy, 6th ed. Philadelphia, Lippincott Williams & Wilkins, 2006:301.]

between the cerebral cortex and the hypothalamus. Specifically, the limbic system is important in the control of emotion, behavior, drive, and memory.

1. **Anatomy**
   a. The **hippocampal formation** is made up of three structures: the **hippocampus,** the **dentate gyrus,** and the **subiculum.** These structures are seated under the **parahippocampal gyrus** along the **medial temporal lobe.** Its primary functions are in learning, memory, and recognition of novelty. Afferent connection is via the entorhinal cortex, and efferents travel through the **fornix.**
   b. The **amygdaloid complex** lies underneath the **parahippocampal uncus** near the tip of the inferior horn of the lateral ventricle. It is made up of several nuclei that are grouped into the **basolateral group** and the **corticomedial group.** Essentially, the amygdaloid complex serves as an integration center for multiple afferents to allow for appropriate behavioral output:
      i. **Afferent** input includes the olfactory lobe, cortex, hypothalamus, thalamus, and brainstem tegmentum.
      ii. **Efferent** output includes the hypothalamus, septal area, hippocampal formation, thalamus, cortex, contralateral amygdala, and brainstem tegmentum.
      iii. Via these connections, the amygdala modulates endocrine activity, sexuality, reproduction, autonomic responses, and emotion.

2. **Clinical correlates of limbic system activity**
   a. After bilateral destruction of the anterior temporal lobes, including the amygdaloid complexes, **Klüver-Bucy syndrome** results. This syndrome involves the triad of **docility, hyperorality,** and **hypersexuality.**
   b. Damage to the amygdala also results in
      i. **Decreased conditioned fear response**
      ii. Decreased ability to recognize the **meaningfulness of facial and vocal expressions of anger** in others
   c. Damage to the **hippocampus** results in an **inability to convert recent memories into long-term memory and store them.** Neuronal death within the hippocampus is specifically associated with Alzheimer disease
   d. The **amygdala** and **hippocampus** are reduced in volume in patients with **schizophrenia** (see Chapter 19).

Chapter 7

The Sensory Nervous System: The Somatosensory System, Vision, and Hearing

Brain & Behavior

I. Somatosensory System

Patient Snapshot 7-1

A 58-year-old homeless woman with a history of prostitution presents to the emergency room with a complaint of worsening clumsiness and frequent falling. On neurologic examination, the patient is asked to stand with her toes and heels together and her eyes closed. As she closes her eyes the patient begins to sway violently and has to be braced so that she does not fall (a positive Romberg test). When the patient performs the same test with her eyes open, she has no difficulties. The resident reasons that the patient's vision compensates for her lack of proprioception. The resident then orders the rapid plasma reagent (RPR) and Venereal Disease Research Lab (VDRL) studies to test for infection with *Treponema pallidum*. The results of these studies, both positive, indicate that the patient has syphilitic damage to the proprioceptive tracts of the spinal cord, specifically the dorsal columns and the cells of the dorsal root ganglia.

A. Proprioception

1. **Proprioception** is the ability to sense the position of one's extremities without the aid of vision. It has two components: stationary **limb position sense** and the sense of limb movement or **kinesthesia.** Proprioceptive signals are predominantly a component of the **medial lemniscal system.**

2. The two major types of **receptors** for the proprioceptive system—**muscle spindles** and **Golgi tendon organs**—are summarized in Table 7-1.
   a. **Muscle spindles** are encapsulated mechanoreceptors that contain **intrafusal muscle fibers** (Fig. 7-1). They are innervated by sensory and γ-motor fibers and are situated **parallel** to the main muscle mass. They function to detect changes in **muscle length** (e.g., the muscle stretch reflex) and the **velocity of muscle stretch.**
   b. **Golgi tendon organs** are encapsulated mechanoreceptors, situated near the tendinous attachments to muscles, in **series** to the muscle mass (Fig. 7-1). They are innervated by sensory fibers alone and serve to detect changes in **tension** and thus the **force of muscular contraction.**
   c. There are also receptors in joint capsules, which detect changes in joint flexion–extension, and in the skin (e.g., Ruffini endings, Merkel cells), which detect skin stretch.

3. **Anatomy of the pathway** (Fig. 7-2)
   a. **Upper limbs.** The ascending pathways for proprioception travel with those for discriminative touch via the **dorsal columns.**
      i. Ascending fibers in the cord are located in the ipsilateral **cuneate fasciculus** and terminate in the ipsilateral **cuneate nucleus** at the cervicomedullary junction.

87

TABLE 7-1	SUMMARY OF THE TWO MAJOR TYPES OF PROPRIOCEPTIVE RECEPTORS	
Characteristic	**Muscle Spindle**	**Golgi Tendon Organ**
Structure	Encapsulated	Encapsulated
Connection with muscle	Parallel	Series
Motor innervation	γ-Motor fibers	NA
Sensory innervation	Ia, II	Ib
Function	Detects change in muscle length and the velocity of stretch	Detects muscle tension and the force of contraction

NA, not applicable.

ii. Axons from the cuneate nucleus **decussate** as **internal arcuate fibers** in the caudal medulla and form the contralateral **medial lemniscus.** These fibers synapse in the **ventral posterolateral (VPL) nucleus** of the **thalamus** in the diencephalon.

iii. Thalamic efferents traverse the **internal capsule** and synapse in the appropriate location along the **postcentral gyrus** and **paracentral lobule** of the parietal lobe.

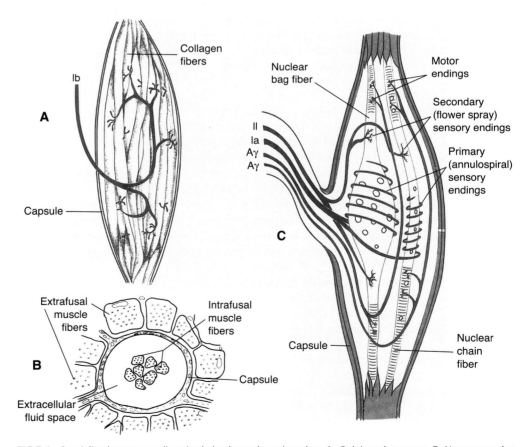

FIG 7-1. Specialized sensory endings in skeletal muscle and tendon. **A.** Golgi tendon organ. **B.** Neuromuscular spindle (transverse section). **C.** Sensory and motor innervation of a muscle spindle. [Reprinted with permission from Kiernan JA. Barr's The Human Nervous System, 8th ed. Baltimore, Lippincott Williams & Wilkins, 2005.]

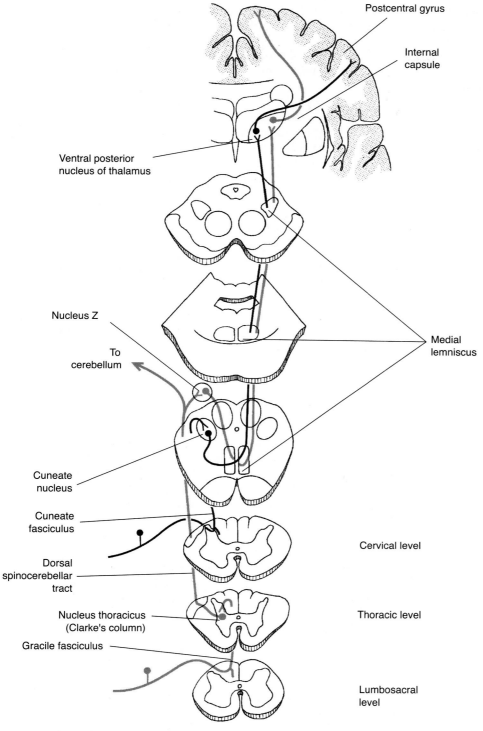

FIG 7-2. Pathways for conscious proprioception. The pathway from the lower limb is shown originating from the medial aspect of the hemisphere; that from the upper limb is shown originating from the lateral aspect. [Reprinted with permission from Kiernan JA. Barr's The Human Nervous System, 8th ed. Baltimore, Lippincott Williams & Wilkins, 2005.]

   b. Lower limbs. The lower limbs possess two pathways.
      i.   Ascending fibers in the cord are located in the ipsilateral **gracile fasciculus** and terminate at the ipsilateral **gracile nucleus.**
      ii. The **law of lamination** states that fibers arising most distally possess locations close to the midline and that more proximally entering fibers

laminate around them. Thus the **gracile fasciculus** lies medial to the **cuneate fasciculus.**

    c. **Head**

        i. Peripheral sensory fibers arising from unipolar neurons in the **mesencephalic trigeminal nucleus** traverse the **trigeminal nerve (CN V1–V3).**

        ii. One group of peripheral fibers comes from the **teeth** to detect **pressure during biting,** a sense related to muscle proprioception. Other groups separate among the three divisions of the nerve to serve as proprioceptive afferents for the ocular, facial, and bulbar muscles.

        iii. Central fibers project to the **trigeminal motor nucleus** to participate in reflex action and join the **dorsal trigeminothalamic tract.**

B. Discriminative touch. The **discriminative touch** modality, or fine touch, allows for the **localization** of sensory stimuli to the skin and the awareness that two unique stimuli in close anatomic proximity are in fact unique (**two-point discrimination**). It also contributes to the recognition of **textures** and **moving patterns** of stimuli.

    1. **Meissner corpuscles** are the sensory receptors that contribute most to discriminative touch (Fig. 7-3A).

        a. These encapsulated receptors are present in hairless skin and are most numerous in the fingertips. They are innervated by three to four myelinated axons and are situated in the skin with their long axes perpendicular to the skin surface.

        b. The primary function of Meissner corpuscles is to detect **mechanical deformation** of the skin.

    2. **Anatomy of the pathway** (Fig. 7-3B)

        a. The anatomy of the discriminative touch pathway for the body mirrors that for proprioception *minus* the accessory pathway for the lower limbs.

        b. Discriminative touch for the head involves the following:

            i. Afferent sensory fibers of unipolar neurons (situated in the trigeminal ganglion) travel as part of the **trigeminal nerve (CN V1–V3).**

            ii. These fibers synapse in the **pontine trigeminal nucleus** and the pars oralis of the **spinal trigeminal nucleus.**

            iii. The majority of fibers from these nuclei project to the contralateral **VPL** nucleus of the thalamus via the ventral trigeminothalamic tract.

            iv. Thalamic efferents synapse along the **postcentral gyrus.**

    3. The anatomy of the **vibratory sense pathway** is identical to that for discriminative touch, with the exception of its receptor, the Pacinian corpuscle. Pacinian corpuscles are found throughout the body, especially the dermis, and are structures with an external capsule of concentric lamellae surrounding the terminal end of a large myelinated nerve fiber.

C. Pain. Pain is one of the most frequent complaints for which patients see their physicians. This sensory modality ascends to the cortex by way of the **spinothalamic tract.** Pain is a complex sensory modality that is influenced by a number of factors (e.g., descending tracts and afferents of other sensory modalities).

    1. Receptors for pain are known as **nociceptors.** These are unencapsulated nerve endings of the smallest myelinated **group A fibers** (group Aδ; fast conducting) and of unmyelinated **group C fibers** (slower conducting). Because of these two fiber types, pain can be perceived in two temporally and qualitatively distinct ways. Like pain, the sensation of hot and cold is via free nerve endings.

        a. Initial **sharp** and **localized** pain travels via the group A fibers.

        b. After a delay of a few tenths of a second, a second wave of more **diffuse** and **disagreeable** pain is felt through transmission by group C fibers. The delay

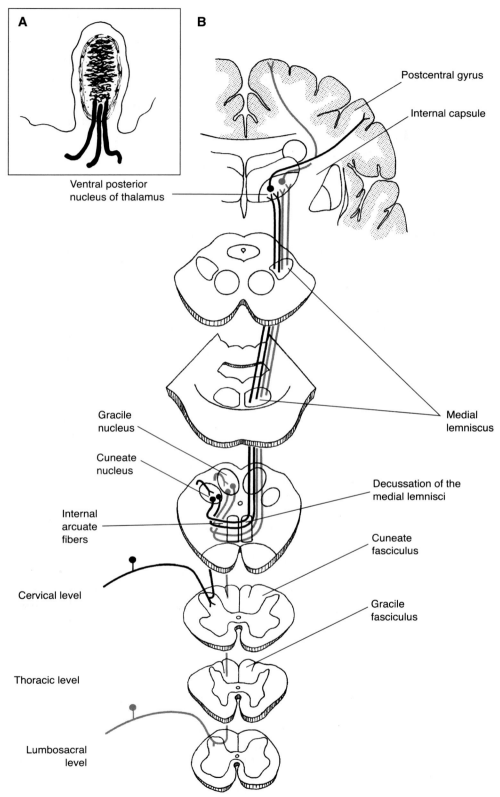

FIG 7-3. Elements of discriminative touch sensation. **A.** A Meissner corpuscle for sensory innervation of the skin. **B.** The medial lemniscus system for discriminative touch. The pathway from the lower limb is shown originating from the medial aspect of the hemisphere; that from the upper limb is shown originating from the lateral aspect. [Reprinted with permission from Kiernan JA. Barr's The Human Nervous System, 8th ed. Baltimore, Lippincott Williams & Wilkins, 2005.]

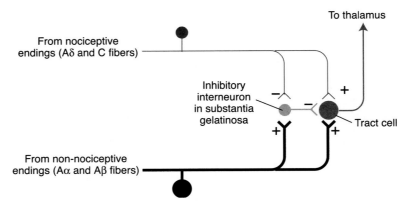

FIG 7-4. The gate control theory of pain. Whereas non-nociceptive primary sensory neurons stimulate the inhibitory interneurons, nociceptive afferents inhibit them. An increase in non-nociceptive input reduces the rate of firing of the spinothalamic tract neuron. [Reprinted with permission from Kiernan JA. Barr's The Human Nervous System, 8th ed. Baltimore, Lippincott Williams & Wilkins, 2005.]

in signal transmission is explained by the slower conduction velocities in group C fibers, largely the result of the absence of myelination.

2. The **gate control theory of pain** explains how spinal cord neurons receive and interpret peripheral signals to determine if afferent signals should be sent to the brain as pain (Fig. 7-4). The anatomic mechanism of this theory involves the following:

    a. The large-diameter afferents for touch and deep pressure (non-nociceptive Aα and Aβ fibers) synapse on spinal cord interneurons that have inhibitory output to nociceptive tracts.

    b. If sufficient stimulus for other sensory modalities exists, it can overwhelm nociceptive signals and block pain.

    c. Example: After suffering a mild cutaneous injury (e.g., stubbed toe) that stimulates nociceptive afferents, stroking the injured and surrounding areas to activate other tactile sensory modalities briefly relieves the pain.

3. **Anatomy of the pathway** (Fig. 7-5)

    a. Painful stimuli reach the brain via the following course:

        i. Axons for pain (and temperature) from neurons in the dorsal root ganglia enter the **propriospinal tract** (also known as the dorsolateral tract of Lissauer) and can ascend or descend one or two segments before synapsing on second-order neurons of the **dorsal horn.**

        ii. Axons from these second-order neurons decussate immediately in the **ventral white commissure** and then travel up the contralateral side of the cord in the **lateral funiculus.**

        iii. Above the **olivary nucleus,** axons of the spinothalamic tract join axons of other tracts to form the **spinal lemniscus.**

        iv. Spinothalamic axons terminate primarily on third-order neurons in the **VPL** nucleus of the thalamus.

        v. Finally, VPL nucleus axons pass through the **posterior limb of the internal capsule** on their way to projecting to the primary somatosensory cortex.

    b. Two **spinal reflexes** mediate responses to pain.

        i. The **flexor reflex** is at least a bisynaptic reflex in the spinal cord. After a painful stimulus, it results in **flexor withdrawal** of the receptive limb.

        ii. The **crossed extensor reflex** was explored in Chapter 5.

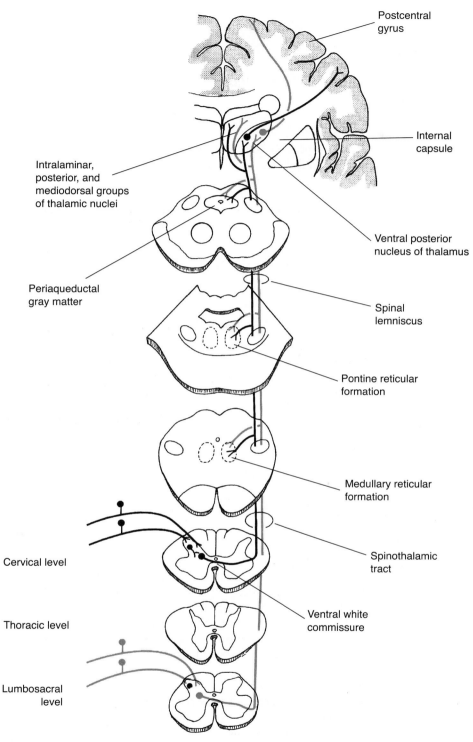

FIG 7-5. Spinothalamic system for pain, temperature, light touch, and pressure. The pathway from the lower limb is shown originating from the medial aspect of the hemisphere; that from the upper limb is shown originating from the lateral aspect. [Reprinted with permission from Kiernan JA. Barr's The Human Nervous System, 8th ed. Baltimore, Lippincott Williams & Wilkins, 2005.]

II. Vision

Vision requires the transmission of signals from **photoreceptors** of the retina to neurons of the **visual cortex.**

Patient Snapshot 7-2

A 64-year-old man reports to his primary-care physician with a complaint of decreased vision while driving and photophobia. These problems started insidiously and have slowly progressed. The patient has a history of infertility and currently complains of impotence and decreased sexual interest. On detailed physical examination, the primary-care physician identifies bitemporal hemianopsia on visual field testing. He also notes gynecomastia and some discharge from the man's breasts. Given the patient's constellation of signs and symptoms, the physician is concerned about the possibility of a prolactin-secreting pituitary adenoma (e.g., prolactinoma). Such a tumor, if large enough, would compress the optic chiasm from below, interfering with axons transmitting the temporal visual fields. An MRI study is performed, which confirms the presence of a large sellar turcica mass, consistent with a pituitary macroadenoma. The patient is immediately referred to a neurosurgeon, who schedules the patient for transsphenoidal pituitary surgery.

A. **Photoreceptors** are light-sensitive cells that convert light stimuli into changes in membrane potential via photo-responsive pigment. Two types of photoreceptors are present in the retina: **rods** and **cones.** Table 7-2 summarizes the differences between these photoreceptor cells.

1. **Rods** outnumber cones 20 to 1. They are absent from the central portion of the **fovea** and make up the dominant proportion of photoreceptors in the periphery. Rods are most sensitive to dim light, based on the chemistry of their visual pigment, **rhodopsin.**

2. **Cones** are critical for color vision. They are similar histologically to rods but contain **cone opsins** as their visual pigment. There are three cone opsins (red, blue, and green). Each cone contains one type of opsin, making cones maximally sensitive to one wavelength of light. Cones are most numerous at the **fovea,** and their numbers diminish toward the periphery.

3. **Anatomy of the pathway**
   a. The output of the retina is derived from the axons of **ganglion cells,** which form the **optic nerves.**
   b. Fibers from the optic nerves partially cross at the **optic chiasm,** an anatomic feature required for **binocular vision.** Specifically, fibers serving the **nasal** retinas decussate to join contralateral fibers serving the **temporal** retinas. Collectively, these fibers form the **optic tracts.**
   c. Fibers from the optic tract terminate at the **lateral geniculate body,** a small swelling beneath the pulvinar of the thalamus.

TABLE 7-2	SUMMARY OF THE RETINAL PHOTORECEPTORS	
Characteristic	Rods	Cones
Structure	Long, uniform shape to outer segments	Short, cone-shaped outer segments
Location	Most numerous at the periphery	Most numerous at the macula
Photoreceptive pigment	Rhodopsin	Three cone opsins (blue, green, red)
Function	Vision in dim light, contrast	Color vision
Number	130×10^6	6.5×10^6

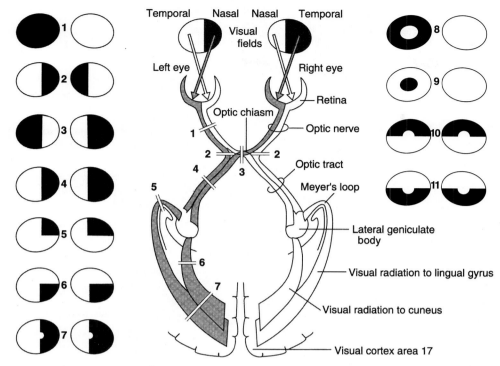

FIG 7-6. The visual pathway from the retina to the visual cortex showing visual field defects. *1,* ipsilateral blindness; *2,* binasal hemianopia; *3,* bitemporal hemianopia; *4,* right hemianopia; *5,* right upper quadrantanopia; *6,* right lower quadrantanopia; *7,* right hemianopia; *8,* left constricted field as a result of end-stage glaucoma (bilateral constricted fields may be seen in hysteria); *9,* left central scotoma as seen in optic (retrobulbar) neuritis in multiple sclerosis; *10,* upper altitudinal hemianopia as a result of bilateral destruction of the lingual gyri; *11,* lower altitudinal hemianopia as a result of bilateral destruction of the cunei. [Reprinted by permission from Fix JD, High-Yield Neuroanatomy, 3rd ed. Philadelphia, Lippincott Williams & Wilkins, 2005.]

    d. The **geniculocalcarine tract** (or optic radiations) conducts fibers from the lateral geniculate to the **calcarine sulcus** and the visual cortex.

    e. A subset of fibers in this tract, known as the **Meyer loop,** travels forward around the temporal horn of the lateral ventricle. These fibers serve the upper half of the visual field.

    f. The remaining fibers traverse the parietal lobe and serve the lower half of the visual field.

    g. The **calcarine sulcus** is the primary visual cortex and is located on the occipital lobe.

    h. **Visual association cortex** is located around the primary cortex on the occipital, parietal, and temporal lobes. It is important for the integration of information for recognition of objects, color perception, depth, and motion.

    i. Understanding of visual pathway anatomy facilitates understanding of the visual field deficits that can result from various lesions (Fig. 7-6).

B. Three **reflex pathways** modulate the function of the visual system via pupillary function and accommodation.

    1. The **pupillary light reflex** consists of pupillary constriction in response to light hitting the retina (Fig. 7-7).

        a. The **afferent limb** is the **optic nerve,** with fibers projecting to the **olivary pretectal nucleus** in the midbrain.

        b. Fibers from the pretectal nucleus project to the **Edinger-Westphal nucleus** of the oculomotor nerve.

        c. Preganglionic parasympathetic fibers from the Edinger-Westphal nucleus, by way of the oculomotor nerve, synapse in the **ciliary ganglion** in the orbit.

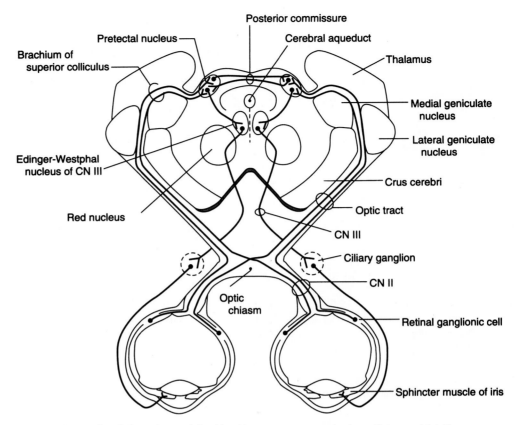

FIG 7-7. The pupillary light pathway. Light shined into one eye causes both pupils to constrict. The response in the stimulated eye is called the direct pupillary light reflex. The response of the opposite eye is called the consensual pupillary light reflex. *CN,* cranial nerve. [Reprinted by permission from Fix JD, High-Yield Neuroanatomy, 3rd ed. Philadelphia, Lippincott Williams & Wilkins, 2005.]

      d. Postganglionic parasympathetic fibers from the ciliary ganglion innervate the **sphincter pupillae muscle** of the iris.

  2. **Pupillary dilation** in response to stimuli such as pain or fear is mediated by the sympathetic nervous system.

      a. Impulses originate from the **amygdala and hypothalamus (paraventricular nucleus)** and project to the **ciliospinal center** of the intermediolateral cell column of the spinal cord (T1–2).

      b. Preganglionic sympathetic fibers from the ciliospinal center traverse the sympathetic trunk to the **superior cervical ganglion (SCG)**.

      c. Postganglionic sympathetic fibers from the SCG travel along with the carotid vascular system to innervate the **dilator pupillae muscle** of the iris.

      d. Lesioning any portion of this pathway results in ipsilateral **Horner syndrome (ptosis, myosis, and anhydrosis)**.

  3. The **accommodation-convergence reaction** is responsible for adjusting sight to a near object. It has three components: convergence of the eyes, pupillary constriction, and rounding of the lens.

      a. Impulses begin in the **visual association cortex** and project to the **superior colliculus** and **pretectal nucleus.**

      b. Fibers from these areas project to the
          i. **Rostral Edinger-Westphal nucleus** (pupillary constriction)
         ii. **Caudal Edinger-Westphal nucleus** (ciliary muscle contraction and lens rounding)
        iii. **Medial rectus subnucleus of the oculomotor nerve**

      c. **Argyll Robertson pupil** or **light-near dissociation** can result from neurosyphilis. What is detected on neurologic examination is pupillary constriction in response to light but not accommodation. Lesions are often found in the **pretectal area.**

III. Hearing

The special sense of hearing results from the **conversion of pressure waves** from air, to liquid, to electrical impulses, which are transmitted to several locations in the central nervous system.

Patient Snapshot 7-3

A 44-year-old woman is referred to a neurologist because she has developed progressively decreased hearing in her left ear. The neurologist performs a thorough neurologic examination, with special focus on the cranial nerves (CNs). On examination of the patient's hearing, the neurologist conducts the Weber and Rinne tests. On the Weber test, the patient indicates that she hears the tuning fork vibrating more in her right ear. The results of the Rinne test are normal bilaterally, as the patient claims she can hear the tuning fork vibrate in the air long after she can hear it vibrating against her mastoid bone. The neurologist is concerned about the possibility of an intracranial mass and sends the patient for an MRI study of the brain. The MRI study shows a 2.0-cm lesion at the cerebellopontine angle suspicious for a vestibular schwannoma (see Fig. 18-3).

A. Cochlea. The **cochlea** contains the **organ of Corti,** the structure that converts the mechanical pressure stimuli into electrical impulses (Fig. 7-8).

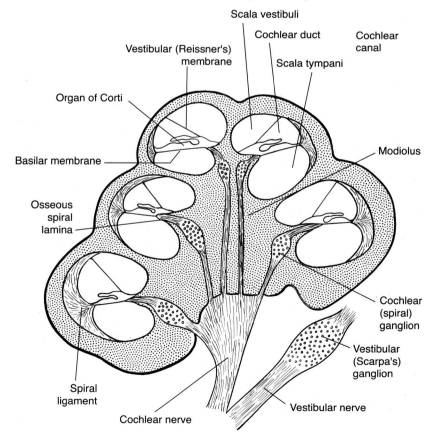

FIG 7-8. A section through the cochlea. [Reprinted with permission from Kiernan JA. Barr's The Human Nervous System, 8th ed. Baltimore, Lippincott Williams & Wilkins, 2005.]

1. There are two types of sensory cells known as **hair cells**, both of which are innervated by peripheral processes of **spiral ganglion bipolar cells.**

    a. There exists a single row of ~7000 **inner hair cells**, the principal sensory cells. Movement of the hairs (microvilli) results in the opening of an ion channel and depolarization. Connections to inner hair cells make up approximately 90% of the **cochlear division of the vestibulocochlear nerve.**

    b. Connections to the nearly 25,000 **outer hair cells** make up only 5–10% of the cochlear division of the vestibulocochlear nerve. Outer hair cells serve to lower the excitation threshold of the inner hair cells.

2. **Anatomy of the pathway** (Fig. 7-9)

    a. **Bipolar cells** of the **spiral ganglion** are the origin of the auditory pathway; they send peripheral fibers to hair cells and central fibers to the **cochlear nuclei** as the **cochlear nerve** (**CN VIII**).

    b. Some cochlear division nerve fibers bifurcate on entering the brainstem and project both ipsilaterally (ventral nucleus) and contralaterally (dorsal

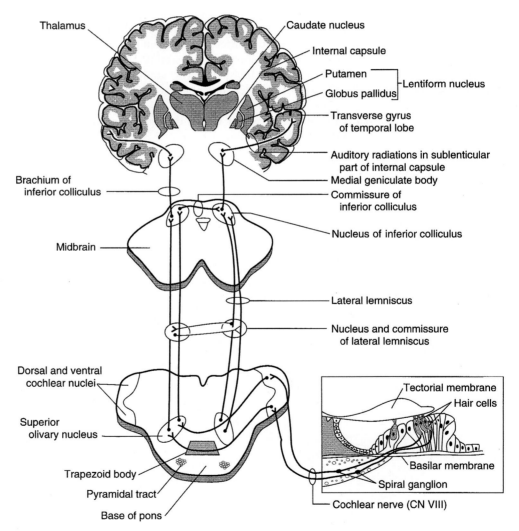

FIG 7-9. Peripheral and central connections of the auditory system. This system arises from the hair cells of the organ of Corti and terminates in the transverse temporal gyri of Heschl of the superior temporal gyrus. It is characterized by the bilaterality of projections and the tonotopic localization of pitch at all levels. For example, high pitch (20,000 Hz) is localized at the base of the cochlea and in the posteromedial part of the transverse temporal gyri. *CN,* cranial nerve. [Reprinted by permission from Fix JD, High-Yield Neuroanatomy, 3rd ed. Philadelphia, Lippincott Williams & Wilkins, 2005.]

nucleus) to the **superior olivary nuclei.** The **trapezoid body** in the pons is the region of auditory fiber decussation.

    c. Olivary fibers project to the **inferior colliculus** via the **lateral lemniscus.**

    d. Collicular fibers project to the **medial geniculate body** through the brachium of the inferior colliculus.

    e. Finally, fibers from the medial geniculate pass through the **internal capsule** via the **auditory radiations** to the **primary auditory cortex** of the temporal lobe.

3. The **auditory association cortex** of the dominant temporal lobe (usually on the left) is known as the **Wernicke area** and is critical for understanding spoken and written language (see Chapter 5).

B. Hearing deficits. Two forms of hearing deficits are clinically identified.

    1. Hearing loss that results from interference with the passage of sound to the receptive cells is called **conductive hearing loss.** Some causes include **obstruction, otitis media,** and **otosclerosis.**

    2. **Sensorineural hearing loss** results from disease to any of the following structures: cochlea, cochlear nerve, and the central auditory pathways. Some causes are **Ménière disease, vestibular schwannoma,** and age-related hearing loss **(presbycusis).**

C. Examination. Using a **tuning fork,** patients can be examined for the two types of hearing loss.

    1. The **Weber test** is conducted by placing a vibrating tuning fork on the vertex of the cranium. A normal individual will hear the vibration equally well on both sides.

        a. With **unilateral conductive hearing loss,** the vibration lateralizes to the affected ear.

        b. With **partial unilateral sensorineural hearing loss,** the vibration **lateralizes to the unaffected ear.**

    2. The **Rinne test** is conducted by first placing a vibrating tuning fork on the mastoid process until vibration is no longer perceived, and then holding the tuning fork in front of the ear. A normal individual will hear air vibration after bone vibration has ceased.

        a. With **unilateral conductive hearing loss,** air vibration is not heard after bone vibration ceases.

        b. With **partial unilateral sensorineural hearing loss,** air vibration is heard after bone vibration ceases.

        c. Table 7-3 summarizes the results of these tests under several conditions.

TABLE 7-3	RESULTS OF THE WEBER AND RINNE TESTS	
Deficit[a]	**Weber Test**	**Rinne Test**
None	No lateralization	AC > BC, both ears
Conductive loss left ear	Lateralizes to left ear	BC > AC, left ear AC > BC, right ear
Conductive loss right ear	Lateralizes to right ear	BC > AC, right ear AC > BC, left ear
Sensorineural loss left ear	Lateralizes to right ear	AC > BC, both ears
Sensorineural loss right ear	Lateralizes to left ear	AC > BC, both ears

[a]Conductive loss is middle-ear deafness (e.g., otosclerosis, otitis media). Sensorineural loss is nerve deafness (e.g., presbycusis).

AC, air conduction; BC, bone conduction.

Adapted with permission from Fix JD, High-Yield Neuroanatomy, 3rd ed. Philadelphia, Lippincott Williams & Wilkins, 2005:84.

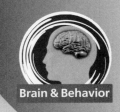
Brain & Behavior

Chapter 8
The Sensory Nervous System: Balance, Olfaction, and Gustation (Taste)

I. Balance

As bipeds, a sense of balance is critical to human functioning. The maintenance of balance (posture and equilibrium, coordination of eye and head movement) is under the control of the **vestibular system,** the receptors for which originate in the inner ear. It is important to note that the *visual* and *proprioceptive systems* also have roles in balance, but this discussion is limited to the vestibular system.

A. Vestibular system includes two subsystems: one for detection the position of the head with respect to gravity (the **static labyrinth**), and one for the detection of angular head acceleration (the **kinetic labyrinth**).

  1. The **static labyrinth** has two components: the **utricle,** which is oriented horizontally, and the **saccule,** which is oriented vertically.

      a. The utricle and saccule each contain specialized epithelia (maculae) that contain the sensory **hair cells.** There are two types of hair cells, each possessing numerous hair-like projections (stereocilia) and a long kinocilium. All the hair-like projections are embedded in a gelatinous **otolithic membrane** that contains **otoliths** (Fig. 8-1).

      b. Because the otoliths have a higher specific gravity than the endolymph, changes in head position cause changes in the position of the otolithic membrane and bending of the hairs.

      c. Bending **toward** the kinocilium causes excitation, whereas bending **away** from the kinocilium triggers inhibition. Changes in the **patterns of action potentials** from this system provide the information that indicates the head's position.

      d. The static labyrinth can respond somewhat to linear head acceleration given its structure. Prolonged, fluctuating stimulation of the static labyrinth is known to cause **motion sickness.**

  2. The **kinetic labyrinth** is composed of the three **semicircular ducts.** Each duct is responsible for the detection of acceleration in its plane of orientation. The **anterior** and **posterior ducts** are oriented in the vertical plane (with ~90° horizontal between them; like a door opened at two positions), whereas the **lateral duct** is oriented at 30° to the horizontal.

      a. Each duct contains an **ampulla** at its end, in which the **crista ampullaris** sits.

          i. The crista is the sensory epithelium and is structurally similar to the maculae of the static labyrinth, with hair cells projecting stereocilia/kinocilium into the gelatinous **cupula** (Fig. 8-2).

          ii. The cupula is the same specific gravity as endolymph, so the kinetic labyrinth *does not* respond to changes in head position.

      b. With *acceleration* in a particular plane, endolymph lags behind because of inertia. Thus the cupula swings in the direction **opposite** the motion of the head (Fig. 8-3A&B).

      c. As movement achieves equilibrium (constant velocity), the endolymph catches up and retains its normal position (Fig. 8-3C).

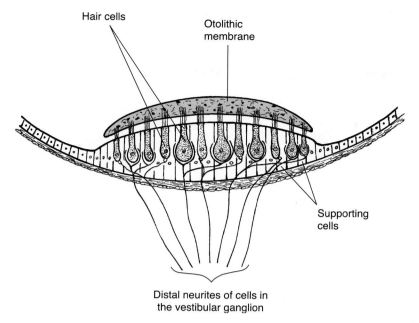

FIG 8-1. Structure of the macula utriculi. [Reprinted with permission from Kiernan JA. Barr's The Human Nervous System, 8th ed. Baltimore, Lippincott Williams & Wilkins, 2005.]

d. When the head *decelerates,* coming to a stop, the endolymph continues to move in the direction of head motion, causing the cupula to swing **in the direction** of head motion (Fig. 8-3D).

e. Action potentials are generated in a fashion similar to those in the static labyrinth. Again, the **pattern** of electrical impulses from the semicircular ducts indicates the nature of head acceleration.

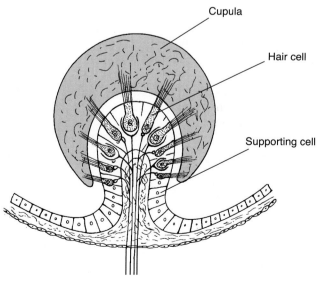

Distal neurites of cell in
the vestibular ganglion

FIG 8-2. Structure of the crista ampullaris. [Reprinted with permission from Kiernan JA. Barr's The Human Nervous System, 8th ed. Baltimore, Lippincott Williams & Wilkins 2005.]

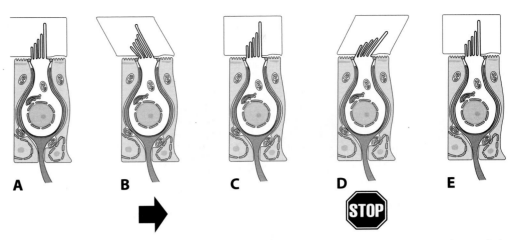

FIG 8-3. The response of hair cells in the crista ampullaris with linear acceleration. **A.** At rest, the cupula is also at rest. **B.** With acceleration to the right (*arrow*) the cupula lags behind, resulting in hair cell activity. **C.** Once constant velocity is reached (acceleration = 0), the cupula returns to the rest position. **D.** On stopping, or deceleration, the inertia of the cupula causes the hair cells to bend and trigger activity. **E.** The cupula returns to the rest position.

B.   Anatomy of the pathway (Fig. 8-4)

   1.   The **vestibular nerve** (**CN VIII**) is formed by central processes of bipolar neurons in the vestibular ganglion. The nerve enters the brainstem, and its fibers terminate at the **vestibular nuclei** and the cerebellum.

   2.   There are **four vestibular nuclei** (**lateral, superior, middle,** and **inferior**), all situated near the dorsum of the brainstem at the pontomedullary junction. The vestibular nuclei efferents project to the following structures (Fig. 8-5):

   a.   The **flocculonodular lobe** of the cerebellum

   b.   CN III, CN IV, and CN VI: the **medial longitudinal fasciculus** (MLF) connects the vestibular nuclei to the nuclei of these cranial nerves. This pathway is responsible for the **vestibulo-ocular reflexes** (see I.B.3).

   c.   The **spinal cord:** projections from the lateral nucleus at the **lateral vestibulospinal tract terminate** in the cervical/lumbar ventral horns to control **postural muscle tone** and **maintain balance.** Fibers from the medial nucleus

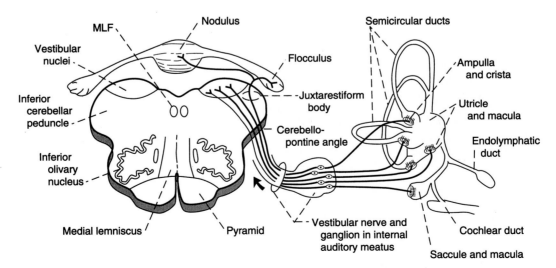

FIG 8-4. Peripheral connections of the vestibular system. The hair cells of the cristae ampullaris and the maculae of the utricle and saccule project through the vestibular nerve to the vestibular nuclei of the medulla and pons and the flocculonodular lobe of the cerebellum (vestibulocerebellum). *MLF,* medial longitudinal fasciculus. [Reprinted with permission from Fix JD. High-Yield Neuroanatomy, 3rd ed. Philadelphia, Lippincott Williams & Wilkins, 2005.]

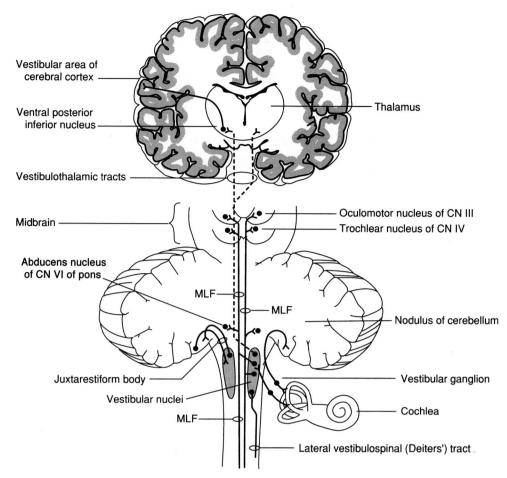

Vestibular area of cerebral cortex

Ventral posterior inferior nucleus

Vestibulothalamic tracts

Midbrain

Abducens nucleus of CN VI of pons

Juxtarestiform body

Vestibular nuclei

MLF

Thalamus

Oculomotor nucleus of CN III
Trochlear nucleus of CN IV

MLF

MLF

Nodulus of cerebellum

Vestibular ganglion

Cochlea

Lateral vestibulospinal (Deiters') tract

FIG 8-5. The major central connections of the vestibular system. Vestibular nuclei project through the ascending medial longitudinal fasciculus (*MLF*) to the ocular motor nuclei and subserve the vestibulo-ocular reflexes. Vestibular nuclei also project through the descending MLF and lateral vestibulospinal tracts to the ventral horn motor neurons of the spinal cord and mediate postural reflexes. *CN,* cranial nerve. [Reprinted with permission from Fix JD. High-Yield Neuroanatomy, 3rd ed. Philadelphia, Lippincott Williams & Wilkins, 2005.]

descend via the **MLF** to modulate cervical motor neurons so **head motion is controlled** to assist equilibrium and fixed gaze.

   d. The **postcentral gyrus** by way of the **thalamus** (ventral posteromedial nucleus): important for the conscious awareness of position and head movement

   e. The **flocculonodular lobe** of the cerebellum is known as the **vestibulocerebellum** and is the target of remaining vestibular afferents. The efferent fibers from the cerebellum largely terminate back on the vestibular nuclei.

  3. **Vestibulo-ocular reflexes** are under the control of the vestibular system.

   a. The **doll's eyes phenomenon** is a vestibulo-ocular reflex that does not require voluntary eye movement. It is often tested in comatose patients to determine if the vestibular pathways in the brainstem are intact. It is tested by passively rotating the head and observing **conjugate** eye movements in the **opposite** direction.

   b. **Nystagmus** is an oscillating eye movement that has fast and slow components. The direction of the **fast component** is designated the direction of the nystagmus. The **slow component** is the reflex correction by the vestibular system to restore direction of gaze.

     i. In **postrotatory nystagmus,** the fast phase is directed opposite the rotation and the slow phase is directed toward the side of rotation.

     ii. In **vestibular nystagmus,** the fast phase is directed toward the side of rotation and the slow phase is directed opposite the rotation.

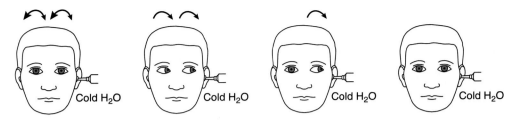

Normal conscious subject   **Brainstem intact**   **MLF (bilateral) lesion**   **Low brainstem lesion**

FIG 8-6. Cold caloric responses in the unconscious patient. When the brainstem is intact, the eyes deviate toward the irrigated side; with bilateral transaction of the medial longitudinal fasciculus (*MLF*), the eye deviates to the abducted side. Destruction of the caudal brainstem results in no deviation of the eyes. *Double-headed arrow,* nystagmus; *single-headed arrow,* deviation of the eyes to one side. [Reprinted with permission from Fix JD. High-Yield Neuroanatomy, 3rd ed. Philadelphia, Lippincott Williams & Wilkins, 2005.]

      iii. **Caloric testing** is performed to determine whether the vestibular system is intact (Fig. 8-6). The external meatus is irrigated with warm or cold water and eye movement is noted. Nystagmus results in a conscious patient with an intact vestibular pathway. **Cold water** triggers nystagmus directed **away** from the irrigated ear; **warm water** triggers nystagmus directed **toward** the irrigated ear. (Remember: **COWS**—cold, opposite/warm, same.)

   c. **Negative results** with the doll's eye and caloric testing indicate a devastating brainstem lesion.

II. Olfaction

Olfaction is the sense of smell, and the parts of the brain responsible for this sense are collectively called the **rhinencephalon**. The olfactory system also plays an important role in how we perceive **taste.**

Patient Snapshot 7-1

A 23-year-old woman is brought to the emergency department after sustaining a head injury in a snowmobile accident. The findings of the physical examination and trauma-series CT scans indicate that she has a skull fracture in the region of the anterior cranial fossa. A blood-tinged watery nasal discharge indicates cerebrospinal fluid (CSF) rhinorrhea. After 7 days of unconsciousness in the intensive care unit, the patient awakens and complains of an inability to smell anything. Neurological examination confirms her complaint. Her neurologist explains that the head injury included fractures of the cribriform plate and ethmoid bone, causing a leak of CSF and damage to the olfactory tract, resulting in anosmia, the inability to smell.

A. Olfactory cells. The **olfactory cells** lie in a pseudostratified columnar epithelium within the nasal cavity.
   1. **Olfactory cells** are bipolar neurons. They send out a modified dendrite into the mucus on the surface of the nasal epithelium. It is this dendrite, through the modified cilia it possesses, that senses chemical odorants.
   2. Olfactory cells are continuously produced via mitosis, to replace those lost by desquamation.
   3. There are approximately **3000** different **types of odorant receptors,** and each neuron possesses several different kinds.

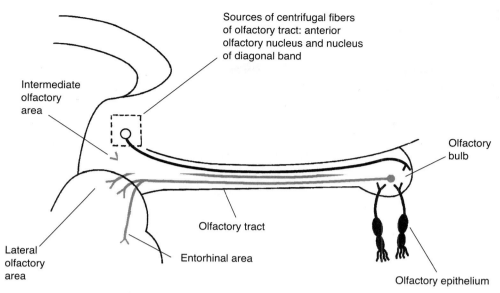

FIG 8-7. Components of the olfactory tract. [Reprinted with permission from Kiernan JA. Barr's The Human Nervous System, 8th ed. Baltimore, Lippincott Williams & Wilkins, 2005.]

4. In general, an olfactory impulse begins with binding of an odorant to a receptor, which depolarizes the olfactory neuron.

B. Anatomy of the pathway (Fig. 8-7)

1. The axons of the olfactory epithelium gather into bundles on each side, thus forming the **olfactory nerves.**

2. Olfactory nerves make their way into the cranial vault by passing through the **cribriform plate** of the ethmoid bone. After doing so, they all join together at the **olfactory bulb** to synapse on its mitral cells: excitatory glutamatergic interneurons.

3. Mitral cell axons project through the **olfactory tract,** which expands to become the **olfactory trigone** just before reaching the **anterior perforated substance.** From there, the pathway diverges:

   a. Most fibers enter the **lateral olfactory stria** and are directed toward the **lateral olfactory area.**

      i. The lateral olfactory area is composed of the **uncus, entorhinal area cortex,** some **limen insulae cortex,** and part of the **amygdala.**

      ii. These regions are collectively known as the **primary olfactory area** and are believed to be responsible for the conscious awareness of smell.

      iii. These regions send fibers to the **olfactory association cortex,** located on the lateral part of the cortical orbital surface.

   b. The remaining fibers enter the anterior perforating substance, a part of the **intermediate olfactory area.**

4. **Centrifugal fibers,** originating from the contralateral olfactory bulb and the **nucleus of the diagonal band** in the anterior perforating substance, are important for modulating the **sensitivity** of the olfactory system.

III. Gustation

The **sense of taste** is called gustation. Unlike vision, olfaction, audition, and balance, gustation is mediated by more than one cranial nerve on the basis of embryologic development. Because of the limited number of flavors that can be identified by the gustatory system, olfaction plays a critical role in taste.

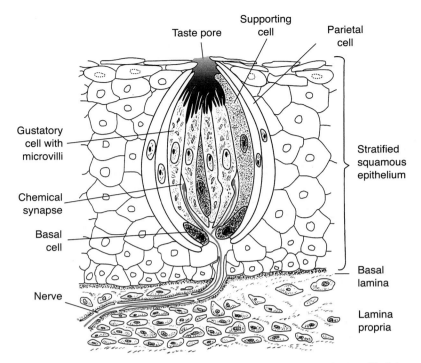

FIG 8-8. Structure of a taste bud. The chemical sensors are the apical microvilli of the taste cells. Chemical synapses communicate with the sensory axons. [Reprinted with permission from Kiernan JA. Barr's The Human Nervous System, 8th ed. Baltimore, Lippincott Williams & Wilkins, 2005.]

A. Taste buds. The receptive apparatus for taste is the **taste bud** (Fig. 8-8). Taste buds are located on the **soft palate,** the **epiglottis,** and the dorsal surface of the **tongue.** Taste buds respond to different chemical stimuli (flavors), and these are distributed anatomically over the tongue.

1. Buds that respond to **sweet** tastes are most abundant at the tip of the tongue.
2. **Sour** things are best tasted on the lateral edges of the tongue.
3. **Bitter** tastes are perceived at the back of the tongue.
4. Foods that taste **salty** are sensed in the middle of the tongue.
5. **Metallic**-tasting items can be sensed over the entirety of the tongue.

B. Anatomy of the pathway. **CN VII, CN IX,** and **CN X** transmit gustatory information (Fig. 8-9).

1. The **facial nerve (CN VII)** possesses axons that innervate taste buds on the **anterior two thirds** of the tongue and the **soft palate** via the **chorda tympani branch** and the **greater petrosal branch,** respectively.
   a. These axons are transmitted from pseudounipolar cells in the **geniculate ganglion,** and they enter the brainstem as the **nervus intermedius.**
   b. Once in the brainstem, the axons join the **tractus solitarius,** turn caudally, are joined by taste fibers from CN IX and CN X, and terminate in the rostral part of the **solitary nucleus.**
2. The **glossopharyngeal nerve (CN IX)** and **vagus nerve (CN X)** possess gustatory unipolar neurons, with cell bodies in the **inferior glossopharyngeal ganglion** and the **inferior ganglion of the vagus nerve.**
   a. Peripheral fibers innervate taste buds on the **posterior third** of the tongue, the **pharyngeal mucosa,** and the **epiglottis (vagus).** Centrally projecting fibers make up part of the solitary tract and terminate in the **solitary nucleus.**

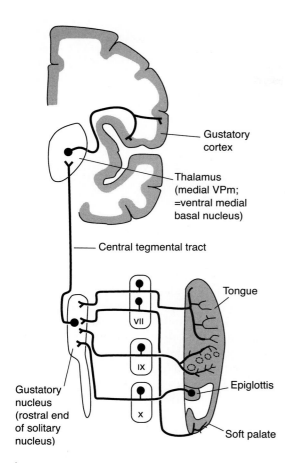

Gustatory
cortex

Thalamus
(medial VPm;
=ventral medial
basal nucleus)

Central tegmental tract

Tongue

VII

IX

X

Epiglottis

Gustatory
nucleus
(rostral end
of solitary
nucleus)

Soft palate

FIG 8-9. Central pathway for gustation: from taste buds to the ipsilateral cerebral cortex. [Reprinted with permission from Kiernan JA. Barr's The Human Nervous System, 8th ed. Baltimore, Lippincott Williams & Wilkins, 2005.]

b. Fibers from the gustatory center in the solitary nucleus project rostrally to the ipsilateral **ventral posteromedial** (VPM) **nucleus** of the thalamus. This nucleus projects to the **cortical area for taste,** an area of the postcentral gyrus adjacent to that for general tongue sensation.

Chapter 9

Somatic Motor and Autonomic Nervous Systems

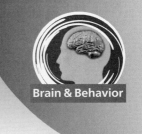

Brain & Behavior

I. Somatic Motor Systems

Patient Snapshot 9-1

On early morning rounds, the neurology stroke service team stops to see a 62-year-old female patient who has had a cerebrovascular accident secondary to a hypertensive bleed. On examination, the chief resident finds that the patient has a positive Babinski sign (dorsiflexion of the great toe and fanning of the remaining toes on noxious sensory stimulus to the lateral aspect of the foot) and absent superficial abdominal reflexes on the left. He attributes these findings to an upper motor neuron (UMN) lesion of the right corticospinal tract. A medical student who continues the examination finds that the patient has dense paralysis of the left arm and leg, including spasticity and exaggerated deep tendon reflexes. The medical student states that this picture is likely to result from an UMN lesion to extrapyramidal tracts (all descending tracts not belonging to the corticospinal tract). The attending views the patient's CT scan and identifies a hemorrhagic lesion to the right internal capsule, where the descending corticospinal (pyramidal) tract and extrapyramidal tract fibers reside.

A. The motor systems begin their descent to the body from the following locations in the brain: the **cerebral cortical motor areas,** the **basal ganglia,** and the **cerebellum.** Each has a different role in regulating motor function.

   1. The major descending motor system is the **pyramidal system,** which includes the **corticospinal and corticobulbar tracts.** It begins in the brain at the **primary motor area,** the **premotor area,** and the **somatosensory cortex.** The pyramidal system functions to control **voluntary skilled motor activity.**

      a. Control of the body's skeletal muscles by the cerebral cortex is primarily via the **contralateral** hemisphere. The body is represented on the precentral gyrus in a somatotopic fashion (or **homunculus**).

      b. The primary motor area receives input from other areas, including the **premotor area, supplemental motor area, cingulate motor area, somatosensory cortex, cerebellum,** and **basal ganglia.**

      c. **Corticospinal** fibers descend through the following brain structures (Fig. 9-1):

         i. The **posterior limb of the internal capsule**

         ii. The middle three fifths of the **crus cerebri** in the midbrain

         iii. The **base of the pons**

         iv. The **medullary pyramids** (thus the term *pyramidal tract*)

      d. Approximately 90% of corticospinal fibers **decussate** (cross) in the caudal medulla, giving rise to the **lateral corticospinal tract.** The remaining fibers descend ipsilaterally, giving rise to the **ventral corticospinal tract.**

         i. Lateral corticospinal fibers descend in the **lateral funiculus,** terminating mostly in the **ventral horn** of the spinal cord.

         ii. Ventral corticospinal fibers decussate at the level of their termination. Therefore, eventually all corticospinal tract fibers cross to the contralateral side, the only difference being the location of decussation (lateral = medulla; ventral = segment of termination).

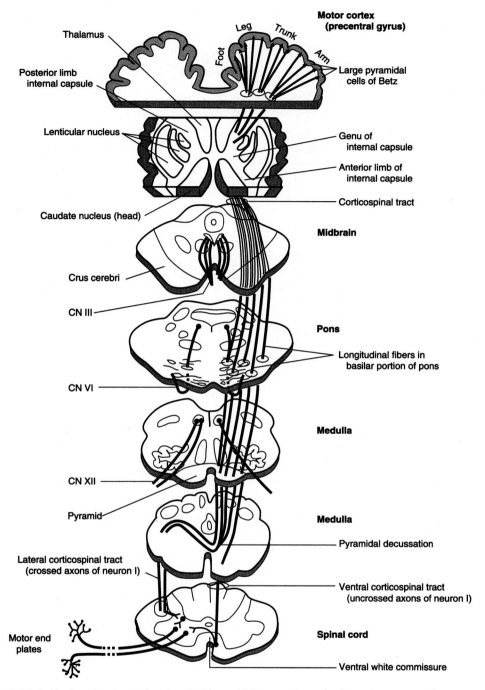

FIG 9-1. The lateral and ventral corticospinal (pyramidal) tracts—the major descending motor pathways—mediate volitional motor activity. The cells of origin are located in the premotor, the motor, and the sensory cortices. *CN,* cranial nerve. [Reprinted with permission from Fix JD. High-Yield Neuroanatomy, 3rd ed. Baltimore, Lippincott Williams & Wilkins, 2005.]

  e. Corticobulbar fibers terminate at or near the motor nuclei of cranial nerves. Unlike corticospinal fibers, corticobulbar fibers can be either crossed or uncrossed. Clinical diagnosis of facial nerve (cranial nerve [CN] VII) dysfunction illustrates this point (Fig. 9-2).

   i. The facial nucleus in the pons has two divisions: one for the upper face and one for the lower face. The upper division is innervated by UMNs

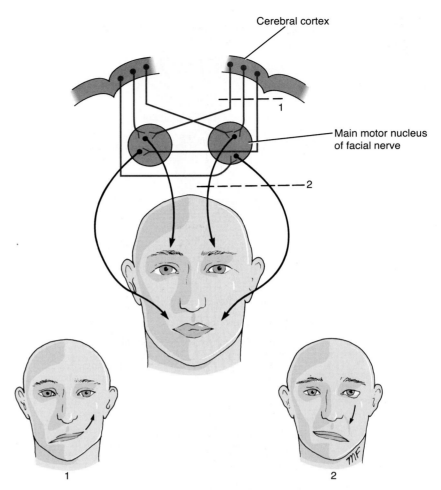

FIG 9-2. Innervation to the facial nerve nuclei and facial expression defects associated with lesions of upper motor neurons (*1*) such as the corticobulbar fibers and of lower motor neurons (*2*) such as the facial nerve itself. [Reprinted with permission from Snell RS. Clinical Neuroanatomy, 6th ed. Baltimore, Lippincott Williams & Wilkins, 2006.]

<blockquote>
from corticobulbar fibers originating from both the contralateral and the ipsilateral motor cortices.

ii. In contrast, the lower division is exclusively innervated by corticobulbar UMNs originating from the contralateral motor cortex.

iii. Therefore, damage to the corticobulbar UMNs on one side results in paralysis of facial muscles in only the contralateral lower face.

iv. A lesion to the facial nerve—a lower motor neuron (LMN) lesion—results in paralysis of facial muscles for the ipsilateral upper and lower face.
</blockquote>

2. All the remaining descending tracts are collectively known as the **extrapyramidal tracts.** These include the following:

a. The **reticulospinal tract** descends from the reticular formation to terminate on interneurons of the **ventral horn.** This pathway functions to control coordinated movements of muscles supplied by different levels of the cord.

b. The **vestibulospinal tract** originates in the lateral vestibular nucleus and terminates at the **ventral horn.** The function of this tract is to facilitate activity of extensor muscles and inhibit the activity of flexor muscles for the maintenance of balance.

c. Fibers arising from the **red nucleus** decussate in the midbrain and descend as the **rubrospinal tract** in the lateral white column of the spinal cord. This

TABLE 9-1	UPPER MOTOR NEURON VERSUS LOWER MOTOR NEURON SIGNS AND SYMPTOMS
Lesion Site	**Signs and Symptoms**
Upper motor neuron	
Pyramidal tracts	Positive Babinski sign
	Absent superficial abdominal reflexes
	Absent cremasteric reflex
	Loss of performance of fine-skilled voluntary movements (especially of distal limbs)
	Severe paralysis without fasciculations or major atrophy (except disuse atrophy)
Extrapyramidal tracts	Spasticity/hypertonicity
	Exaggerated deep tendon reflexes
Lower motor neuron	Flaccid paralysis
	Profound atrophy
	Loss of deep tendon reflexes
	Muscular fasciculations
	Muscular contractures

tract, via connections to the cerebral cortex and cerebellum, facilitates the activity of flexor muscles and inhibits that of the extensors.

3. Clinically, it is diagnostically useful to recognize and distinguish the signs and symptoms that result from UMN and LMN lesions (Table 9-1).

Patient Snapshot 9-2

A 70-year-old man who has had a stroke is in the intensive care unit (ICU). The patient's poststroke course has been complicated by left-sided hemiplegia. The ICU nurse observes that the when the patient awakened he showed uncoordinated, vigorous, and aimless movements of the left trunk and left upper extremity. The neurologist notes that these observations indicate hemiballismus, a neurologic sign that results from a destructive lesion to the contralateral subthalamic nucleus, a component of the basal ganglia.

B. **The basal ganglia** are a collection of nuclei that are important for the initiation and execution of voluntary movement, stereotyped movement, and reflexes (see Chapter 5).
   1. **Anatomy.** Several structures make up this system:
      a. The **corpus striatum** is made up of the **striatum** and the **lentiform nucleus.**
         i. The **caudate nucleus** and the **putamen** make up the striatum.
         ii. The **globus pallidus** and the **putamen** make up the lentiform nucleus.
         iii. Therefore, the components of the corpus striatum are the caudate, the putamen, and the globus pallidus.
      b. The **subthalamic nucleus (STN)**
      c. The **substantia nigra**
   2. Two signaling pathways explain the function of the basal ganglia (Fig. 9-3).
      a. Simplified, the **direct loop** is composed of the following:
         i. Excitatory glutamatergic input from the cortex stimulates the **striatum**
         ii. Increased striatal output triggers inhibition (via γ-aminobutyric acid [GABA] and substance P) of its target, the tonically active pars interna of the **globus pallidus.**

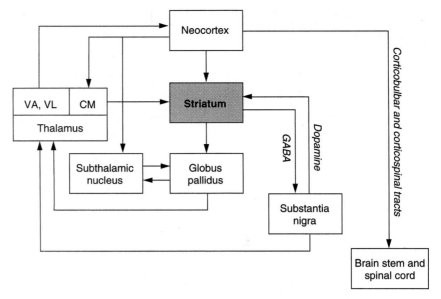

FIG 9-3. Major afferent and efferent connections of the striatal system. The striatum receives major input from three sources: the thalamus, neocortex, and substantia nigra. The striatum projects to the globus pallidus and substantia nigra. The globus pallidus is the effector nucleus of the striatal system and projects to the thalamus and subthalamic nucleus. The substantia nigra also projects to the thalamus. The striatal motor system is expressed through the corticobulbar and corticospinal tracts. *CM,* centromedian nucleus; *GABA,* γ-aminobutyric acid; *VA,* ventral anterior nucleus; *VL,* ventral lateral nucleus. [Reprinted with permission from Fix JD. High-Yield Neuroanatomy, 3rd ed. Baltimore, Lippincott Williams & Wilkins, 2005.]

   iii. Decreased pallidal output results in less inhibition (via GABA) of the **thalamus.**
   iv. The final output of the thalamus is increased.
  b. The **indirect loop** is composed of the following:
   i. **Dopaminergic** activity of the **substantia nigra** excites the GABAergic/ enkephalinergic neurons and inhibits the GABAergic/substance P neurons of the striatum.
   ii. The GABAergic/enkephalinergic neurons inhibit the pars externa of the **globus pallidus.**
   iii. This decreases GABAergic inhibition of the **STN.**
   iv. Increased glutamatergic activity of the STN excites the pars interna of the **globus pallidus.**
   v. The result is increased inhibition of the **thalamus** and decreased excitation of the cortex.

Patient Snapshot 9-3

A 46-year-old African American man is referred to a neurologist by his primary-care physician because of a chief complaint of worsening clumsiness of his left upper extremity. The patient first noticed the problem nearly 8 months before presentation. On questioning by the neurologist, the patient notes that his left arm shakes when he attempts fine motor tasks such as buttoning his shirt. Moreover, sometimes when he walks he reels over to the left. On detailed neurological examination, the physician notes hypotonia and looseness of the patient's left arm and leg on passive movement. With heel-to-toe walking, the patient sways to his left side. When asked to touch his nose with his left index finger, the patient overshoots his target and his hand is tremulous. The remainder of the examination is unremarkable. Given these findings, the neurologist hypothesizes that a lesion of the left cerebellar hemisphere could cause all of the patient's

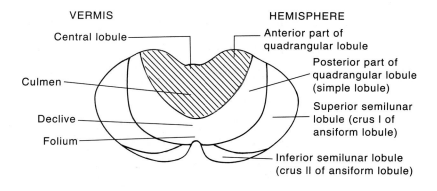

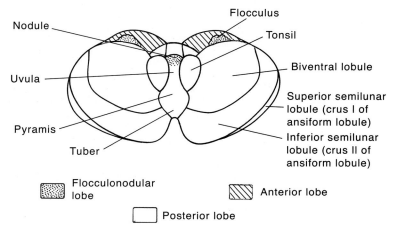

FIG 9-4. Anatomy of the cerebellum. (The lingula, not seen in the figure, is a small, flattened portion of the superior vermis beneath the central lobule and adherent to the superior medullary velum.) [Reprinted with permission from Kiernan, JA. Barr's The Human Nervous System, 8th ed. Baltimore, Lippincott Williams & Wilkins, 2005.]

problems—namely, unilateral clumsiness, tremor, muscle incoordination, and hypotonia. When an MRI study of the brain is obtained, a lesion of the left cerebellar hemisphere consistent with an astrocytoma is identified (see also Table 18-3). .

C. **The role of the cerebellum** in motor function is to maintain equilibrium, coordinate muscle contraction, and synergize muscle action.
  1. **Gross anatomy** (Fig. 9-4)
     a. The cerebellum is divided into a midline **vermis** and **hemispheres.**
     b. It is also divided into lobes: the **anterior, posterior,** and **flocculonodular lobes.**
     c. Three large white matter tracts, called **peduncles,** conduct afferent and efferent fibers (Table 9-2):
        i. The **superior cerebellar peduncle** contains the primary output of the cerebellum.
        ii. The **middle cerebellar peduncle** contains only afferent fibers.
        iii. The **inferior cerebellar peduncle** contains afferent and efferent fibers.
     d. The cerebellum possesses four deep nuclei (Fig. 9-5):
        i. **Fastigial nucleus**
        ii. **Globose nucleus**
        iii. **Emboliform nucleus** (the globose and emboliform nuclei make up the **interposed nuclei**)
        iv. **Dentate nucleus**

TABLE 9-2	CONTENTS OF THE CEREBELLAR PEDUNCLES	
Peduncle	**Afferents**	**Efferents**
Inferior cerebellar peduncle	Olivocerebellar fibers	Cerebellovestibular fibers
	Dorsal spinocerebellar tract	Cerebelloreticular fibers
	Cuneocerebellar fibers	
	Vestibulocerebellar fibers	
	Arcuate nucleus	
	Trigeminal sensory nuclei	
	Precerebellar reticular nuclei	
Middle cerebellar peduncle	Pontocerebellar fibers	No efferents
Superior cerebellar peduncle	Ventral spinocerebellar tract	Cerebellothalamic fibers
	Trigeminothalamic fibers	Cerebellorubral fibers
	Tectocerebellar fibers	
	Noradrenergic fibers from locus ceruleus	

Adapted with permission from Kiernan, JA. Barr's The Human Nervous System, 8th ed. Baltimore, Lippincott Williams & Wilkins, 2005.

2. **Histology.** The cerebellar cortex has three cells layers (Fig. 9-6).
   a. The outer **molecular layer,** which contains stellate and basket cells, Purkinje cell dendrites, parallel fibers (axons from granule neurons), and climbing fibers
   b. The single-cell **Purkinje cell layer**
      i. Purkinje cell axons are the only **efferent output** of the cerebellum.
      ii. They are GABAergic and inhibitory to their targets, the **deep cerebellar nuclei** (a minority of Purkinje axons leave the cerebellum to synapse on the vestibular nuclei).
      iii. Purkinje cells receive excitatory input from **climbing fibers** (of the olivocerebellar tract) and **parallel fibers.**

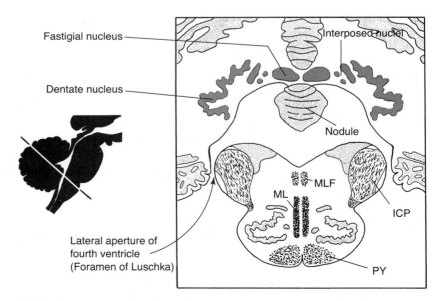

FIG 9-5. The central nuclei of the cerebellum, as seen in a transverse section that also passes through the open part of the medulla. *ICP,* inferior cerebellar peduncle; *ML,* medial lemniscus; *MLF,* medial longitudinal fasciculus; *PY,* pyramid. [Reprinted with permission from Kiernan, JA. Barr's The Human Nervous System, 8th ed. Baltimore, Lippincott Williams & Wilkins, 2005.]

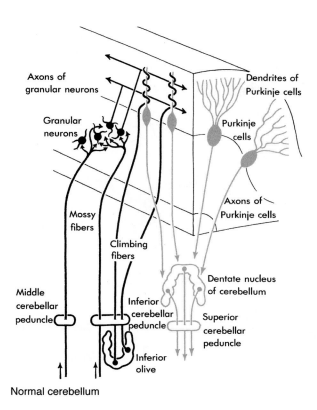

FIG 9-6. The normal cerebellar architecture and connections. [Reprinted with permission from Fix JD. High-Yield Neuroanatomy, 3rd ed. Baltimore, Lippincott Williams & Wilkins, 2005.]

   c.   The inner **granule cell layer,** which contains granule and Golgi cells
    i. Granule neurons are the target of afferent excitatory **mossy fibers** (of the spinocerebellar, pontocerebellar, and vestibulocerebellar tracts).
    ii. Granule cell axons, **parallel fibers,** form excitatory synapses on Purkinje neurons.
3. **Functional anatomy.** The cerebellum has three functional divisions (Fig. 9-7).
  a. The **vestibulocerebellum** is composed of the **flocculonodular lobe.**
    i. Afferent input comes primarily from the **ipsilateral vestibular nuclei.**
    ii. Efferent output is via the **fastigial nucleus** and the **inferior cerebellar peduncle** to the **vestibular nuclei** and **reticular formation.**
    iii. The vestibulocerebellum is important for modulating muscle activity in response to vestibular stimuli.
  b. The **spinocerebellum** is made up of the **vermis of the anterior lobe** and the adjacent **paravermal areas.**
    i. Four afferent systems are known: **somatic sensory systems** (touch/pressure receptors for the body and head), **precerebellar reticular nuclei, inferior olivary complex,** and tracts connected to the **special senses** (from the superior and inferior colliculi). Afferent signals terminate **ipsilaterally.**
    ii. Output is via the **fastigial** and **interposed** nuclei and traverses the **inferior** and **superior cerebellar peduncles.** Targets of output include the **reticular nuclei, red nucleus, inferior olivary nucleus,** and **thalamus.**
    iii. The spinocerebellum modulates muscle tone and synergy of muscle activity for adequate posture.
  c. The **pontocerebellum** is composed of the **lateral hemispheres** and the **superior vermis** of the posterior lobe.
    i. Afferent fibers from contralateral **pontine nuclei** constitute nearly the entire **middle cerebellar peduncle.**

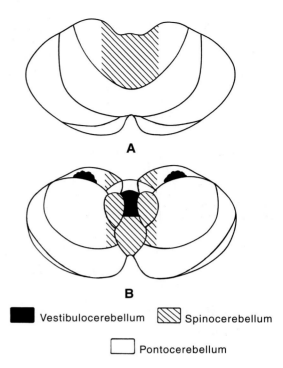

FIG 9-7. Functional regions of the cerebellum from the superior **(A)** and inferior **(B)** surfaces. [Reprinted with permission from Kiernan, JA. Barr's The Human Nervous System, 8th ed. Baltimore, Lippincott Williams & Wilkins, 2005.]

■ Vestibulocerebellum ▨ Spinocerebellum
▢ Pontocerebellum

      ii. Efferent fibers synapse in the **dentate nucleus,** traverse the **superior cerebellar peduncle,** and terminate at the **ventral lateral nucleus** of the thalamus.

      iii. The pontocerebellum functions to ensure smooth and precise muscle movements.

    d. Cerebellar dysfunction can result in **hypotonia, clumsiness, intention tremor, ataxia,** and **dyssynergia.**

  4. Recent data suggest that the cerebellum does more than coordinate movement. It may have roles in **cognitive** and **sensory tasks**—for instance, the recognition of faces and words.

II. Autonomic Nervous System

Patient Snapshot 9-4

A 52-year-old Hispanic woman presents to her primary-care physician with multiple progressive complaints, including tremor, stiffness, difficulty walking, and falling spells. The physician is at first concerned that the patient has Parkinson disease. However, the physician also finds that the patient also has urinary incontinence and that her falling spells are triggered primarily by attempts to get up from a seated or supine position. The physical examination is noteworthy for orthostatic hypotension, a resting tremor that dissipates with intended movement, bradykinesia, cogwheel rigidity, and a shuffling gate. He recognizes this combination of signs and symptoms as being consistent with Shy-Drager syndrome, a combination of a parkinsonian disorder with autonomic dysfunction. The Parkinson symptoms are caused by the loss of neurons within the basal ganglia, and the autonomic symptoms (orthostatic hypotension, urinary incontinence) are primarily the result of a loss of preganglionic sympathetic neurons within the intermediolateral cell column.

A. **The autonomic nervous system (ANS)** functions to maintain physiologic and endocrine equilibria. **Afferent** sensory fibers from sensory neurons on the viscera and organs monitor the local environment. **Efferent** motor fibers, via a two-neuron connection (**preganglionic** and **postganglionic neurons**) terminate on smooth muscle, cardiac muscle, and glands. The ANS is divided into the **sympathetic nervous system (SNS)** and the **parasympathetic nervous system (PNS).**
  1. **Sympathetic nervous system**
     a. **Functions** (Table 9-3)
        i. The SNS stimulates activities that are accompanied by the expenditure of energy.

TABLE 9-3	ACTIONS OF THE SYMPATHETIC AND PARASYMPATHETIC NERVOUS SYSTEMS	
Structure	**Sympathetic Functions**	**Parasympathetic Functions**
Eye		
Radial muscle of iris	Pupillary dilation (mydriasis)	
Circular muscle of iris	NA	Pupillary constriction (miosis)
Muscle of ciliary body	NA	Near vision accommodation
Lacrimal gland	NA	Stimulates secretion
Salivary glands	Viscous secretion	Watery secretion
Sweat glands		
Thermoregulatory	Increases secretion	NA
Apocrine (stress)	Increases secretion	NA
Heart		
Sinoatrial node	Accelerates automaticity	Decreases automaticity (vagus)
Atrioventricular node	Speeds conduction velocity	Slows conduction velocity
Contractility	Increases	Decreases (atria only)
Vascular smooth muscle		
Skin, splanchnic vessels	Contraction	NA
Skeletal muscle vessels	Relaxation	NA
Bronchiolar smooth muscle	Relaxation	Contraction
Gastrointestinal		
Smooth muscle		
Walls	Relaxation	Contraction
Sphincters	Contraction	Relaxation
Secretion and motility	Decrease	Increase
Genitourinary (smooth muscle)		
Bladder wall	Marginal effects	Contraction
Sphincter	Contraction	Relaxation
Penis, seminal vesicles	Ejaculation	Erection
Adrenal medulla	Secretion of epinephrine and norepinephrine	NA
Metabolic functions		
Liver	Gluconeogenesis and glycogenolysis	NA
Adipocytes	Lipolysis	NA
Kidney	Renin release	NA

NA, not applicable.

Adapted with permission from Fix JD. High-Yield Neuroanatomy, 3rd ed. Baltimore, Lippincott Williams & Wilkins, 2005:130.

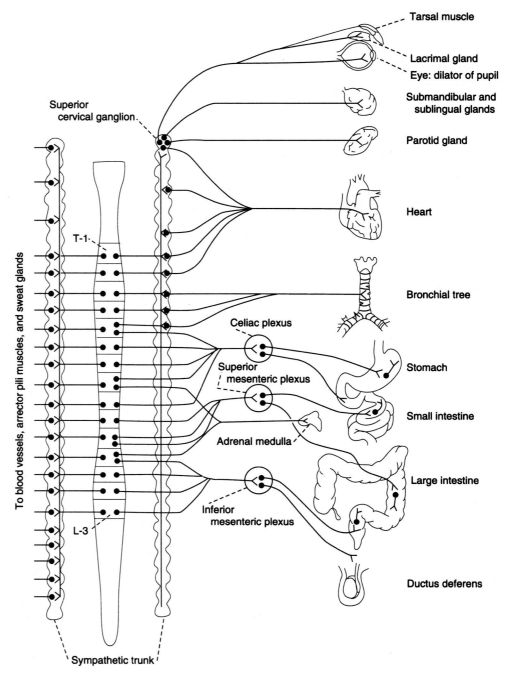

FIG 9-8. The sympathetic (thoracolumbar) innervation of the autonomic nervous system. The entire sympathetic innervation of the head is through the superior cervical ganglion. Gray communicating rami are found at all spinal levels; white communicating rami are found only in spinal segments T1–L3. [Reprinted with permission from Fix JD. High-Yield Neuroanatomy, 3rd ed. Baltimore, Lippincott Williams & Wilkins, 2005.]

    ii. It regulates the **fight-or-flight,** or emergency, responses—for example, increased rate/force of cardiac contraction, increased arterial blood pressure, and redirection of blood flow to the skeletal muscles.

  b. Anatomy (Figs. 9-8 and 9-9)

    i. The first-order efferent, or **preganglionic, neurons** have their cell bodies in the **lateral gray columns** of the spinal cord from **T1** to **L2–3.** The origin of first-order neurons within the thoracic and lumbar spinal cord explains why the SNS is also known as the **thoracicolumbar** autonomic nervous system.

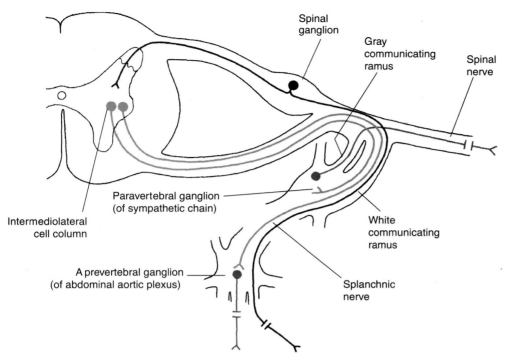

FIG 9-9. Visceral efferent and afferent neurons associated with a thoracic segment of the spinal cord. Visceral sensory axons pass through autonomic ganglia, but their cell bodies are located in dorsal root ganglia. Preganglionic neurons have their nuclei within the intermediolateral cell column. Postganglionic neurons have their nuclei within the paravertebral and prevertebral ganglia. Sensory (pain) neuron supplying internal organs of the abdomen have their nuclei within the spinal ganglia. [Reprinted with permission from Kiernan JA. Barr's The Human Nervous System, 8th ed. Baltimore, Lippincott Williams & Wilkins 2005.]

    ii. Their myelinated axons exit the ventral roots and traverse the **white rami communicans** to reach the sympathetic ganglia of the **paravertebral trunk.**

       (a) Some fibers travel rostrally or caudally to synapse with postganglionic neurons in cervical or lumbar ganglia.

       (b) Other preganglionic fibers leave the sympathetic trunk without synapsing: the **splanchnic nerves.** These fibers synapse on the **celiac, superior mesenteric,** and **inferior mesenteric ganglia** as well as cells of the adrenal medulla.

    iii. Unmyelinated axons of the postganglionic neurons exit the sympathetic trunk via the **gray rami communicans** and join spinal nerves to reach their targets.

    iv. **Afferent** sensory fibers enter the sympathetic trunk from their targets, exit via white rami communicans, join general sensory nerves, and have their cell bodies in the dorsal root ganglia.

  c. **Neurotransmitters** (Fig. 9-10)

    i. **Acetylcholine** (ACh) is the neurotransmitter released by the preganglionic neurons, both SNS and PNS. Its action is terminated rapidly by the enzyme **acetylcholinesterase.**

    ii. Receptors on all postganglionic neurons are **nicotinic ACh receptors.**

    iii. There are two neurotransmitters for the SNS released by postganglionic neurons:

       (a) The majority of postganglionic neurons release **norepinephrine,** which acts on postsynaptic α- or β-adrenergic receptors. Norepinephrine is removed from the synaptic cleft by **reuptake.**

       (b) Postganglionic fibers that synapse on sweat glands release **ACh,** which acts on **muscarinic ACh receptors.**

    iv. Actions of the SNS on the adrenal gland result in the release of **epinephrine.**

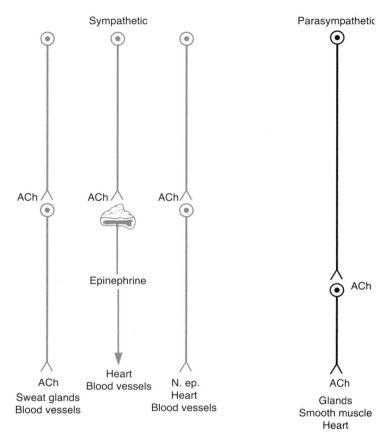

FIG 9-10. Efferent parts of the autonomic nervous system and the chemical transmitter substances released at the nerve endings. *ACh,* acetylcholine; *N. ep.,* norepinephrine. [Reprinted with permission from Snell RS. Clinical Neuroanatomy, 6th ed. Baltimore, Lippincott Williams & Wilkins, 2006.]

2. **Parasympathetic nervous system**
    a. **Functions** (Table 9-3)
        i.   The PNS controls smooth muscle and glands to conserve and restore energy.
        ii. It regulates **rest-and-digest** activities—for example, the PNS triggers a slower heart rate, pupillary constriction, and peristalsis.
    b. **Anatomy.** Like the SNS, the PNS is a two-neuron pathway (Fig. 9-11). The **preganglionic neurons** of the PNS make up the **craniosacral outflow.** The preganglionic axons synapse on **postganglionic neurons,** which are often located in the walls of the target organs (Table 9-4).
    c. **Neurotransmitters** (Fig. 9-10)
        i.   Like the SNS, the preganglionic neurons form **cholinergic** synapses with the postganglionic neurons. The receptors are **nicotinic.**
        ii. Unlike the majority of the SNS, the sole neurotransmitter of postganglionic neurons is **ACh,** the target of which is the **muscarinic** receptor.
3. The ANS also conducts afferent fibers in the form of **general visceral afferents (GVAs).** GVA fibers carry signals in response to visceral organ distension and pain.
    a. Some visceral pain is reasonably well localized to the area of the stimulus. For instance, bladder distension is often perceived as discomfort at the site of the bladder. In general, pain impulses carried by the PNS are better localized than those carried by the SNS.
    b. In contrast, visceral pain is often perceived at a site some distance away from the stimulus.
        i.   This is known as **referred pain** and is most notable among the visceral structures innervated by the SNS.

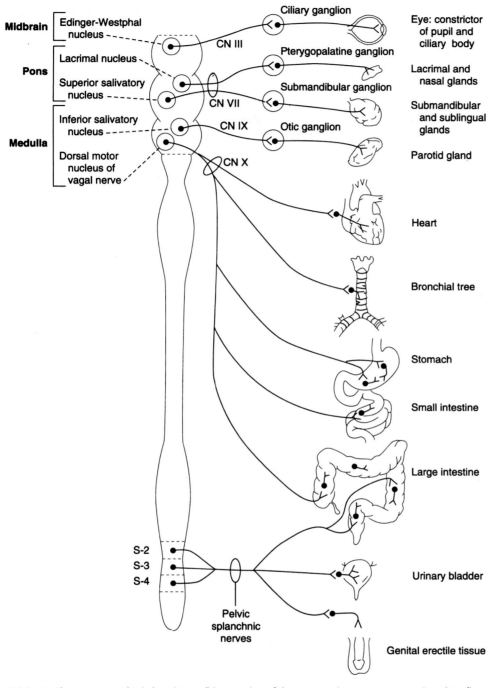

FIG 9-11. The parasympathetic (craniosacral) innervation of the autonomic nervous system. Sacral outflow includes segments S1–4. Cranial outflow is mediated through cranial nerve (*CN*) III, CN VII, CN IX, and CN X. [Reprinted with permission from Fix JD. High-Yield Neuroanatomy, 3rd ed. Baltimore, Lippincott Williams & Wilkins, 2005.]

    ii.   For example, pain originating from the heart owing to myocardial ischemia is transduced to the CNS via afferent cardiac branches of the sympathetic trunk. These afferent branches enter the spinal cord by way of the dorsal roots of the upper four thoracic nerves. Instead of feeling the pain at the heart, it is often **referred** to the skin areas supplied by the corresponding spinal nerves (e.g., the left anterior chest wall; the skin on the medial side of the upper part of the arm).

TABLE 9-4	LOCATIONS AND FUNCTIONS OF PARASYMPATHETIC NERVOUS SYSTEM COMPONENTS	
Preganglionic Origin	**Postganglionic Origin**	**Target(s)**
Edinger-Westphal nucleus (CN III)	Ciliary ganglion	Pupilloconstrictor of iris
		Ciliary muscle
Superior salivatory nucleus (CN VII)	Submandibular ganglion	Sublingual and submandibular glands
	Pterygopalatine ganglion	Tear glands and glands of nasal mucosa
Inferior salivatory nucleus (CN IX)	Otic ganglion	Parotid gland
Dorsal motor nucleus of vagus	Cardiac ganglion	SA and AV nodes
	Visceral plexuses	Wall of pulmonary tree
		Smooth muscles of gastrointestinal glands up to splenic flexure
		Kidney
S2–4 spinal segments	Intramural ganglion	Distal colon
	Hypogastric plexus	Rectum
		Anal sphincter
	Intramural ganglion (vesical plexus)	Urinary bladder
		Urethral sphincter
	Hypogastric plexus (pelvic plexus)	Genitals

AV, atrioventricular; *CN,* cranial nerve; *SA,* sinoatrial.

Adapted with permission from Fix JD. High-Yield Neuroanatomy, 3rd ed. Baltimore, Lippincott Williams & Wilkins, 2005:100.

B. Central control of the ANS

1. The **hypothalamus** is important for regulating the ANS. It integrates many different afferents (e.g., neocortex, hippocampus, amygdala) to modulate homeostasis via the ANS.

2. Hypothalamic efferents to the autonomic nuclei in the brainstem and spinal cord reach them directly or via relays through the reticular formation.

3. **Horner syndrome** results from a lesion to the sympathetic pathway from the CNS to head structures. Classically, Horner syndrome involves the triad of ipsilateral **ptosis** (drooping eyelid), **miosis** (pupil constriction), and **anhydrosis** (absence of sweating).

Chapter 10

Cell/Tissue Structure and Function

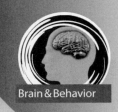

Brain & Behavior

I. Axonal Transport

Because neuronal cell bodies are sometimes located long distances from the ends of their axons, a mechanism must be in place for transporting materials from the cell body to the distal processes and back. **Molecular motor proteins** (e.g., members of the **kinesin superfamily of proteins**), **adaptor molecules**, and **scaffolding proteins** are required to traffic such materials.

Patient Snapshot 10-1

A 27-year-old man is bitten by a bat while on a camping trip. Because the bite barely breaks the skin, the man refuses to go to the emergency room. During the next day or two the man feels somewhat ill and notices some funny feelings and muscle jumping around the site of the wound. Almost 3 weeks later, his girlfriend notices that the man is agitated, confused, and combative. He has a seizure and is brought to the emergency room where the history of the bat bite is revealed. While in the emergency room the man is found to have a high fever and evidence of autonomic instability, including profound salivation. Physical examination also reveals upper motor neuron disease and cranial nerve palsies. Despite intensive therapy in the intensive care unit, the man dies 8 days later. An autopsy reveals the presence of rabies virus in the central nervous system (CNS). The pathology resident reasons that the rabies virus from the bat's saliva traveled to the CNS via the retrograde transport machinery in the neuronal processes near the bite location.

A. **Anterograde transport** involves the movement of materials from the cell body to the distal axonal processes. **Kinesin** is the best described of the molecular motor proteins responsible for anterograde transport. Anterograde transport comes in two forms, distinguished by the rate of transport:
   1. **Fast anterograde transport** can transport materials at a rate of **100–400 mm/day.** Examples of transported substances include proteins, neurotransmitters, and their precursors.
   2. **Slow anterograde transport** is largely responsible for moving large structural proteins (e.g., neurofilaments, microtubules). The rate of this form of transport is **0.1–3 mm/day.**

B. Conversely, **retrograde transport** is responsible for moving material from the distal axon back to the cell body. All retrograde transport moves at approximately the same speed, around two thirds the rate of fast anterograde transport. **Dynein** is the motor protein responsible for retrograde transport. Examples of transported substances are **activated growth factor receptors, pinocytotic vesicles,** and **expired organelles.**

C. **Retrograde transport** is used by several pathogens to gain entry into the CNS—for example, **tetanus toxin, polio virus, rabies virus,** and **herpes simplex virus.**

II. Excitable Properties of Neurons, Axons, and Dendrites, Including Channels

A. **The action potential.** The nature of neuronal electrical excitability is shown in Figure 10-1.

1. Like other biologic membranes, a neuron's membrane is **semipermeable,** allowing only certain substances to diffuse through.

2. In the **resting state,** the **resting membrane potential** is established by the **Na$^+$/K$^+$-ATPase pump** and the slow leak of **K$^+$ ions** out of the cell (Fig. 10-1A). Thus the inside of the cell is **negatively charged** relative to the outside of the cell (**resting membrane potential is about −80 mV**). The neuron is **polarized.**

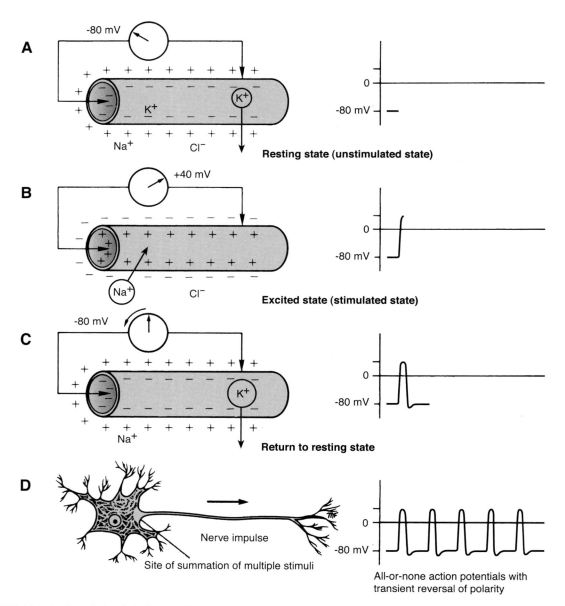

A — Resting state (unstimulated state)

B — Excited state (stimulated state)

C — Return to resting state

D — Nerve impulse / Site of summation of multiple stimuli / All-or-none action potentials with transient reversal of polarity

FIG 10-1. Ionic and electrical changes that occur in a neuron when it is stimulated. [Reprinted from Snell RS. Clinical Neuroanatomy, 6th ed. Baltimore, Lippincott Williams & Wilkins, 2006.]

3. Action potentials are generated at the **axon hillock** by the passive spread of electrical potential through dendrites and the cell body. Whether an action potential is generated depends on the nature (timing, amplitude, and localization) of the inputs a neuron receives.

   a. An excitatory stimulus at a synapse results in depolarization and an **excitatory postsynaptic potential (EPSP).**

   b. An inhibitory stimulus at a synapse results in hyperpolarization and an **inhibitory postsynaptic potential (IPSP).**

4. As the incoming excitatory and inhibitory signals are processed and summed, an **action potential** results when the EPSP is greater than the IPSP and the axon hillock becomes depolarized to a certain voltage, known as the **threshold potential.**

   a. When this occurs, the neuronal membrane becomes permeable to Na^+ ions owing to the opening of voltage-gated Na^+ channels, which flood into the cell, causing it to **depolarize.**

   b. At the peak of the action potential, the membrane potential can be approximately +40 mV (Fig. 10-1B).

5. If the magnitude of the EPSP is not sufficient to depolarize the neuron to the threshold potential, an action potential will not occur. Thus generation of an action potential is an **all-or-none phenomenon.**

   6. The period of Na^+ permeability is brief (fractions of a second), after which voltage-gated Na^+ channels become inactivated and the neuronal membrane develops increased permeability to K^+ **ion efflux** (Fig. 10-1C). This drives the membrane potential back toward the resting state.

7. Near the end of the action potential, K^+ **ion efflux** can continue, producing a short period of **hyperpolarization** and a membrane potential more negative than in the resting state.

8. The action potential is propagated via the passive spread of depolarization from one region to another. This depolarization opens downstream voltage-gated Na^+ channels; and, via a domino-like effect, the action potential is transmitted.

B. Ion channels are responsible for the transit of Na^+ and K^+ ions across the lipid bilayer of the plasma membrane.

   1. These ion channels are composed of protein molecules that **span** the entire width of the plasma membrane and form a **central pore** through which the ions can travel.

   2. The Na^+ and K^+ ion channels responsible for the action potential are **voltage gated.**

   a. For example, if a stimulus is sufficient to raise the membrane potential to about −60 mV, the proteins of the Na^+ channels in the region of the potential change will undergo a **conformational change.**

   b. This change results in the central canal of the channel being opened and in the influx of Na^+ ions.

   3. The behavior of these ion channels is responsible for the following properties of neuronal excitability:

   a. A stimulus sufficient to depolarize the axon hillock to the threshold potential will elicit **the same size action potential** regardless of the magnitude of depolarization. Stronger stimuli are reflected in an increase in the **frequency of action potentials** generated, not the size of the action potentials.

   b. The **absolute refractory period** is the time after an action potential during which another action potential cannot be triggered regardless of the strength of the inciting stimulus.

      i. The absolute refractory period results from a conformational change in the voltage-gated Na^+ channels to an inactive state before returning to the resting state.

      ii. This inactive state of the voltage-gated Na^+ channels is responsible for the unidirectional nature of action potentials.

    c. During the **relative refractory period,** an action potential can be triggered; but a stronger stimulus than usual is required because of the ensuing **K⁺ efflux,** which causes the inside of the cell to become briefly **hyperpolarized.** In this brief hyperpolarized state, a greater EPSP is required to sufficiently depolarize the cell to the threshold potential.

C. **Axons** are the longest processes that arise from neuronal cell bodies. They are responsible for transmitting electrical impulses away from the cell body. Each neuron, by definition, has only one axon.
    1. Axons arise from a region of the neuronal cell body known as the **axon hillock.** The first 50–100 μ of the axons is known as the **initial segment** and is the most excitable portion of the axon.
    2. Axons have a tubular structure with a smooth surface that remains nearly uniform in diameter until their termination.
    3. Near their termination, axons can branch widely to form **axon terminals.**
    4. The cytoplasm of the axon (or **axoplasm**) differs in its constituents from those of the cell body. It *does not* contain Nissl substance or Golgi.

D. **Dendrites** are distinct from axons; they are **shorter,** are **highly branched,** and can possess **dendritic spines** along their surface to increase their surface area. Although a neuron can have only one axon, it can have many dendrites.
    1. Dendrites can be thought of as extensions of the cell body that function to increase its surface area for the reception of synapses.
    2. The cytoplasm of dendrites closely resembles that of the cell body.
    3. In general, dendrites transmit impulses **toward** the cell body.

III. Glia and Myelin

Patient Snapshot 10-2

A 34-year-old executive assistant presents to her primary-care physician with neurologic complaints. After obtaining a history and performing a physical examination, the physician finds that the patient has horizontal diplopia, bilateral fingertip numbness, and an unsteady gait. He orders a brain MRI study; the T2-weighted images reveal several regions of hyperintensity bilaterally in the frontal periventricular areas and brainstem. The patient's symptoms worsen over the following couple of weeks to include right arm clumsiness, abnormal eye movements, and inappropriate mood. The primary-care physician refers the woman to a neurologist who suspects the she may have multiple sclerosis (MS), an inflammatory demyelinating disease defined by the presence of multiple lesions separated in space and time. The pathology of MS is believed to involve autoimmune processes, but the exact cause is unknown. The symptoms are a result of the loss of myelin sheaths around axons, leading to the slowing of action potentials and ultimately blockade. The physician treats the patient with a course of corticosteroids with much improvement. Over the next several years, the patient has several relapsing–remitting episodes of similar neurologic symptoms (see also Chapter 18).

A. **Glia** are the non-neuronal supporting cells of the nervous system and are intimately related to neurons and their processes. There are several types of glial cells, each with unique morphology and function (Fig. 10-2; Table 10-1).
    1. **Astrocytes** are supporting cells that possess small cell bodies and numerous processes.
        a. There are two general morphologic types: **fibrous** (largely populating white matter) and **protoplasmic astrocytes** (largely populating gray matter).

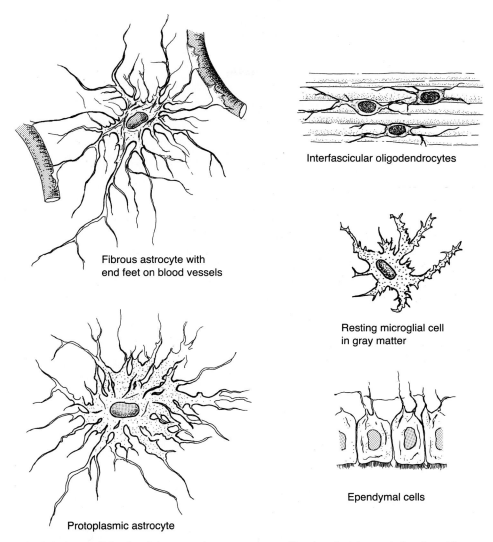

FIG 10-2. Neuroglial cells of the central nervous system. [Reprinted with permission from Kiernan AJ. Barr's The Human Nervous System, 8th ed. Baltimore, Lippincott Williams & Wilkins, 2005.]

    b. They contain abundant **glial fibrillary acidic protein** (**GFAP**), the presence of which can be used as a marker.

    c. Astrocytes have several important functions in the nervous system, including forming the **blood–brain barrier,** forming the external and internal glial-limiting membranes and facilitating the uptake of **neurotransmitters** and **extracellular K$^+$ ions.**

    d. Astrocytes can serve as phagocytes. After injury to the nervous system, astrocytes proliferate to fill the space left by dead neurons. This process is known as **replacement gliosis.**

2. **Oligodendrocytes** are cells of the CNS that are responsible for the production of **myelin** (see III.B). They have small nuclei with a few long, thin processes.

3. **Schwann cells** are the myelin-producing counterpart of the oligodendrocytes for the peripheral nervous system (PNS). They are tubular cells with elongated nuclei.

4. **Microglia** are derived from the monocyte/macrophage lineage of cells. They are the primary phagocytic cells of the CNS.

5. **Ependymal cells** are the cuboidal/columnar cells that line the ventricular system of the brain. There are three general types:

TABLE 10-1	LOCATION AND FUNCTION OF GLIAL CELLS	
Cell Type	**Location**	**Function(s)**
Astrocytes		
Fibrous	White matter	Construct supportive scaffold for CNS
		Help make up blood–brain barrier
		Modulate contents of extracellular space
		Scavenge neurotransmitters
		Alter neuronal metabolism and polarization
Protoplasmic	Gray matter	Phagocytosis of debris
		Glycogen storage
		Production of trophic substances
Oligodendrocytes	Along myelinated nerves	Produce myelin in CNS
		Influence neuronal physiology
Microglia	Throughout the CNS	Active only in disease or injury to phagocytose debris
Ependyma		
Ependymocytes	Line ventricles and central canal	Circulate and absorb CSF
Tanycytes	Line floor of third ventricle	Move substances from CSF to hypophyseal-portal system
Choroidal epithelial cells	Cover surface of choroid plexus	Synthesize and release CSF

CNS, central nervous system; CSF, cerebrospinal fluid.
Adapted with permission from Snell RS. Clinical Neuroanatomy, 6th ed. Baltimore, Lippincott Williams & Wilkins, 2006: 53.

    a. **Ependymocytes** make up the majority of ependymal cells. They are **lining cells** *without* tight junctions and are not in direct contact with the cerebrospinal fluid (CSF).

    b. **Tanycytes** make up most of the floor of the third ventricle. It is believed that they are somehow involved in **regulating endocrine function** in response to hypothalamic signals.

    c. **Choroidal epithelial cells** make up the lining of the choroid plexus. These cells possess **tight junctions,** and their function is to **regulate the composition of the CSF.**

B. **Myelin sheaths** envelope the axons of many neurons in the nervous system. These sheaths are laid down beginning near the origin of an axon and terminate before their branching ends (Fig. 10-3).

    1. Myelin sheaths are formed by two different types of neuroglial cells, depending on the location of the axon.

        a. In the **CNS,** myelin sheaths are formed by **oligodendrocytes.** One oligodendrocyte can myelinate **many** axons simultaneously.

        b. **Schwann cells** are responsible for myelinating axons in the **PNS.** Unlike oligodendrocytes, Schwann cells myelinate only a single axon.

        c. Myelination of the nervous system begins in the **late fetal period** and continues through adolescence (see Chapter 1).

    2. **Structure**

        a. Myelin sheaths are composed of closely opposed layers of neuroglial **plasma membranes.**

        b. Myelin sheaths are not continuous but are interrupted by unmyelinated regions called **nodes of Ranvier.** These areas represent spaces between the myelin formed by different oligodendrocytes or Schwann cells.

    3. The **function** of the myelin sheath and its corresponding nodes of Ranvier is to allow for faster action potential conduction along axons.

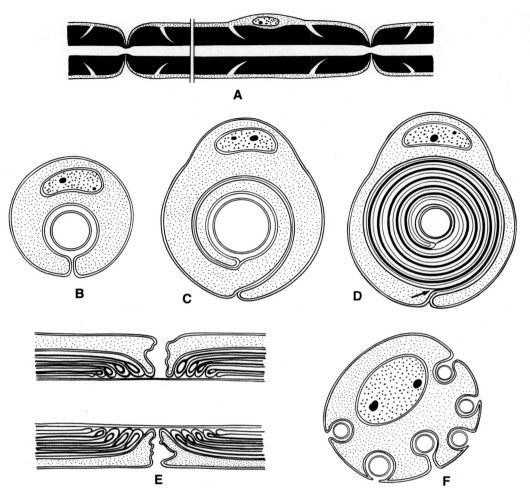

FIG 10-3. A. The myelin sheath and Schwann cell as they are seen (ideally) by light microscopy. **B–D.** Successive stages in the development of the myelin sheath from the plasma membrane of a Schwann cell. **E.** Ultrastructure of a node of Ranvier (longitudinal section). **F.** Relation of a Schwann cell to several unmyelinated axons. [Reprinted with permission from Kiernan AJ. Barr's The Human Nervous System, 8th ed. Baltimore, Lippincott Williams & Wilkins, 2005.]

a. Faster action potential occurs because nearly all ion movement is restricted to the nodes of Ranvier. As a result, the action potential jumps electrically from one node to the next, an arrangement known as **saltatory conduction.**

b. A second factor that contributes to increased velocity of action potentials is **axonal diameter.** The larger the axonal diameter, the faster the conduction of the action potential.

Chapter 11
Brain Homeostasis and Biochemistry of Behavior

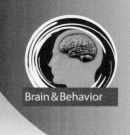
Brain & Behavior

I. Brain Homeostasis

Patient Snapshot 11-1

While on rounds at the children's hospital, the neurology team is consulted about a 5-day-old boy who has been lethargic, feeding poorly, and demonstrating muscle spasms. Because the boy appears jaundiced, the team requests measurement of the level of indirect (unconjugated) bilirubin in the infant's serum. The level of indirect bilirubin is found to be 48 mg/mL, and the diagnosis of kernicterus (toxic level of bilirubin in the brain, leading to neuronal dysfunction and cell death) is made. The medical student on the team tells the neurology attending about an elderly man whose case he reviewed on surgical service the month before. The man had obstructive jaundice from pancreatic cancer. Although the man also had high levels of indirect bilirubin, in contrast to the newborn, those high levels did not lead to neurologic sequelae. The attending explains the discrepancy in presentation between the elderly man and the newborn: In a newborn, unconjugated bilirubin can enter the central nervous system (CNS) and cause kernicterus because the blood–brain barrier is not fully developed. In contrast, an elderly man with pancreatic cancer has a developed and intact blood–brain barrier, so unconjugated bilirubin cannot cross it, and no neurologic sequelae will be observed.

A. Brain metabolism

1. Although the brain makes up only about **2%** of total body weight, **15%** of cardiac output is required to supply it with the glucose and oxygen it needs. These high metabolic requirements are reflected in the ability of the brain's vasculature to autoregulate in response to changes in energy demand.

   a. Brain arterioles alter their diameter in response to **systemic blood pressure.** When blood pressure goes down, these arterioles constrict; when blood pressure rises, they dilate. Therefore, cerebral blood flow is **maintained at a constant level** within a large range of blood pressures (mean arterial pressures of 60–150 mm Hg).

   b. Cerebral arterioles also change their caliber in response to changes in **levels of blood gases** (**carbon dioxide** and **oxygen**), and **pH**. With hypercarbia, they dilate, and with hypocarbia they constrict. Clinically, decreased arterial oxygen levels (hypoxemia) triggers vasodilation of the cerebral arterioles.

2. **Neuronal activity, energy expenditure,** and **cerebral blood flow** are closely related.

   a. Approximately 85% of cerebral glucose is used by **astrocytes** rather than neurons.

   b. One function of astrocytes is to take up and metabolize neuronally released synaptic **glutamate.** In coordination with these activities, astrocytes take up glucose, perform aerobic glycolysis, and produce **lactate**.

   c. Astrocytic lactate is transferred to the neurons; and in the presence of oxygen it is converted to **pyruvate.** Pyruvate serves as a substrate for the tricarboxylic acid cycle and oxidative phosphorylation.

   d. Therefore, both **glucose** and **lactate** can serve as energy sources for the brain.

3. **Clinical considerations.** Positron emission tomography (PET) and functional MRI (fMRI) allow clinicians and scientists to evaluate brain function via changes in brain metabolism (see also Table 17-1).

a. PET imaging involves detection of positrons emitted from a radioactive tracer. Specifically, a positron-emitting isotope is attached to 2-deoxyglucose (2-DG), and the tracer is injected into a patient. 2-DG is taken up by metabolically active astrocytes and neurons, and positron emission from the active brain regions can be detected.

b. fMRI involves detecting the difference in the magnetic signature of oxyhemoglobin and deoxyhemoglobin in the cerebral vasculature. As mentioned, the highly active brain regions receive more blood and thus more oxyhemoglobin. The ratio of oxyhemoglobin to deoxyhemoglobin indicates which brain regions are most active.

B. The blood–brain barrier

1. Structure

    a. Three layers exist between the lumen of brain capillaries and the extracellular space of neurons (Fig. 11-1):

      i. **Endothelial cells,** which make up the capillary wall

      ii. A **basement membrane,** which surrounds the capillaries on which the endothelial cells lie

      iii. **Astrocyte foot processes,** which adhere to the outer surface of the capillary wall

    b. Between the endothelial cells of the capillary wall are **tight junctions.** Research suggests that these tight junctions between endothelial cells make up the blood–brain barrier.

2. Function

    a. Permeability of substances through the blood–brain barrier depends on two primary features.

      i. A substance's ability to pass through the blood–brain barrier is **inversely related** to its **size.**

      ii. Permeability is **directly related** to a compound's **lipid solubility.**

    b. Thus gases and water are easily able to pass into the CNS, whereas large organic molecules are almost completely excluded.

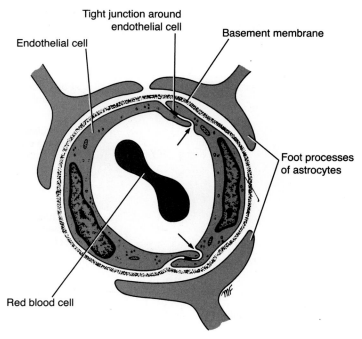

FIG 11-1. Cross section of a capillary of the central nervous system in the area of the blood–brain barrier. [Reprinted with permission from Snell RS. Clinical Neuroanatomy, 6th ed. Baltimore, Lippincott Williams & Wilkins, 2006.]

3. **Clinical considerations**
   a. The blood–brain barrier of a newborn is **not fully developed.** As such, drugs and toxins usually excluded by the adult can pass into the CNS of a newborn and cause negative effects (see Patient Snapshot 11-1).
   b. Although tumor cells produce growth factors that trigger the formation of new blood vessels (**angiogenesis**), when angiogenesis occurs in association with a brain tumor, the newly formed endothelial cells *do not create tight junctions* between themselves. Rather, the new vascular territories become regions of disruption of the blood–brain barrier and can be detected with certain imaging techniques (e.g., MRI studies with contrast); thus systemic chemotherapeutic agents can be used for the treatment of CNS cancers.

C. **Choroid plexus**
   1. The choroid plexus is a structure of specialized function that projects into the **lateral, third,** and **fourth ventricles** of the brain.
   2. It possesses infoldings of blood vessels of the **pia mater** that are covered by modified ciliated ependymal cells.
   3. **Function.** The choroid plexus produces and secretes cerebrospinal fluid (CSF) into the ventricular system. **Tight junctions** between the cells of the choroid plexus form, in part, the blood–CSF barrier.

D. **CSF biology**
   1. CSF is a colorless fluid, largely devoid of cells, that flows through the ventricles and into the subarachnoid space. Approximately **130 mL** of CSF are contained within the ventricles and subarachnoid space.
   2. **Functions** of the CSF
      a. **Support** and **cushion** the CNS, thus protecting it against concussive injury
      b. **Transport** hormones and hormone-releasing factors
      c. **Remove** metabolic waste products through absorption
   3. **Circulation** of the CSF (Fig. 11-2)
   4. The **composition** of the CSF is clinically relevant for the diagnosis of treatable medical emergencies (Table 11-1). Important characteristics are as follows:

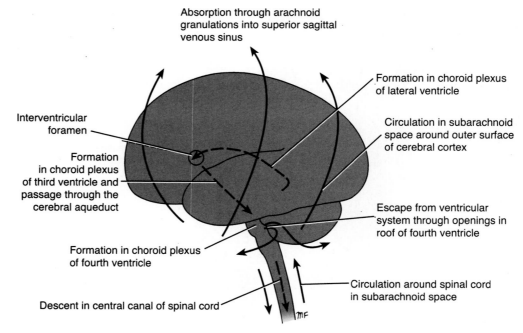

FIG 11-2. Circulation of the cerebrospinal fluid. *Dashed line,* the course taken by the fluid within the cavities of the central nervous system. *Solid line,* the course taken by the fluid around the brain and spinal cord. [Reprinted with permission from Snell RS. Clinical Neuroanatomy, 6th ed. Baltimore, Lippincott Williams & Wilkins, 2006.]

TABLE 11-1	STEREOTYPICAL CEREBROSPINAL FLUID PROFILES IN IMPORTANT INTRACRANIAL PATHOLOGY			
Cerebrospinal Fluid	Normal[a]	Bacterial Meningitis	Viral Meningitis	Subarachnoid Hemorrhage
Color	Clear and colorless	Cloudy	Clear or cloudy	Frankly bloody, xanthochromic
Cell count/mm^3	<5/μL and mostly lymphocytes	>1000/μL with a polymorphonuclear predominance	<250/μL with a lymphocytic predominance	Red blood cells present
Protein	<45 mg/dL	Elevated; >500 mg/dL	Slightly elevated; <150 mg/dL	Normal or slightly elevated
Glucose	~66% of blood glucose 50–75 mg/dL	Reduced; <45 mg/dL	Usually in normal range	Usually in normal range

[a]Infants: cell count = <20 cells/mm^3; protein = 20–170 mg/dL.

Adapted from Fix JD. High-Yield Neuroanatomy, 3rd ed. Baltimore, Lippincott Williams & Wilkins, 2005:24.

a. **Mononuclear cells** normally number <5/μL.

b. Red blood cells, or **erythrocytes,** in the CSF may indicate **intracranial bleeding** (e.g., a subarachnoid hemorrhage).

c. CSF **glucose** concentration is usually 50–75 mg/dL (or **approximately two thirds** of the blood glucose level). Glucose levels are often within the **normal** range in patients with **viral meningitis** and **greatly decreased** in patients with **bacterial meningitis** (see also Chapter 18).

d. CSF **protein** concentration is normally in the range of 15–45 mg/dL. Protein levels are delectably **increased** in patients with **bacterial meningitis** and normal to slightly increased in patients with viral meningitis.

e. Normal CSF **pressure** (also called *opening pressure* during a lumbar puncture) in the lateral decubitus position is measured by using a water manometer. It normally ranges from 6 to 15 cm H$_2$O. Space-occupying lesions (e.g., brain tumors) and meninigitis can elevate the measured CSF opening pressure.

II. Neurotransmitters and Neuromodulators (Table 11-2)

Patient Snapshot 11-2

A 32-year-old man with a diagnosis of paranoid-type schizophrenia has been treated with haloperidol for 2 years. Prior treatment with atypical antipsychotics, such as risperidone, did not adequately control his psychotic symptoms. For the past several weeks symptoms of paranoia and auditory hallucinations have reoccurred, so his psychiatrist increases the dose of haloperidol. Today, the patient's mother, parkinson calls the psychiatrist to report that since the haloperidol was increased, the patient seems slower than usual and has a fine resting tremor in his arms and hands. Also, he is drooling and complaining of generalized stiffness. The psychiatrist recognizes that the patient's parkinsonian symptoms are a side effect of haloperidol. Such symptoms are caused by a decrease in dopaminergic activity in the substantia nigra, resulting from dopamine receptor antagonism that can occur with high doses of high-potency antipsychotic medications, such as haloperidol. Although the patient's symptoms were partly controlled with benztropine, an anticholinergic agent, the psychiatrist decides to change the patient's medication to an atypical anticholinergic that has fewer parkinsonian side effects (see also Patient Snapshot 22-1).

TABLE 11-2	NEUROTRANSMITTERS AND NEUROMODULATORS
Compound	**Functions and Location**
Amino acids	
Glutamate	Excitatory neurotransmitter ubiquitous throughout CNS
GABA	Inhibitory neurotransmitter ubiquitous throughout CNS
Glycine	Inhibitory neurotransmitter in spinal cord and brainstem
Amines and related compounds	
Acetylcholine	Excitatory neurotransmitter released by motor neurons, all preganglionic, and some postganglionic autonomic neurons
	Transmitter/modulator used by neurons in nuclei of reticular formation and nuclei of basal forebrain that project to cerebral cortex
Dopamine	Transmitter for neurons of hypothalamus, substantia nigra, and ventral tegmental area
	Has modulatory actions in corpus striatum, limbic system, and prefrontal cortex
Norepinephrine	Neurotransmitter of majority of postganglionic sympathetic neurons, actions of which depend on receptor subtype targeted
	Release from neurons of locus ceruleus and parts of reticular formation have modulatory effects throughout brain and spinal cord
Histamine	Excitatory neurotransmitter of neurons in tuberomammillary nucleus of hypothalamus
	Neurons possess long, branched axons that project to most regions of brain and are believed to have a role in consciousness
Serotonin	Neuromodulator released by neurons in brainstem's midline, also with long, branched axons that project to many brain regions
	Has a role in various systems, including sleep, mood, and pain

CNS, central nervous system.

Adapted with permission from Kiernan JA. Barr's The Human Nervous System, 8th ed. Baltimore, Lippincott Williams & Wilkins, 2004:28.

A. **Biogenic amines**
1. **Overview**
   a. The biogenic amines, or monoamines, include **catecholamines, indolamines, ethylamines,** and **quaternary amines.**
   b. According to the **monoamine theory of mood disorder,** lowered monoamine activity results in depression.
   c. **Metabolites of the monoamines** are often measured in psychiatric research and diagnosis because they are more easily measured in body fluids than the actual monoamines (Table 11-3).
2. **Dopamine**
   a. Dopamine, a catecholamine, is involved in the pathophysiology of **schizophrenia** and other psychotic disorders, **Parkinson disease, mood disorders,** the conditioned fear response, and the rewarding nature of drugs of abuse.
   b. **Metabolism.** The amino acid tyrosine is converted to the precursor for dopamine by the enzyme tyrosine hydroxylase.
   c. **Receptor subtypes.** At least five dopamine receptor subtypes (D1–D5) have been identified; the major site of action is **D2** for traditional antipsychotic agents; **D1, D4,** and **D2** are the sites for the newer atypical antipsychotic agents (see also Chapter 22).

TABLE 11-3	METABOLITES OF MONOAMINES AND ASSOCIATED NEUROPATHOLOGY	
Neurotransmitter	**Concentration of Metabolite in Plasma, Cerebrospinal Fluid, or Urine**	**Associated Psychopathology**
Dopamine	↑Homovanillic acid	Schizophrenia and other conditions involving psychosis
	↓Homovanillic acid	Parkinson disease
		Treatment with antipsychotic agents
Norepinephrine	↑Vanillylmandelic acid	Adrenal medulla tumor (pheochromocytoma)
	↓3-Methoxy-4-hydroxyphenylglycol	Severe depression and attempted suicide
Serotonin	↓5-Hydroxyindolacetic acid	Severe depression and attempted suicide
		Aggressiveness and violence
		Impulsiveness and fire setting
		Tourette syndrome
		Alcohol abuse
		Bulimia

Reprinted with permission from Fadem B. BRS Behavioral Science, 4th ed. Baltimore, Lippincott Williams & Wilkins, 2005:32.

    d. Dopaminergic tracts
       i. The **nigrostriatal tract** is involved in the regulation of muscle tone and movement.
         (a) This tract is affected in **Parkinson disease.**
         (b) Treatment with antipsychotic drugs, which block postsynaptic dopamine receptors receiving input from the nigrostriatal tract, can result in Parkinson-like (parkinsonian) symptoms (see Patient Snapshot 11-2).
      ii. Dopamine acts on the **tuberoinfundibular** tract to **inhibit** the secretion of prolactin from the anterior pituitary.
         (a) Blockade of dopamine receptors by antipsychotic drugs prevents the inhibition of prolactin release and results in elevated prolactin levels.
         (b) This elevation, in turn, results in symptoms such as breast enlargement, galactorrhea, and sexual dysfunction.
      iii. The **mesolimbic–mesocortical tract** is associated with psychotic disorders.
         (a) This tract may have a role in the **expression of emotions** because it projects into the limbic system and prefrontal cortex.
         (b) In schizophrenia, hyperactivity of the mesolimbic tract is associated with the **positive symptoms** and hypoactivity of the mesocortical tract is associated with the **negative symptoms** (see Chapter 19).
3. Norepinephrine, a catecholamine, has a role in **mood, anxiety, arousal, learning,** and **memory.**
    a. Metabolism
       i. Like dopaminergic neurons, noradrenergic neurons synthesize dopamine.
      ii. **Dopamine-hydroxylase,** present in noradrenergic neurons, converts dopamine to norepinephrine.
    b. Localization. Most noradrenergic neurons (~10,000 per hemisphere in the brain) are located in the **locus ceruleus.**
4. Serotonin, an indolamine, plays a role in **mood, sleep, sexuality,** and **impulse control;** elevation of serotonin is associated with improved mood and sleep but

decreased sexual function (particularly delayed orgasm). Very high levels are associated with psychotic symptoms. Decreased serotonin is associated with poor impulse control, depression, and poor sleep.

    a. Metabolism. The amino acid **tryptophan** is converted to serotonin (also known as 5-hydroxytryptamine [5-HT]) by the enzyme **tryptophan hydroxylase** and by an amino acid decarboxylase.

    b. Localization. Most serotonergic cell bodies in the brain are found in the raphe nuclei.

5. Histamine

    a. Histamine is an ethylamine.

    b. Histamine-receptor blockade with drugs, such as antipsychotics and tricyclic antidepressants, is associated with common side effects, such as **sedation** and **increased appetite** leading to weight gain.

6. Acetylcholine (ACh), a quaternary amine, is the transmitter used by motor neurons at the neuromuscular junction.

    a. Degeneration of cholinergic neurons is associated with dementia of the **Alzheimer type, Down syndrome,** and **movement** and **sleep** disorders (e.g., decreased rapid eye movement [REM] sleep).

    b. Metabolism. Cholinergic neurons synthesize ACh from acetyl coenzyme A and choline (which must be transported to neurons from the body's circulation through the blood–brain barrier) using choline acetyltransferase. **Acetylcholinesterase** (**AChE**) breaks ACh down into choline and acetate. The choline is recycled via reuptake by presynaptic neurons.

    c. The **nucleus basalis** (of Meynert) is a brain area involved in production of ACh.

    d. Blocking the action of AChE with drugs such as donepezil (Aricept), rivastigmine (Exelon), and galantamine (Reminyl) may **delay the progression of Alzheimer disease** but cannot reverse function already lost (see Chapter 4).

    e. Blockade of **muscarinic ACh** receptors with drugs such as antipsychotics and tricyclic antidepressants results in the classic anticholinergic adverse effects seen with use of these drugs, including **dry mouth, blurred vision, urinary hesitancy,** and **constipation.**

7. Amino acid neurotransmitters are involved in most synapses in the brain and include glutamate, **γ-aminobutyric acid** (GABA), and **glycine.**

    a. Glutamate is the **primary excitatory neurotransmitter** of the CNS and may be associated with **epilepsy, schizophrenia, neurodegenerative illnesses** such as Alzheimer disease, and mechanisms of cell death.

        i. Metabolism. Glutamate is a nonessential amino acid and by definition can be synthesized by cells that require it. Its synthetic pathways involve production from glycolytic and citric acid cycle intermediates (e.g., from α-ketoglutarate).

        ii. Several classes of glutamate receptors have been identified on the basis of their selective activation on exposure to certain drugs and their second messenger systems: **N-methyl-D-aspartate** (NMDA) receptors, **kainate receptors,** and **metabotropic** glutamate receptors.

        iii. Co-activation of kainate and NMDA receptors has a role in **long-term potentiation,** which is believed to be involved in **learning and memory.**

    b. GABA

        i. GABA is the **principal inhibitory neurotransmitter** in the CNS.

        ii. Metabolism. GABA is formed via the decarboxylation of glutamate by **glutamate decarboxylase.** GABA is removed from the synapse by reuptake and is eliminated by the enzyme GABA transaminase.

        iii. GABA is closely involved in the action of the antianxiety agents **benzodiazepines** (e.g., diazepam [Valium]) and **barbiturates** (e.g., secobarbital [Seconal]).

    c. Glycine is an inhibitory neurotransmitter that works on its own and as a regulator of glutamate activity.

8. **Neuropeptides**
   a. **Endogenous opioids**
      i. **Enkephalins** and **endorphins** are opioids produced by the brain itself that function to decrease pain and anxiety. They also have a role in addiction and mood.
      ii. **Placebo effects** may be mediated by the endogenous opioid system. Prior treatment with an opiate receptor antagonist such as **naloxone** may block placebo effects.
   b. Other neuropeptides have been implicated in the following conditions:
      i. **Schizophrenia:** cholecystokinin (CCK) and neurotensin
      ii. **Mood disorders:** somatostatin, substance P, vasopressin, oxytocin, and vasoactive intestinal peptide (VIP) .
      iii. **Huntington disease:** somatostatin and substance P
      iv. **Alzheimer disease:** somatostatin and VIP
      v. **Anxiety disorders:** substance P and CCK
      vi. **Physical** and **mental pain, aggression:** substance P

III. Biochemistry of Behavior

A. Synapses and neurotransmitters
1. Information in the nervous system is transferred across a **synaptic cleft** (i.e., the space between the axon terminal of the presynaptic neuron and the dendrite of the postsynaptic neuron).
2. When the presynaptic neuron experiences an action potential that reaches its axon terminals, the **neurotransmitter** is released from the terminals, diffuses across the synaptic cleft, and binds to receptors on the postsynaptic neuron.
3. Neurotransmitters are **excitatory** if they increase the chances that a neuron will fire and **inhibitory** if they decrease these chances.

B. Presynaptic and postsynaptic receptors are proteins present in the membrane of the neuron that can recognize specific neurotransmitters.
1. The upregulation or downregulation in the number of receptors or in the affinity of receptors for specific neurotransmitters (**neuronal plasticity**) can control the responsiveness of neurons.
2. **Second messengers.** When bound by neurotransmitters, postsynaptic receptors may alter the physiology of neurons via second-messenger signaling cascades, which include **cyclic adenosine monophosphate** (cAMP), **lipids** (e.g., diacylglycerol), **Ca^{2+}**, and **nitric oxide.**

C. Regulation of neurotransmitter activity
1. The **concentration** of neurotransmitters in certain synaptic networks has been closely related to **mood** and **behavior.** A number of mechanisms affect this concentration.
2. After release by the presynaptic neuron, neurotransmitters are **removed** from the synaptic cleft by mechanisms, including
   a. **Reuptake** by presynaptic neurons or astroglia
   b. **Degradation** by enzymes such as monoamine oxidase (MAO) and acetylcholinesterase
3. Availability of specific neurotransmitters is associated with common psychiatric conditions (Table 11-4). Normalization of neurotransmitter availability by pharmacologic agents is associated with symptom improvement in some of these disorders:
   a. **Antidepressants**—heterocyclics, selective serotonin reuptake inhibitors (SSRIs), and MAO inhibitors (MAOIs)—ultimately **increase** the presence of

TABLE 11-4	PSYCHIATRIC CONDITIONS AND ASSOCIATED NEUROTRANSMITTER ACTIVITY
Psychiatric Condition	**Neurotransmitter Activity**
Depression	↓Norepinephrine
	↓Serotonin
	↓Dopamine
Mania	↑Dopamine
Schizophrenia	↑Dopamine
	↑Serotonin
	↑Glutamate
Anxiety	↓γ-Aminobutyric acid
	↓Serotonin
	↑Norepinephrine
Alzheimer disease	↓Acetylcholine
	↑Glutamate

Reprinted with permission from Fadem B. BRS Behavioral Science, 4th ed. Baltimore, Lippincott Williams & Wilkins, 2005:32.

serotonin and norepinephrine in the synaptic cleft (see Chapter 22) and relieve depression by at least two mechanisms.

   i. **Heterocyclics** block reuptake of serotonin and norepinephrine; **SSRIs,** such as fluoxetine (Prozac), selectively block reuptake of serotonin by the presynaptic neuron.
   ii. **MAOIs** prevent the degradation of serotonin and norepinephrine by MAO.

  b. Benzodiazepines and barbiturates **increase** the affinity of GABA for its binding site, allowing more chloride to enter the neuron. The chloride-laden neurons are thus **hyperpolarized** and action potentials are inhibited. This is believed to be the basis for their efficacy at decreasing anxiety.

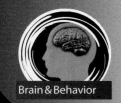

Section III
FACTORS INFLUENCING PATIENT BEHAVIOR

Chapter **12**

Biopsychosocial Factors Influencing Patient Behavior

The behavior of an individual is the result of biologic (e.g., genetic), psychological (e.g., psychodynamic factors and learning), and social/environmental (e.g., family and culture) influences. Because these influences interact at a molecular level, it is difficult to separate their relative importance on behavior. For example, psychological and social/environmental experiences can both disrupt and enhance synaptic connections, producing chemical and structural alterations in the brain. This suggests a way that negative social influences, such as abuse in childhood, or positive life experiences, such as psychotherapy, have the potential to alter brain biology and ultimately behavior.

I. Genetic Factors in Behavior

Patient Snapshot 12-1

A family physician confirms that a 22-year-old woman is in her first trimester of pregnancy. During the discussion after the examination, the woman tells the doctor that she recently learned that her father, whom she believed had died years ago, was in fact alive in a long-term-care psychiatric hospital. The patient explains that her father was hospitalized and diagnosed with schizophrenia at the age of 24 after he reported hearing voices telling him that he was the messiah. She asks her physician if she or her unborn child is at increased risk for developing the same illness. The physician tells the patient that, while the cause of schizophrenia is multifactorial, the risk is higher for relatives of patients than for the general population (see Table 19-3).

A. **Research tools**
1. **Family risk studies** compare how frequently a behavioral trait or disorder occurs in the relatives of an affected individual (**the proband**) with how frequently it occurs in the general population.
2. **Twin studies**
   a. **Adoption studies** using **monozygotic (MZ) twins** and **dizygotic (DZ) twins** reared in different homes are used to differentiate the effects of genetic factors from environmental factors in the occurrence of disorders.
   b. If there is a genetic component to the cause, a disorder may be expected to have a higher **concordance rate** in MZ twins than in DZ twins (if concordant, the disorder occurs in both twins).

B. **Temperament and intelligence**
1. **Temperamental traits,** such as reactivity to stimuli and activity level, have a strong genetic component (see Chapter 1). These traits interact with social/environmental experiences to form an individual's personality.
2. Children tend to have the same **intelligence** as their **biologic parents,** even if they are adopted (see Chapter 17).

C. **Psychiatric and neuropsychiatric disorders**
1. **Mental retardation** may be associated with specific genetic abnormalities (see Table 3-3)
2. **Schizophrenia** and **bipolar disorder** each occur in about 1% of the general population. People with a close genetic relationship to patients with schizophrenia or bipolar disorder are more likely than those with more distant relationships to develop the disorder (see Chapter 19).
3. **Personality disorders (PDs)** are diagnosed when individuals have significant difficulties in social or occupational functioning because of their personality characteristics (see Chapter 20). These disorders have a genetic relationship to other psychiatric disorders. For example, patients with schizotypal personality disorder are likely to have relatives with schizophrenia.
4. **Neuropsychiatric disorders** such as dementia of the Alzheimer type, Huntington disease, Tourette syndrome, Parkinson disease, and amyotrophic lateral sclerosis have a genetic component (see Chapter 4).
5. **Alcohol abuse** (see Chapter 14)
   a. The concordance rate for alcoholism is about **twice as high for MZ twins** as it is for DZ twins.
   b. Alcoholism is four times more prevalent in the **biologic children** (particularly males) of individuals with alcoholism than of those without alcoholism.

II. Psychodynamic Factors in Behavior

Patient Snapshot 12-2

A 31-year-old internist loses her left arm above the elbow as a result of an osteosarcoma (malignant bone tumor). After the amputation, the internist tells colleagues that the loss of her arm was unfortunate but ultimately beneficial to her medical practice because it helps her better understand the experience of her amputee patients. This physician is using the unconscious defense mechanism of rationalization, a seemingly reasonable explanation—the loss was ultimately beneficial for her practice—for her personally unacceptable feelings of grief at the loss of her arm. Although this has helped her in the short term to cope with the loss, excessive use of defense mechanisms such as rationalization can prevent individuals from dealing with their true feelings about negative life events and can ultimately hamper full recovery.

A. **Psychoanalytic theory** is based on Freud's concept that the behavior of an individual is determined by forces derived from **unconscious mental processes.**
1. Psychoanalysis and related therapies are **treatments** based on this concept (see Chapter 23).
2. Freud's early (topographic: unconscious, preconscious, and conscious mind) and later (structural: id, ego, and superego) **theories of the mind** were developed to explain his ideas (Table 12-1).

Theory	Component of the Mind	Characteristics and Functions
TABLE 12-1		**FREUD'S TOPOGRAPHIC AND STRUCTURAL THEORIES OF THE MIND**
Topographic	Unconscious	Contains repressed thoughts and feelings
		Uses primary process thinking (seen also in young children and psychotic adults)
		Has no logic or concept of time
		Involves primitive drives, wish fulfillment, and pleasure
	Preconscious	Contains memories that are not immediately available but can be retrieved readily
	Conscious	Contains thoughts that an individual is currently aware of
		Operates in conjunction with preconscious but cannot access unconscious directly
Structural	Id	Present at birth and controlled by primary process thinking
		Contains instinctual sexual and aggressive drives
		Acts in concert with pleasure principle
		Is not influenced by external reality
		Operates almost completely on an unconscious level
	Ego	Begins developing immediately after birth
		Controls expression of instinctual drives, mainly by use of defense mechanisms, to adapt to requirements of external world
		Maintains a relationship to external world
		Evaluates what is valid (reality testing) and then adapts to that reality
		Maintains satisfying interpersonal or object relationships
		Operates on unconscious, preconscious, and conscious levels
	Superego	Is developed by about age 6 years
		Is associated with conscience, empathy, and morality
		Operates on unconscious, preconscious, and conscious levels

Adapted with permission from Fadem B, Simring S. High-Yield Psychiatry, 2nd ed. Baltimore, Lippincott Williams & Wilkins, 2003.

B. Neuroanatomic substrates of Freud's structural theory
   1. The **id** is associated with the motivation to **pursue pleasure** (e.g., substance abuse). Such motivation is primarily a function of the **cingulate gyrus-nucleus accumbens** circuit (see Chapter 6).
   2. The **ego** is associated with facilitation of problem solving and decision making. Such executive function is found mainly in the **dorsolateral prefrontal** circuit (see Chapter 6).
   3. The **superego** is associated with setting limits on risk taking and anticipating potential punishment or embarrassment. Such functions are contained largely in the **orbitofrontal-amygdala** circuit (see Chapter 6).

C. Defense mechanisms
   1. **Definition.** Defense mechanisms are **unconscious mental techniques** used by the ego to keep conflicts out of the conscious mind, thus decreasing anxiety and maintaining a person's sense of safety, equilibrium, and self-esteem (Table 12-2).
   2. Altruism, humor, sublimation, and suppression are considered **mature defense mechanisms** because they have a positive social outcome—for example, using sublimation, a man whose wife was killed by a drunk driver channels his anger into counseling people who have been cited for driving under the influence of alcohol.

TABLE 12-2		DEFENSE MECHANISMS
Defense Mechanisms	**Definition**	**Patient Snapshot**
Acting out	Avoiding unacceptable emotions by behaving in an attention-getting, often negative manner	A depressed 16-year-old boy with no history of conduct problems steals a car after his parents divorce
Altruism	Assisting others to avoid negative personal feelings	A man with a poor self-image gives one fifth of his annual salary to charity
Denial	Not accepting aspects of reality that one finds unbearable	An active 50-year-old man insists that a laboratory report that shows that he has had a myocardial infarction is in error
Displacement	Moving emotions from an unacceptable situation to one that is tolerable	A surgical resident with unacknowledged anger toward her husband is abrasive to male medical students on her service
Dissociation	Mentally separating part of one's personality or mentally distancing oneself from others	A soldier has no memory of a battle in which his best friend was killed
Humor	Expressing feelings without causing discomfort	A man who is uncomfortable about his pattern baldness makes jokes about hair restoration techniques
Identification (with the aggressor)	Patterning one's behavior after that of someone more powerful (may be positive or negative)	A woman who was physically abused in childhood by her mother abuses her own children
Intellectualization	Using the mind's higher functions to avoid experiencing emotion	A physician explains technical details of treatment options for his own terminal illness
Isolation of affect	Failing to experience feelings associated with a stressful life event, although one logically understands significance of event	Although he was very close to her, a man whose mother recently died relates the circumstances of her death dispassionately
Projection	Attributing one's own unacceptable feelings to others; associated with paranoid symptoms and ordinary prejudice	A woman who has unacknowledged and unacceptable feelings for men other than her husband believes (without evidence) that her husband is cheating on her
Rationalization	Distorting one's perception of an event so that its negative outcome seems reasonable	A job candidate who is not hired says, "I'm glad. That was a dead-end job anyway."
Reaction formation	Adopting opposite attitudes to avoid unacceptable emotions (unconscious hypocrisy)	A woman bakes cookies for her brother who sexually abused her
Regression	Reverting to behavior patterns seen in someone of a younger age	A woman hospitalized for cancer surgery insists that her husband not leave her room
Splitting	Putting people (or even same person at different times) into categories of either perfect or awful because of intolerance of ambiguity	A hospitalized patient tells you that all nurses on night shift are cold and insensitive but that all those on day shift are warm and friendly
Sublimation	Expressing an unacceptable feeling in a socially useful way	A medical student with strong destructive impulses decides to do a residency in surgery
Suppression	Deliberately pushing unacceptable emotions out of conscious awareness	An emergency room resident chooses to put his feelings of horror and pity aside to deal with medical needs of victims of a fire
Undoing	Believing that one can magically reverse events caused by wrong behavior in past by adopting right behavior	A woman diagnosed with lung cancer owing to smoking buys books on nutrition, stops smoking, and starts working out

Adapted with permission from Fadem B, Simring S. High-Yield Psychiatry, 2nd ed. Baltimore, Lippincott Williams & Wilkins, 2003.

D. Transference reactions
  1. Definitions
    a. Transference and countertransference **are unconscious mental attitudes based on important past personal relationships** (e.g., with parents).
    b. These phenomena **increase emotionality** and may thus alter judgment and behavior in patients' relationships with their doctors (transference) and doctors' relationships with their patients (countertransference).

   2. Transference
   a. In **positive transference,** the patient has confidence in the doctor. If intense, the patient may overidealize the doctor or develop sexual feelings toward the doctor.
   b. In **negative transference,** the patient may become resentful or angry toward the doctor if the patient's desires and expectations are not realized. This may lead to nonadherence with medical advice (see Chapter 16).
   3. Countertransference. Feelings about a patient who reminds the doctor of a close friend or relative can **interfere with the doctor's medical judgment.**

III. Learning and Behavior

Learning is a relatively **permanent change** in behavior that occurs as a result of exposure to social and environmental life experiences. Neural areas involved in learning include temporal structures, such as the **hippocampus** and **amygdala,** and the **cerebellum.**

A. Methods of learning
   1. Methods of learning include simple forms (**habituation** and **sensitization**) and more complex types (**classical conditioning** and **operant conditioning**).
   2. Learning methods are the basis of **behavioral treatment techniques,** such as systematic desensitization, aversive conditioning, flooding, biofeedback, token economy, and cognitive therapy (see Chapter 23).

B. Habituation and sensitization
   1. In **habituation,** repeated stimulation results in a decreased response (e.g., a child who receives weekly allergy injections cries less and less with each injection). The **neural mechanism** of habituation involves **depression** of synaptic neurotransmission with repeated exposure to a stimulus.
   2. In **sensitization,** repeated stimulation results in an increased response (e.g., a child who is afraid of insects feels more anxiety each time he encounters an insect). The **neural mechanism** of sensitization involves **enhancement** of synaptic transmission with repeated exposure to a stimulus.

C. Classical conditioning. In classical conditioning, a **natural or reflexive response** (behavior) is elicited by a **learned stimulus** (a cue from an internal or external event)—that is, an individual must learn to associate one stimulus with another (e.g. **associative learning**).
   1. Neural associations
   a. The **hippocampus** is particularly important in **associative learning.**
   b. The **cerebellum** also participates in classical conditioning, specifically in associations involving **motor skills.**
   2. Elements of classical conditioning
   a. An **unconditioned stimulus** (UCS) is something that automatically, without having to be learned, produces a response (e.g., the odor of food).
   b. An **unconditioned response** (UCR) is a natural, reflexive behavior that does not have to be learned (e.g., salivation in response to the odor of food).
   c. A **conditioned stimulus** (CS) is a neutral stimulus that produces a response after learning (e.g., the sound of the lunch bell).
   d. A **conditioned response** (CR) is a behavior that is learned by an association that is made between a CS and an UCS (e.g., salivation in response to the lunch bell).
   3. Response acquisition, extinction, and **stimulus generalization**
   a. In **acquisition,** the CS quickly follows and thus becomes paired with the UCS (the bell is rung just after the food is presented) and the CR (salivation in response to the lunch bell) is learned.

      b. In **extinction,** the CR decreases if the CS (the sound of the lunch bell) is not paired with the UCS (the odor of food) for a period of time.

      c. In **stimulus generalization,** a new stimulus (a church bell) that resembles the CS (the lunch bell) causes the CR (salivation).

   4. **Aversive conditioning.** An unwanted behavior (setting fires) is paired with an aversive stimulus (a painful electric shock). An association is created between the unwanted behavior (fire setting) and the aversive stimulus (pain), and the fire setting ceases.

   5. **Learned helplessness**

      a. An animal receives a series of painful electric shocks from which it is **unable to escape.**

      b. By classical conditioning, the animal learns that there is an association between an aversive stimulus (painful electric shock) and the inability to escape.

      c. Subsequently, the animal makes no attempt to escape when shocked or when faced with any new aversive stimulus; instead the animal becomes **hopeless** and **apathetic.**

      d. Learned helplessness in animals may be a model system for **depression** (often characterized by hopelessness and apathy) in humans. **Antidepressant medications** delay the onset of learned helplessness in animals.

D. **Operant conditioning** (also termed instrumental conditioning and trial-and-error learning). Like classical conditioning, operant conditioning is a form of associative learning and is under similar neurologic control.

   1. **Principles**

      a. Behavior is determined by its consequences for the individual. The consequence (reinforcement or punishment) occurs immediately after the behavior.

      b. In operant conditioning, a behavior that is **not part of the individual's natural repertoire** can be learned through reinforcement or punishment.

Patient Snapshot 12-3

A worried mother reports that her 4-year-old daughter often hits her 2-year-old brother. The mother relates that sometimes she scolds the older child but sometimes she just removes the younger child and says nothing to the older child. No matter what she does, the child's negative behavior toward the 2-year-old persists and is getting worse. The doctor explains that the older child's hitting behavior has been learned by reinforcement—that is, when she hits her brother she gets attention from her mother. Also, because the child never knows when the reward (attention) will come (variable ratio reinforcement), the hitting behavior persists for a long time (is resistant to extinction) even when the mother ignores it. The doctor then advises the mother to continue protecting the younger child but avoid giving the older child attention (scolding) for her unacceptable behavior toward the 2-year-old. If the mother does not reinforce the behavior, it will disappear in time (extinction). In addition, the mother should reinforce the 4-year-old's good behavior and hence increase it by giving her attention and praise (positive reinforcement) when she is kind toward her brother.

   2. **Features**

      a. The likelihood that a **behavior** will occur is **increased by positive** and **negative reinforcement** and **decreased by punishment** and **extinction** (Table 12-3).

      b. The pattern, or **schedule, of reinforcement** affects how quickly a behavior is learned and how quickly a behavior becomes extinct when it is not rewarded (Table 12-4).

      c. **Resistance to extinction** is the force that prevents the behavior from disappearing when a reward is withheld.

   3. **Shaping and modeling**

      a. Shaping involves **rewarding close approximations** of the wanted behavior until the correct behavior is achieved (e.g., a child learning to write is praised when he or she makes a letter, even when it is not formed perfectly).

TABLE 12-3		FEATURES OF OPERANT CONDITIONING[a]	
Feature	**Effect on Behavior**	**Example**	**Comments**
Positive reinforcement	Behavior is increased by reward	Child increases her kind behavior toward her younger brother to get praise from her mother	Reward or reinforcement (praise) increases desired behavior (kindness toward brother)
			A reward can be praise or attention as well as a tangible reward like candy
Negative reinforcement	Behavior is increased by avoidance or escape	Child increases her kind behavior toward her younger brother to avoid being scolded	Active avoidance of an aversive stimulus (being scolded) increases desired behavior (kindness toward brother)
Punishment	Behavior is decreased by suppression	Child decreases her hitting behavior after her mother scolds her	Delivery of an aversive stimulus (scolding) decreases unwanted behavior (hitting brother) rapidly but not permanently
Extinction	Behavior is eliminated by nonreinforcement	Child stops her hitting behavior when behavior is ignored by her mother	Extinction is more effective than punishment for long-term reduction in unwanted behavior
			There may be an initial increase in hitting behavior before it disappears

[a]Refer to Patient Snapshot 12-3

Adapted with permission from Fadem B, Simring S. High-Yield Psychiatry, 2nd ed. Baltimore, Lippincott Williams & Wilkins, 2003.

TABLE 12-4		SCHEDULES OF REINFORCEMENT	
Schedule	**Reinforcement**	**Example**	**Effect on Behavior**
Continuous	Presented after every response	A teenager receives a candy bar each time she puts $1 into a vending machine. One time she puts $1 in and nothing comes out. She never buys candy from the machine again.	Behavior (putting in $1 to receive candy) is rapidly learned but disappears rapidly (has little resistance to extinction) when not reinforced (no candy comes out)
Fixed ratio	Presented after a designated number of responses	A man is paid $10 for every five hats he makes. He makes as many hats as he can during his shift.	Fast response rate (many hats are made quickly)
Fixed interval	Presented after a designated amount of time	A student has an anatomy quiz every Friday. He studies for 10 min on Wednesday nights, and for 2 hr on Thursday nights.	Response rate (studying) increases toward end of each interval (week) When graphed, response rate forms a scalloped curve
Variable ratio	Presented after a random and unpredictable number of responses	After a slot machine pays off $5 for a single quarter, a woman plays $50 in quarters even though she receives no further payoff.	Behavior (playing machine) continues (highly resistant to extinction) even though it is reinforced (winning money) only after a large but variable number of responses
Variable interval	Presented after a random and unpredictable amount of time	After 5 min of fishing in a lake, a man catches a large fish. He then spends 4 hr waiting for another bite	Behavior (fishing) continues (highly resistant after to extinction) even though it is reinforced (a fish is caught) only varying time intervals

Adapted with permission from Fadem B. BRS Behavioral Science, 4th ed. Baltimore, Lippincott Williams & Wilkins, 2004:58.

b. **Modeling** is a type of observational learning (e.g., an individual behaves in a manner similar to that of someone he or she admires).

IV. Family and Cultural Factors in Behavior

Patient Snapshot 12-4

A 40-year-old Hispanic American woman who has been diagnosed with hypertension tells her physician that a healer, used by many members of her community, told her that because hypertension is a hot illness and corn is a cold food, eating corn can lower her blood pressure. Provided that eating corn poses no danger to this patient, the physician should incorporate her belief about corn and the food itself into the medical treatment plan.

A. **Marriage and children**

1. A good marriage is an important predictor of mental and physical health. Married people are **mentally** and **physically healthier, live longer,** and have **higher self-esteem** than nonmarried people.
2. About **half** of all marriages in the United States end in **divorce.**
   a. **Factors associated with divorce** include young age, short courtship, lack of family support, premarital pregnancy, divorce in the family, differences in religion or socioeconomic background, and serious illness or death of a child.
   b. **Children in single-parent families** are at **increased risk** for failure in school, depression, drug abuse, suicide, criminal activity, and divorce.

B. **Cultural influences on behavior.** There are approximately **300 million people** in the United States. The population is made up of many **minority subcultures** and a **large white middle class,** which is the major cultural influence.

1. Although ethnic groups are **not homogeneous** (their members have different backgrounds and, if immigrants, different reasons for emigrating), these groups often have **characteristic ways of dealing with illness.**
2. A patient's belief system has much to do with **adherence** and response to medical treatment (see Chapter 16).

C. **Culture shock**

1. Culture shock is a **strong emotional response** (which may involve **psychiatric symptoms**) related to geographic relocation and the need to adapt to unfamiliar social and cultural surroundings. Culture shock is reduced when groups of immigrants of a particular culture live in the same geographic area.
2. **Young immigrant men** appear to be at **higher risk for culture shock,** including symptoms such as paranoia and depression, than other sex and age groups.

D. **American subcultures.** Although people in ethnic, religious, and cultural groups share some characteristics, there is more variability than sameness among the individuals within such groups. Thus physicians must **avoid stereotyping** their patients by these parameters. With this caveat, selected characteristics of some of the larger cultural groups in the United States are given in Table 12-5

TABLE 12-5	SELECTED HEALTH-RELATED CHARACTERISTICS OF ETHNIC SUBCULTURES IN THE UNITED STATES
Subculture (appropriate number)	**Characteristics**
Hispanic/Latino American (37 million)	Value nuclear family and having many children
	Respect elderly, protect them from negative medical diagnoses, and make medical decisions for them
	May seek healthcare from folk healers in community
	Emphasis on herbal and botanical remedies
	Dramatic presentation of symptoms
	Less likely to get mammograms and more likely to have cervical cancer than white or African Americans
	Hot and cold dietary influences are deemed important (Patient Snapshot 12-3)
African American (36 million)	Average income approximately half that of white American families
	Decreased access to healthcare services
	Increased risk of illness (e.g., hypertension, stroke, obesity, asthma, tuberculosis, diabetes, prostate cancer, and AIDS) and early death
	Higher death rates from heart disease and most forms of cancer
	When compared with whites, lower suicide rate across age groups; equal suicide rate in teenagers
	Religion and strong extended kinship networks important in social and personal support
Asian American (10 million)	Respect elderly, protect them from negative medical diagnoses, and make medical decisions for them
	Care for one's elderly parents
	Emphasis on education
	May express emotional pain as physical illness
	Use of folk remedies (e.g., coining: pressing medicated oil into skin using edge of a coin)
	Some believe that one's spiritual core lies in thoracic area rather than brain; this makes concept of brain death and organ transplant less acceptable
Native American (2.7 million)	Blurred distinction between physical and mental illness
	Illness may be caused by engaging in forbidden behavior or witchcraft
	Low income
	High rates of alcoholism and suicide, particularly among teenagers
Middle Eastern/North African American (1.2 million)	Most follow Muslim religion
	Female modesty and purity are valued
	Females often prefer a female physician
	Some are Christian (e.g., Coptic Christian); fewer are Jewish
White American (227 million)	When of English-speaking descent (Irish, English, Welsh, Scottish), are likely to be stoic and uncomplaining
	When of Mediterranean descent (Italian, Greek, Jewish), are likely to visit physicians and report their medical problems

Adapted with permission from Fadem B. BRS Behavioral Science, 4th ed. Baltimore, Lippincott Williams & Wilkins, 2004.

Chapter **13**

Aggression and Physical Abuse

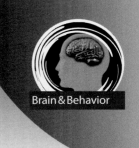
Brain & Behavior

I. Biologic and Social Determinants of Aggressive Behavior

Patient Snapshot 13-1

A 25-year-old man is brought to the hospital with facial injuries after attacking another, much larger man while waiting in the checkout line at the supermarket. The store clerk tells the police that the victim had stepped in front of the attacker in the line, and a fight ensued. In the emergency room, the attacker expresses remorse and states that he has always had a terrible temper and has been involved in similar incidents in the past. Aside from the facial injuries, physical and neurologic examinations are unremarkable. The behavior and history suggest that this man has an impulse control disorder, specifically, intermittent explosive disorder (see Chapter 21). Because this disorder has been linked to neurotransmitter abnormalities such as low serotonin levels, it can be treated with selective serotonin reuptake inhibitors such as fluoxetine (Prozac). Mood stabilizers, such as lithium, and psychotherapy may also benefit this patient.

A. Biologic determinants of aggression
  1. **Neurotransmitters**
     a. **Serotonin** (5-HT) and γ-aminobutyric acid (**GABA**) **inhibit** aggression.
     b. **Dopamine, glutamate,** and **norepinephrine facilitate** aggression.
     c. Low levels of the serotonin metabolite **5-hydroxyindoleacetic acid** (**5-HIAA**) are associated with impulsive aggression.
     d. **5-HT receptors** are found in neuroanatomic areas involved in aggression, such as the amygdala and periaquaductal gray (PAG).
     e. Drugs used to treat inappropriate aggressiveness include **antidepressants** (increase 5-HT), **benzodiazepines** (increase GABA), **antipsychotics** (decrease dopamine), and **mood stabilizers** such as valproate (increase GABA, decrease glutamate).
  2. **Neuroanatomy**
     a. In animal studies, stimulation of the **amygdala, hypothalamus, PAG,** and **ventral tegmental area** is associated with **increased aggression; lesions** of these areas are associated with **decreased aggression.**
     b. Violent people often have a history of **head injury** or show abnormal electroencephalogram (EEG) readings.
  3. **Hormones**
     a. **Androgens** are closely associated with aggression; in most animal species and human societies, males are more aggressive than females; **homicide** involving strangers is **committed** almost exclusively by **men.**
     b. **Androgenic** or **anabolic steroids,** often taken by body builders to increase muscle mass, can result in **high levels of aggression** and even psychosis. Severe depression frequently occurs with withdrawal from these hormones.
     c. Female hormones (**estrogen, progesterone**) and **antiandrogens** may be useful in treating male sex offenders.

148

4. **Substances of abuse**
   a. Low doses of **alcohol** and **barbiturates** inhibit aggression, whereas high doses facilitate it.
   b. While intoxicated, heroin users show little aggression; increased aggression is associated with the use of **cocaine, amphetamines,** and **phencyclidine** (**PCP**).

B. **Social determinants of aggression**
   1. Factors associated with increased aggression include poverty, frustration, physical pain, and exposure to aggression in the media (e.g., violence on television).
   2. At least half of homicides result from the use of **guns**.
   3. In **African American** males **15–24 years of age**, homicide is the **leading cause of death;** it is the second leading cause of death (after accidents) in white males in this age group.
   4. Children at risk for showing aggressive behavior in adulthood frequently have moved and changed schools repeatedly, have been **physically** and/or **sexually abused, mistreat animals,** and cannot defer gratification. Their parents frequently display criminal behavior and abuse drugs and alcohol.

II. Sexual Aggression: Rape and Related Crimes

A. **Rape**
   1. **Rape** is a crime of violence, not of passion, and is known legally as **sexual assault,** or aggravated sexual assault.
   2. Definitions of rape and **sodomy**, characteristics of the **rapist, victim,** and crime, and factors associated with **recovery** are provided in Table 13-1.
   3. When treating a rape victim, the physician should **encourage the patient to notify the police.** The doctor is not required to do this if the victim is a competent adult.

TABLE 13-1	RAPE
Definitions	Sexual contact without consent involving vaginal penetration by a penis, finger, or object; erection and ejaculation do not have to occur
	Sodomy is insertion of penis into oral or anal orifice; victim may be male or female
Characteristics of rapist	Usually <age 25
	Usually same race as victim
	Usually known to victim
	Alcohol use common
Characteristics of victim	Usually between 16 and 24 years of age
	Usually occurs inside victim's home
	Vaginal injuries may be absent, particularly in women who have children
Characteristics of crime	Most rapes are not reported; only 25% are reported to police
	Others tend to blame victim (e.g., for wearing provocative clothing)
Recovery	The emotional recovery period commonly lasts at least 1 year
	Posttraumatic stress disorder (see Chapter 20) may occur
	Group therapy with other rape victims is most effective

Adapted with permission from Fadem B. High-Yield Behavioral Science, 2nd ed. Baltimore, Lippincott Williams & Wilkins, 2001:89.

B. Legal considerations

1. Because **rapists may use condoms** to avoid contracting HIV or to avoid DNA identification and may have difficulty with erection or ejaculation, semen may not be present in the vagina of a rape victim.

2. A victim is **not required to prove that she resisted the rapist** for him to be convicted. A rapist can be convicted even though the victim asks him to use a condom or other form of sexual protection.

3. Certain information about the victim (e.g., previous sexual activity) is generally not admissible as evidence in rape trials.

4. **Husbands can be prosecuted** for raping their wives. It is illegal to force anyone to engage in sexual activity. Even if a woman consents to go on a date with a man and consents to sexual activity not involving intercourse, a man can be prosecuted for rape (**date rape**).

5. Consensual sex may be considered rape if the victim is younger than 16 or 18 years old (depending on state law) or is physically or mentally handicapped (**statutory rape**).

III. Abuse of Children and the Elderly

Patient Snapshot 13-2

A 10-year-old girl is brought to the pediatrician because of frequent and painful urination. Urinalysis reveals a urinary tract infection. This is the child's second visit for the same complaint in 6 months. The physician observes that, while formerly friendly toward him, the child now seems sad and does not make eye contact. The mother states that since she remarried 1 year earlier, the child's behavior seems different and her school performance has been poor. In children, signs of sexual abuse include recurrent urinary tract infections and personality changes—for example, sadness and withdrawal. The physician suspects that the child has been sexually abused by her mother's new husband and, keeping the child and her mother in his office, immediately contacts the state child protective agency.

A. Child and elder abuse

1. Types of child and elder abuse include **physical abuse, emotional** or **physical neglect,** and **sexual abuse.** The elderly may also be exploited for monetary gain.

2. **Abuse-related injuries** must be differentiated from injuries obtained during normal activity. Examples of **accidental** (non-abuse) **injuries** in children include bruises and scrapes on bony prominences (e.g., chin, forehead, knees, elbows) and in the elderly, bruising on extensor surfaces of the limbs.

3. Characteristics of the **physical abuser** and **abused** and signs of abuse in children and the elderly are provided in Table 13-2 and Figure 13-1.

B. Neurologic sequelae of child abuse

1. Severe and **fatal injuries** as a result of abuse are often of the **brain** and occur more often in **infants** than in older children.

2. The **shaken baby** syndrome occurs when an infant is shaken vigorously to stop him or her from crying, causing **deceleration** and **rotational force** of the brain in the skull and leading to brain and eye damage.

3. There may be no external evidence of injury, but CT and MRI scans show **subdural hematoma, low-density brain swelling,** and **multifocal hemorrhage.**

4. Of shaken children presenting with **reduced consciousness,** one third die, one third have severe disability, and one third have moderate to good recovery.

TABLE 13-2	CHILD AND ELDER PHYSICAL ABUSE	
Category	**Child Abuse**	**Elder Abuse**
Characteristics		
Abuser	Substance abuse	Substance abuse
	Poverty and social isolation	Poverty and social isolation
	Closest family member (e.g., the mother) is most likely to abuse	Closest family member (e.g., spouse, daughter, son, or other relative with whom person lives and often supports financially is most likely to abuse)
	Personal history of victimization by caretaker or spouse	
	Delays seeking treatment for victim	Delays seeking treatment for victim
Abused	Prematurity, low birth weight	Some degree of worsening cognitive impairment (e.g., Alzheimer disease)
	Hyperactivity or mild physical handicap; child is perceived as slow or different	Incontinence
	Colicky or fussy infant	Physical dependence on others
	Most are <5 years of age (33%); 25% of cases are 5–9 years of age	Does not report abuse; instead says that he or she fell, causing injury
Signs of abuse		
Neglect	Poor personal care (e.g., diaper rash, dirty hair)	Poor personal care (e.g., urine odor in incontinent person), lack of medication or health aids (e.g., eyeglasses, dentures)
	Lack of needed nutrition	Lack of needed nutrition
Bruises	Particularly in areas not likely to be injured during normal play, such as buttocks or lower back	Often on arms from being grabbed
	Belt or buckle marks, hand prints	
Fractures and burns	Fractures at different stages of healing	Fractures at different stages of healing
	Spiral fractures caused by twisting limbs	Spiral fractures caused by twisting limbs
	Cigarette burns	Cigarette and other burns
	Burns on feet or buttocks from immersion in hot water	
Other signs	Internal abdominal injuries (e.g., ruptured spleen)	Internal abdominal injuries
	Wrist rope burns caused by tying to a bed or chair	Wrist rope burns caused by tying to a bed or chair
	Shaken baby syndrome (retinal detachment and/or hemorrhage and subdural hematoma caused by shaking infant to stop him or her from crying)	Evidence of depleted personal finances (elder's money was spent by abuser and other family members)
	Injuries of mouth caused by forced feeding	Injuries of mouth caused by forced feeding

Adapted with permission from Fadem B. BRS Behavioral Science, 4th ed. Baltimore: Lippincott Williams & Wilkins, 2005:194.

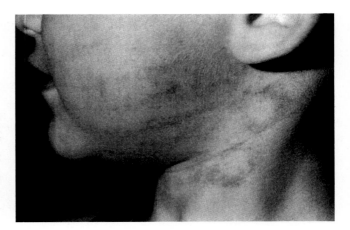

Figure 13-1. A young child with a hand print on the face and neck showing the outline of the fingers of the abuser. [Reprinted with permission from Reece RM, Ludwig S, eds. Child Abuse: Medical Diagnosis and Management, 2nd ed. Baltimore, Lippincott Williams & Wilkins, 2001:28.]

C. **Psychological sequelae of child abuse**
    1. Children who are being abused often seem **sad,** show **personality changes** (e.g., are no longer outgoing and friendly), and **do poorly in school.**
    2. Adults who were abused during childhood are more likely to
        a. Have **dissociative disorders** (e.g., dissociative identity disorder) and **borderline personality disorder** (see Chapters 20 and 21).
        b. Have **post-traumatic stress disorder** and other anxiety disorders (see Chapter 20)
        c. Have **substance abuse** disorders and **depression** (see Chapters 14 and 19)
        d. **Abuse** their own children

D. **Sexual abuse of children**
    1. **Signs**
        a. **Sexually transmitted diseases** (STDs) in children are signs of sexual abuse; children do not contract STDs through casual contact with an infected person or with their bedclothes, towels, or toilet seats.
        b. **Genital** or **anal trauma** is also a sign of sexual abuse.
        c. Young children have only a vague knowledge about sexual activities; specific **knowledge about sexual acts** (e.g., fellatio) in a young child often indicates that the child has been sexually abused.
        d. Recurrent **urinary tract infections** and excessive **initiation of sexual activity** with friends also are signs of sexual abuse.
    2. **Occurrence**
        a. Most sexually abused children are **8–13 years of age,** and 25% are <8 years old.
        b. Approximately 20% of women and 5–10% of men report sexual abuse at some time during their childhood and adolescence.
    3. **Characteristics of the sexual abuser**
        a. Most sexual abusers are **known to the child,** and almost all are **men.** About 50% of these men are relatives (e.g., uncle, father, mother's boyfriend), and 50% are family acquaintances (e.g., neighbor).
        b. **Alcohol** and **drugs** are commonly used by the abuser.
        c. The abuser typically has **marital problems** and **no appropriate alternate sexual partner;** occasionally, he is a pedophile (prefers children to appropriate sexual partners).

E. **Role of the physician in suspected child and elder abuse**
    1. According to the law in every state, **physicians must report** suspected **physical** or **sexual abuse of a child** or **elderly person** (particularly if the elderly person appears to be physically or mentally impaired) to the appropriate family social service agency (state child protective service or state adult protective service) **before** or **in conjunction with treatment** of the patient.

2. The physician is **not required to tell the suspected abuser** of the child or impaired elder that he or she suspects abuse.

3. The physician **does not need family consent** to hospitalize the abused child or elderly person for protection or treatment.

4. Although there is no intention to injure, if a **cultural remedy** such as coining injures a child or elderly person (see Chapter 12), such injury also must be reported to the appropriate agency.

IV. Abuse of Domestic Partners

Patient Snapshot 13-3

A 35-year-old woman comes to the emergency room with contusions on her cheek, a deep laceration above her right eye, and a fractured radius. The woman states that her boyfriend cursed at her and "pushed me around again" because she did not pick up his clothing from the dry-cleaner. After treating her injuries, the physician should make every effort to secure the safety of this patient. That would involve providing information about how to report the abuse to the police and the location of safe houses (places where she can go for protection from the abuser) in the area. Because this patient is a competent adult, it is not appropriate for the physician to report this domestic partner abuse to law enforcement without the patient's permission.

A. Occurrence

1. **Domestic abuse** is a common reason women come to a hospital emergency room. The abuser is almost always male.

2. The abused partner may not report the abuse to the police or **leave the abuser** because she has nowhere to go and because he has **threatened to kill her** if she reports or leaves him. (In fact, she does have a greatly increased risk of being killed by her abusive partner if she leaves.)

B. Evidence of domestic abuse

1. The victim commonly has **bruises** (e.g., blackened eyes) and broken bones.

2. In **pregnant women** (who have a higher risk of being abused), the **injuries** are often in the **"baby zone"** (breasts and abdomen).

3. An **irrational explanation** of how the injury occurred, **delay** in seeking treatment, and appearance of **sadness** in the victim are other indications of domestic abuse.

C. The cycle of abuse involves three phases:

1. **Buildup of tension** in the abuser

2. Abusive behavior (**battering**)

3. **Apologetic** and **loving behavior** by the abuser toward the victim

D. Characteristics of abusers and abused partners

1. **Abusers** often use **alcohol or drugs,** are impulsive, have a low tolerance for frustration, and displace their angry feelings onto their partner.

2. The abused partner is often emotionally or **financially dependent** on the abuser, is pregnant, and blames herself for the abuse.

3. **Both** the abuser and the abused commonly have **low self-esteem.**

E. Role of the physician in suspected domestic partner abuse

1. **Direct reporting by the physician of domestic partner abuse is not appropriate** because the victim is usually a competent adult.

2. A physician who suspects **domestic partner abuse** should
   a. **Document** the abuse.
   b. **Ensure the safety** of the abused person.
   c. Develop an **emergency escape plan** (e.g., locate a safe house for the abused person).
   d. Provide **emotional support** to the abused person.
   e. Refer the abused person to an **appropriate shelter or program.**
   f. **Encourage the abused person to report** the case to law-enforcement officials.

Chapter 14

Substance Abuse

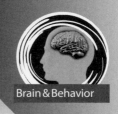

Brain & Behavior

I. The Neurobiology of Substance Abuse

A. Overview

1. The **positive effects** of abused substances such as stimulants, opioids, and sedatives (e.g., alcohol) are mediated by the action of neurotransmitters such as **dopamine** (**DA**) acting on **limbic** and **forebrain structures.**

2. The **neuroanatomic structures** involved in this **reward system** for all drugs of abuse include the following:

   a. The **ventral tegmental area** (**VTA**) in the midbrain, which is the site of origination of DA neurons

   b. The **mesolimbic-mesocortical tract** (**MT**), which projects from the VTA through the hypothalamus

   c. The **nucleus accumbens** (**NA**), which receives projections from one branch of the MT

   d. The **prefrontal cortex,** which receives projections from another branch of the MT

3. **Additional structures** are believed to be involved in the brain reward system with use of opioids and alcohol (Fig. 14-1).

B. Neurotransmitter (NT) associations

1. **Dopamine.** DA is the principal neurotransmitter involved in substance abuse and is increased in the brain by a number of mechanisms.

   a. **Heroin** and **nicotine** stimulate release of DA

   b. **Cocaine** prolongs the action of DA at its receptors by blocking its reuptake

   c. **Amphetamines** both stimulate release and block reuptake of DA.

   d. **Downregulation** of DA receptors with chronic drug use leads to craving and tolerance.

   e. As in **schizophrenia,** increased DA availability may also result in **psychotic symptoms** (see Chapter 19).

2. **γ-Aminobutyric acid** (**GABA**)

   a. **Sedatives** such as alcohol and benzodiazepines work primarily by **increasing** the activity of GABA, an inhibitory neurotransmitter.

   b. Because GABA may in turn **inhibit dopamine,** sedatives indirectly also affect the VTA-NA reward system.

3. **Serotonin** is closely involved in the action of hallucinogenic drugs, such as **lysergic acid diethylamine** (**LSD**), and recreational drugs, such as **ecstasy** (combined amphetamine and hallucinogen).

4. **Glutamate**

   a. Increased activity of **glutamate** is involved in the action of stimulants, opioids, and hallucinogens.

   b. **Phencyclidine** (**PCP**) binds with N-methyl-D-aspartate (NMDA) receptors of glutamate-gated ion channels.

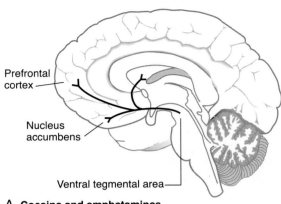

A. **Cocaine and amphetamines**

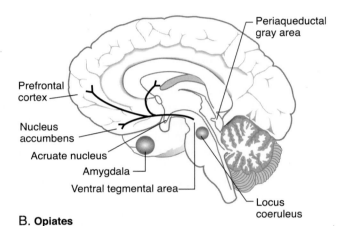

B. **Opiates**

FIG 14-1. Structures purported to be involved in the reward system of the human brain with use of various abused substances. **A.** The system for cocaine and amphetamines includes dopaminergic neurons found in the ventral tegmental area (VTA), which connect to the nucleus accumbens (NA) and prefrontal cortex. **B.** The system for opiates (or opioids) includes not only the VTA, the NA, and the prefrontal cortex but also structures using neurotransmitters that mimic the action of abused opioids, such as the arcuate nucleus, amygdala, locus ceruleus, and periaqueductal gray. **C.** The alcohol system also includes the VTA, the NA, and the prefrontal cortex as well as structures that use γ-aminobutyric acid (GABA), such as the cortex, cerebellum, hippocampus, superior and inferior colliculi, and amygdala. [Reprinted with permission from The brain's drug reward system [Tearoff]. NIDA Notes 1996;11.]

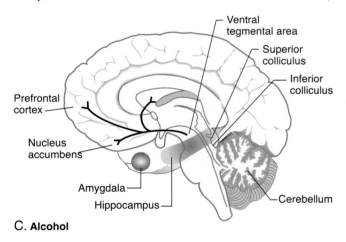

C. **Alcohol**

II. Substance Abuse, Demographics, Tolerance, and Dependence

Patient Snapshot 14-1

A 25-year-old man is brought to the emergency room by his girlfriend. He is physically agitated and is speaking very quickly. The patient states, "I am the most intelligent person in the world and I communicate mentally with Bill Gates every day about the new Microsoft operating system." His pulse is 120 bpm, and his blood pressure is 150/95 mm Hg. Just 1 hour later, the patient is very quiet and shows little response to the doctor's presence. He expresses the wish to be left alone "to die." His pulse and blood pressure are now normal. Because of the patient's rapid change in physical and emotional state, the doctor suspects that he has used a substance. His girlfriend reveals that both she and the patient spent that morning snorting cocaine.

A. Demographics. In decreasing order, alcohol, marijuana, nonmedical use of psychotherapeutic agents (e.g., benzodiazepines), cocaine, and—to a lesser extent—heroin are the most commonly used substances in the United States.

B. Substance abuse is a pattern of abnormal substance use leading to impairment of social, physical, or occupational functioning.

C. Substance dependence is substance abuse plus withdrawal symptoms, tolerance, or a pattern of repetitive use.
  1. Withdrawal is the development of physical or psychological symptoms after the reduction or cessation of intake of a substance.
  2. Tolerance is the need for increased amounts of the substance to achieve the same positive psychological effect.
  3. Cross-tolerance is the development of tolerance to one substance as the result of use of another substance—for example, tolerance to benzodiazepines as a result of prior alcohol use.

D. Positive and negative reinforcement are involved in drug abuse (see Chapter 12).
  1. Positive reinforcement: drug abuse continues to **gain the reward or high.**
  2. Negative reinforcement: drug abuse continues to **avoid uncomfortable withdrawal symptoms.**

E. Effects of use and withdrawal of stimulants, sedatives, opioids, and hallucinogens are listed in Table 14-1.

III. Sedatives

A. Sedatives are **central nervous system** (CNS) **depressants** and include alcohol, benzodiazepines (BZs), and barbiturates.

B. Alcohol
  1. About **10%** of Americans have life problems because of alcohol use.
  2. Alcohol use is associated with **traffic accidents, homicide, suicide, rape, child physical** and **sexual abuse, spouse abuse,** and **elder abuse.**
  3. Positive responses to the **CAGE questions** can help identify those who have a problem with alcohol: Do you ever . . .
    a. Try to **c**ut down on your drinking?
    b. Get **a**ngry when someone comments on your drinking?
    c. Feel **g**uilty about your drinking?
    d. Take a drink as an **e**ye-opener in the morning?
  4. Fetal alcohol syndrome (e.g., facial abnormalities, reduced head size, low height and body weight, and mental retardation) is seen in newborns whose mothers used large amounts of alcohol during pregnancy.

C. Benzodiazepines and barbiturates
  1. BZs and barbiturates are used medically as **sleep aids, antianxiety agents, muscle relaxants, anticonvulsants,** and **anesthetics** and to treat withdrawal from alcohol.

TABLE 14-1	EFFECTS OF USE AND WITHDRAWAL OF PSYCHOACTIVE SUBSTANCES	
Category	**Effects of use**	**Effects of withdrawal**

Sedatives
  Alcohol
  Benzodiazepines
  Barbiturates
	Mood elevation
	Decreased anxiety
	Sedation
	Behavioral disinhibition
	Respiratory depression
	Poor coordination
		Mood depression
		Increased anxiety
		Insomnia
		Tremor
		Psychotic symptoms (e.g., delusions and formication)
		Seizures
		Increased cardiovascular activity (e.g., tachycardia and hypertension)

Opioids
  Heroin
  Methadone
  Opioids used medically
	Mood elevation
	Sedation
	Analgesia
	Respiratory depression
	Constipation
	Pupil constriction (miosis)
		Mood depression
		Anxiety
		Flu-like symptoms (e.g., sweating, muscle aches, fever, rhinorrhea)
		Stomach cramps and diarrhea
		Pupil dilation (mydriasis)
		Piloerection (goose bumps)

Stimulants
  Amphetamines
  Cocaine
  (Similar but less pronounced effects with use of minor stimulants, such as caffeine and nicotine)
	Mood elevation
	Increased alertness
	Agitation and insomnia
	Increased cardiovascular, neurologic, and gastrointestinal activity
	Decreased appetite
	Psychotic symptoms (e.g., tactile hallucinations "cocaine bugs")
	Pupil dilation
	Seizures
	Increased sexuality
		Mood depression
		Lethargy
		Fatigue
		Increased appetite
		Irritability
		Headache
		Pupil constrictions

Hallucinogens
  LSD
  PCP
  Cannabis
  Psilocybin
  Mescaline
  Ketamine
	Mood elevation
	Altered perceptual states (e.g., hallucinations; distortions of time and space)
	Bad trips (panic reactions)
	Flashbacks (re-experiencing effects of drug without using it)
	Cardiovascular symptoms
	Sweating, tremor
	Nystagmus (PCP)
		Few if any withdrawal symptoms

LSD, lysergic acid diethylamide; *PCP,* phencyclidine.

2. Barbiturates have a **low safety margin**—that is, the effective dose is close to the lethal dose.
3. BZs have a **high safety margin,** unless taken in conjunction with other sedatives, such as alcohol.

D. Withdrawal from sedatives
   1. Withdrawal from sedative agents is the most **physically dangerous** of all withdrawal syndromes; hospitalization is required.

2. Withdrawal symptoms can include **seizures, psychotic symptoms** such as hallucinations, and **cardiovascular symptoms** such as hypertension. Alcohol withdrawal delirium (the DTs) has a death rate of 20% in long-term heavy users.

IV. Opioids

A. Opioids (narcotics) include drugs used medically as analgesics (e.g., **morphine**) as well as drugs of abuse (e.g., **heroin**).
   1. Compared to medically used opioids, abused opioids are more potent, cross the blood–brain barrier more quickly, and have **more euphoric action.**
   2. Death from withdrawal of opioids rarely occurs, unless a serious illness is present.

B. Methadone, ʟ-α-acetylmethadol acetate (LAMM), and buprenorphine (Temgesic) are synthetic opioids used to treat heroin addiction; like heroin, all three can cause dependence and tolerance.
   1. All can be taken in **pill or liquid form.**
   2. All have **fewer euphoric effects** than heroin.
   3. Methadone and LAMM are **dispensed by federal health authorities to registered addicts** enrolled in formal treatment programs.
   4. Buprenorphine is a partial opioid receptor agonist.
       a. It can block both withdrawal symptoms and the euphoric action of heroin.
       b. It can be prescribed by a **physician in private practice** who has participated in a special training program; the patient does not have to be enrolled in a formal treatment program.

V. Stimulants

A. Stimulants include major agents such as **amphetamines** and **cocaine** and agents with similar although much smaller effects, such as **caffeine** and **nicotine.**

B. Amphetamines are used in the following situations:
   1. Medically indicated in the treatment of **attention deficit hyperactivity disorder (ADHD)** and **narcolepsy** (see Chapters 3 and 15)
   2. Medically indicated to treat **depression** in the elderly and terminally ill and depression and health-threatening **obesity** in patients who do not respond to other interventions
   3. Illegally acquired and used by students and in professions in which **wakefulness** is desired—for example, overnight truck drivers.

C. Crack and freebase are cheap, smokable forms of cocaine; in the pure form, cocaine is sniffed into the nostrils (snorted).
   1. Cocaine provides an intense but **short-lived** (about 1 hr) elevation of mood.
   2. Hyperactivity and **growth retardation** are seen in newborns whose mothers used cocaine during pregnancy.

VI. Hallucinogens and Related Agents

A. Hallucinogens and related agents include **LSD**, **PCP** (angel dust), **cannabis** (tetrahydrocannabinol, marijuana, hashish), **psilocybin** (from mushrooms), **mescaline** (from cactus), and **ketamine** ("special K") as well as **inhalants** (e.g., gasoline). These agents have the following effects:
1. Produce **altered states of consciousness**
2. Have few or **no withdrawal symptoms**

B. Marijuana
1. Chronic users can have **lung problems** associated with smoking along with decreased interest in work and increased apathy (**the amotivational syndrome**).
2. Although **illegal** in the United States, a few states permit limited medical use to treat glaucoma and cancer treatment–related nausea and vomiting.

C. LSD and PCP
1. Typically, LSD is ingested and PCP is smoked in a marijuana or other cigarette.
2. **Nystagmus** (abnormal eye movements) and episodes of **violent behavior** are associated with use of **PCP.**
3. Consumption of >20 mg of PCP may cause seizures, coma, and even death.

VII. Treatment of Substance Abuse

Patient Snapshot 14-2

 A 45-year-old man who has been using heroin regularly for the past 20 years is arrested and charged with possession of the drug. As part of a plea bargain, the man agrees to go into treatment for heroin addiction and is admitted to the detox

TABLE 14-2	LABORATORY FINDINGS FOR SELECTED DRUGS OF ABUSE	
Class of Substance	**Elevated Levels in Body Fluids (urine, blood)**	**Time after Use That Substance Can Be Detected**
Sedatives	Alcohol (legal intoxication is 0.08–0.15% blood alcohol concentration)	7–12 hr
	γ-Glutamyltransferase	7–12 hr
	Specific barbiturate or benzodiazepine or its metabolite	1–3 days
Opioids	Heroin	1–3 days
	Methadone	2–3 days
Stimulants	Cotinine (nicotine metabolite)	1–2 days
	Amphetamine	1–2 days
	Benzoylecgonine (cocaine metabolite)	1–3 days in occasional users; 7–12 days in heavy users
Hallucinogens and related agents	Cannabinoid metabolites	3–28 days
	Phencyclidine (PCP)	7–14 days in heavy users
	Serum glutamic-oxaloacetic transaminase and creatinine phosphokinase (with PCP use)	>7 days

Adapted with permission from Fadem B. BRS Behavioral Science, 4th ed. Baltimore, Lippincott Williams & Wilkins, 2004:79.

TABLE 14-3	TREATMENT FOR ABUSE OF COMMONLY USED SUBSTANCES[a]	
Substance	**Immediate Treatment/Detoxification**	**Extended Treatment/Maintenance**
Alcohol (or other abused sedative)	Hospitalization Flumazenil to reverse the effects of benzodiazepines Substitute long-acting barbiturate (e.g., phenobarbital) or benzodiazepine (e.g., chlordiazepoxide) in decreasing doses Intravenous diazepam, lorazepam, or phenobarbital if seizures occur For alcohol abuse: thiamine to restore nutritional state	Alcoholics Anonymous or other peer support (12-step) program Disulfiram (Antabuse) Naloxone (Narcan) Naltrexone (ReVia) Acamprosate (Campral) Psychotherapy
Heroin (or other abused opioid)	Hospitalization and naloxone for overdose Clonidine to stabilize autonomic nervous system during withdrawal Substitution of long-acting opioid (e.g., methadone) in decreasing doses to reduce withdrawal symptoms	Methadone, LAMM, or buprenorphine maintenance program Naloxone, naltrexone, or buprenorphine used prophylactically to block effects of abused opioids Narcotics Anonymous or other peer support (12-step) program
Nicotine (or other stimulant such as caffeine)	Identify pattern of use (e.g., after meals) and substitute a "safe" activity (e.g., exercise, having sugar-free gum or candy) Analgesics to control headache due to withdrawal	Education for maintenance of abstinence Substitute nicotine-containing gum, patch, or nasal spray Bupropion (Zyban), an antidepressant indicated for smoking cessation SmokEnders or other peer support (12-step) program Hypnosis to prevent smoking

[a]Treatments are listed in order of utility: highest to lowest.

LAMM, L-α-acetylmethadol acetate. Adapted from Fadem, B. Behavioral Science in Medicine. Baltimore, Lippincott Williams & Wilkins, 2004: 375–376.

unit of a local hospital. Each day in detox, he is given clonidine (a noradrenergic receptor antagonist to decrease withdrawal symptoms) and methadone in decreasing doses. After 1 week, his opioid requirement is significantly lower, and he is released from the hospital and enrolled in a methadone maintenance program. At the program, he is given a dose of methadone dissolved in liquid daily to block further withdrawal symptoms, after which he attends group therapy with other recovering addicts. As part of the program, he also is required to attend biweekly meetings of Narcotics Anonymous. Random urine tests for heroin and other abused substances are administered approximately weekly. Gradually, over the course of 2 years, the methadone dose is lowered until the patient is no longer opioid dependent.

A. **Laboratory findings** can often confirm substance use (Table 14-2).

B. **Treatment of substance abuse** ranges from abstinence and peer support groups to agents that block withdrawal symptoms (Table 14-3).

C. **Dual diagnosis.** Mentally ill–chemically addicted (MICA) patients require treatment for both substance abuse and the comorbid psychiatric illness (e.g., major depression), often in a special unit in the hospital.

Chapter 15

Brain Rhythms and Sleep

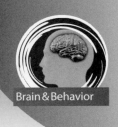

Brain & Behavior

I. Circadian Rhythms

A. Characteristics

1. Behaviors, such as **sleeping** and **waking,** and physiologic processes, such as **regulation of body temperature** and **hormone secretion,** are coordinated by daily **cycles of light and dark.** These behaviors and processes are circadian in nature— that is, they last approximately (circa) one day (dies).

2. **Zeitgebers** (time givers) are environmental cues (e.g., ambient temperature, level of illumination) that entrain circadian cycles.

3. Most circadian physiologic and behavioral cycles can continue even in the **absence of zeitgebers.** However, in their absence, the circadian cycle in humans is closer to **25 hr** than to 24 hr.

B. Biology

1. The **hypothalamus** (**HT**) plays an important role in the control of circadian rhythms. Lesions of the anterior HT disrupt circadian cycles.

2. The **suprachiasmatic nuclei** (**SCN**), small (<0.3 mm^3 each) structures on either side of the midline of the HT bordering the third ventricle, receive afferent fibers from the retina and function as the **brain clock** (see Fig. 6-11).

   a. SCN neurons communicate with classical chemical synapses using **γ-aminobutyric acid** (**GABA**) as their primary neurotransmitter.

   b. SCN neurons also communicate using electrical synapses (**gap junctions**) and input from glial cells.

II. The Electroencephalogram (EEG)

The cerebral cortex produces rapid **electrical rhythms** that can be recorded and measured. These rhythms make up the **EEG.**

A. EEG rhythms

1. The EEG displays voltages generated mainly by the synchronous firing of thousands of **pyramidal neurons** in the cortex.

   a. Voltages are measured between two points on the scalp.

   b. The measurement is repeated in different locations on the scalp (Fig. 15-1).

2. The **amplitude** of the EEG signal is positively correlated with the **number of activated neurons** and the **synchronicity** of their firing.

   a. The **more neurons** that fire and the more synchronous their firing, the **higher the amplitude** of the signal.

   b. Synchronicity of neurons is coordinated both by a central pacemaker located in the **thalamus** and by cortical neurons mutually exciting or inhibiting each other.

3. The **frequency** of the EEG signal is correlated with level of attentiveness (e.g., waking vs. sleeping) and **brain pathology** (e.g., seizures, coma).

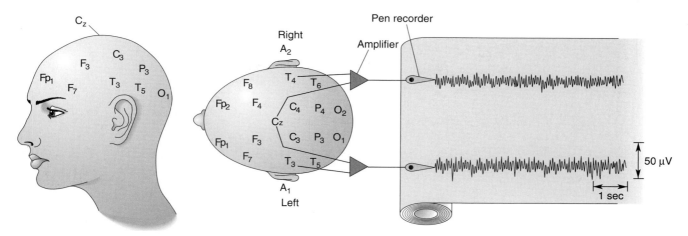

FIG 15-1. The standard positions on the scalp at which electrodes are applied to record the electroencephalogram (EEG). [Reprinted with permission from Baer MF, Connors BW, Paradiso MA. Neuroscience: Exploring the Brain, 3rd ed. Baltimore, Lippincott Williams & Wilkins, 2007:587.]

    a. The **faster** the rhythm, the more **alert** the individual.—for example, with active mental concentration, the fastest rhythms, **beta (β) rhythms** (>14 Hz), are seen.

    b. The **slowest** rhythms, **delta (δ) rhythms** (<4 Hz), are seen in the pathologic state of **coma.**

B. Seizures

Patient Snapshot 15-1

A 17-year-old high school senior is brought to the hospital when he suddenly begins to experience visual hallucinations, altered thinking, and delusions of persecution and grandeur. The patient is awake but seems confused and is diagnosed with complex partial seizures. MRI studies reveal a cystic lesion in the right temporal lobe in the region of the hippocampus. After surgical removal of the lesion, pathologically identified as a dysembryoplastic neuroepithelial tumor, the patient's psychotic symptoms and complex partial seizures disappear over a period of 2 years.[a]

    1. Seizures are a result of abnormal **high-amplitude, low-frequency, synchronous** brain activity. They can be generalized (tonic–clonic or absence) or partial (simple or complex).

        a. A **generalized seizure** involves the entire cerebral cortex and both hemispheres and **consciousness is lost** (Fig. 15-2).

            i. In a **tonic–clonic seizure,** all muscle groups show tonic (ongoing) or clonic (rhythmic) activity.

            ii. In an **absence seizure,** the person seems unaware of the environment and is unable to respond to stimuli; only subtle motor signs (e.g., fluttering of the eyelids) are present.

        b. A **partial seizure** involves one particular area of the cortex.

            i. **Simple** partial seizures do not affect awareness or memory.

            ii. **Complex** partial seizures affect awareness or memory.

            iii. The effects of the seizure depend on where the seizure begins:

                (a) In a **motor area:** movement of one limb may be affected

                (b) In a **sensory area:** an abnormal sensation (i.e., aura) such as an odd taste or smell may occur

[a]Adapted with permission from Escosa BM, Villarejo Ortega FJ, Perez Jimenez MA, Gonzalez Mediero I. [Psychosis in a case of temporal lobe epilepsy associated with a dysembryoplastic neuroepithelia tumour] [Spanish] Rev Neurol. 2004; 38:643–646.

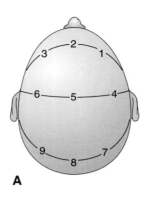

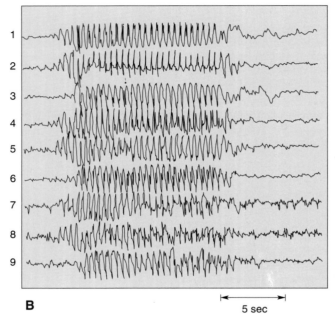

FIG 15-2. EEG of a generalized epileptic seizure. **A.** Placement of the EEG electrodes on the scalp. **B.** EEG results showing a brief absence seizure that begins suddenly, is synchronized across the entire head, generates strong neural rhythms of ~3 Hz, and ends after about 12 sec. [Reprinted with permission from Baer MF, Connors BW, Paradiso MA. Neuroscience: Exploring the Brain, 3rd ed. Baltimore, Lippincott Williams & Wilkins, 2007:594.]

5 sec

      (c) In the cortex of the **temporal lobe** (e.g., the amygdala): abnormal thoughts or behavior may occur (Patient Snapshot 15-1).

  2. **Epilepsy** is a condition involving repeated seizures.

  3. **Neurotransmitters,** particularly GABA, are involved in the production and treatment of seizures.

    a. Drugs that block GABA receptors **promote seizures.**

    b. **Anticonvulsants** counter neural excitability and seizures by at least two mechanisms:

      i. Prolonging the **inhibitory action of GABA** (e.g., benzodiazepines)

      ii. **Decreasing** the **excitability** of neurons (e.g., carbamazepine, phenytoin)

III. Normal Sleep

Patient Snapshot 15-2

During the 26th hr of a marathon radio program aimed at raising money for charity, the hostess, a 24-year-old medical student who has no history of emotional or medical problems begins to have difficulty concentrating and seems confused. By the 50th hr of the marathon, the student is agitated, refuses to drink anything, and states,

"I know someone is trying to poison me." Her colleagues become alarmed and call 911. On the way to the hospital, the student starts shouting that everyone is against her. She is admitted to the hospital and given antipsychotic medication to control her delusions. After sleeping for 12 hr, the student's behavior and mood are normal, and she is released.

A. Overview

1. The **sleep–wake cycle** is the most familiar circadian cycle.
2. The function of sleep is unknown. However, extended sleep deprivation can result in the transient display of psychopathologic states such as **anxiety** or, with even longer deprivation, **psychosis** (Patient Snapshot 15-2).
3. Sleep may be required for life itself. **Fatal familial insomnia,** a rare disorder resulting from mutations in the prion protein gene (PRNP), leads to degeneration of the thalamus that results in the inability to sleep and is, as the name of the disorder implies, fatal within 1–2 years.

B. Sleep state.
During sleep, the EEG shows distinctive changes.

1. Sleep is divided into rapid eye movement (**REM**) sleep and **non-REM** sleep. Non-REM sleep consists of stages 1, 2, 3, and 4.
    a. **REM sleep** takes up about 25% of total sleep time in young adults and is characterized by β and **alpha (α) waves;** dreaming; increased pulse, respiration, and blood pressure; and absence of skeletal muscle movement.
    b. **Stage 1** is the shortest (5% of total sleep time in young adults) and lightest stage of sleep. It is characterized by peacefulness; decreased pulse, respiration, and blood pressure; and episodic body movement **theta (θ) waves** predominate.
    c. **Stage 2** takes up the largest percentage of total sleep time (45% in young adults) and is characterized by **sleep spindles and K-complexes.**
    d. **Stages 3 and 4**, known collectively as **slow wave** or **delta (δ) sleep** (because δ waves predominate) make up about 25% of total sleep time (in young adults) and are the deepest stages of sleep.
2. **Sleep measures** include sleep latency, REM latency, and sleep efficiency
    a. **Sleep latency** is the period of time from going to bed to falling asleep and is normally $<$**20 min.**
    b. **REM latency** is the average time to the first REM period after falling asleep and is normally $\sim$**90 min.**
    c. **Sleep efficiency,** the percentage of time spent sleeping per amount of time spent in bed, typically exceeds **90%.**
3. Mapping the transitions from one stage of sleep to another during the night produces a structure known as **sleep architecture** (Fig. 15-3).
    a. Sleep architecture changes with **age** and in **depression** (Table 15-1).
    b. **Sedative agents,** such as alcohol, barbiturates, and benzodiazepines, are associated also with **reduced REM sleep and δ sleep.**
    c. Most δ sleep occurs during the **first half of the sleep cycle.**
    d. The **longest REM periods** occur during the **second half of the sleep cycle.**
4. During **REM** sleep, **high levels of brain activity** occur, although the body is essentially paralyzed.
    a. **REM** periods of 10–40 min each occur about **every 90 min** throughout the night.
    b. A person who is deprived of REM sleep one night (e.g., because of inadequate sleep or repeated awakenings) has increased REM sleep the next night (**REM rebound**).

C. Neurotransmitters
are involved in the production of sleep.

1. **Increased** levels of **acetylcholine (Ach)** in the reticular formation **increase both total sleep time and REM sleep.** Acetylcholine levels, total sleep time, and REM sleep decrease in normal aging as well as in Alzheimer disease.

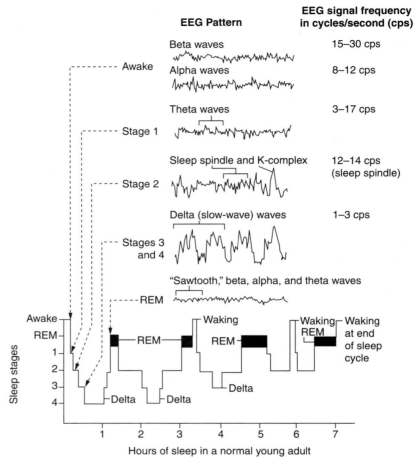

Figure 15-3. Electroencephalographic (EEG) tracings, associated EEG signal frequencies, and sleep architecture in a normal young adult. [Reprinted with permission from Fadem B. Behavioral Science in Medicine. Baltimore, Lippincott Williams & Wilkins, 2004:107.]

2. **Increased** levels of **dopamine decrease total sleep time.** Treatment with antipsychotics, which block dopamine receptors, may improve sleep in patients with psychotic symptoms.
3. **Increased** levels of **norepinephrine decrease both total sleep time and REM sleep.**

TABLE 15-1	SUMMARY OF CHARACTERISTICS OF SLEEP IN YOUNG, DEPRESSED AND ELDERLY PEOPLE		
Sleep Measure	Normal Young Adults	Depressed Young Adults	Normal Elderly Adults
Percentage REM	~25%	>25%	<25%
REM latency	~90 min	<90 min	~90 min
REM pattern	Increased REM toward morning	Decreased REM toward morning	Increased REM toward morning
Percentage delta (δ)	~25%	<25%	<25%
Sleep latency	~10 min	<10 min	>10 min
Sleep efficiency	~100%	<100%	<100%
Nighttime awakenings	1–3 per night	>3 per night	>3 per night

REM, rapid eye movement.

Reprinted with permission from Fadem B. BRS Behavioral Science, 4th ed. Baltimore, Lippincott Williams & Wilkins, 2005:89.

4. **Increased** levels of **serotonin increase both total sleep time and δ sleep.** Damage to the dorsal raphe nuclei, which produce serotonin, decreases both of these measures. Treatment with antidepressants, which increase serotonin availability, can improve sleep in depressed patients.

IV. Sleep Disorders

Patient Snapshot 15-3

The parents of a 5-year-old boy report that the child often screams during the night. They are particularly concerned because during these disturbances, the child sits up, opens his eyes and "looks right through them," and they are unable to awaken him. The child has no memory of these experiences in the morning. Physical examination is unremarkable, and the child is doing well in kindergarten. A sleep study reveals that during these disturbances the child's electroencephalogram is characterized primarily by δ waves. The child is diagnosed with sleep terror disorder.

A. **Overview.** The *Diagnostic and Statistical Manual of Mental Disorders*, 4th edition, text revision (DSM-IV-TR), classifies sleep disorders into two major categories.
   1. **Dyssomnias** are characterized by problems in **the timing, quality, or amount** of sleep. They include insomnia, breathing-related sleep disorder (sleep apnea), and narcolepsy as well as circadian rhythm sleep disorder, nocturnal myoclonus, restless leg syndrome, and the primary hypersomnias (e.g., Kleine-Levin syndrome and menstrual-associated syndrome).
   2. **Parasomnias** are characterized by **abnormalities in physiology or in behavior** associated with sleep. They include bruxism (tooth grinding), sleepwalking, sleep terror, REM sleep behavior, and nightmare disorders.
   3. The sleep disorders are described in Table 15-2 and below.

B. **Insomnia**
   1. **Definition.** Insomnia is **difficulty falling asleep or staying asleep** that occurs 3 times per week **for at least 1 month.**
      a. Insomnia leads to sleepiness during the day or causes problems fulfilling social or occupational obligations.
      b. Insomnia is common; it is present at some time in at least **30% of the population.**
   2. **Psychological causes** of insomnia include the affective and anxiety disorders.
      a. **Major depressive disorder: waking too early** in the morning (terminal insomnia) is the most common sleep abnormality in depressed patients.
      b. **Bipolar disorder: manic or hypomanic** patients show increased sleep latency, sleep fewer hours, and often become exhausted**.**
      c. **Anxious** patients often worry excessively, leading to increased sleep latency.
   3. **Physical causes** of insomnia
      a. **Use of central nervous system (CNS) stimulants** (e.g., caffeine) is the most common cause of insomnia.
      b. **Withdrawal of agents with sedating action** (e.g., alcohol, benzodiazepines, opioids) can result in nighttime wakefulness.
      c. **Medical conditions** causing pain also result in insomnia, as do endocrine and metabolic disorders.

C. **Breathing-related sleep disorder (sleep apnea)**
   1. Patients with sleep apnea **stop breathing** for brief intervals. Low oxygen or high carbon dioxide level in the blood **awakens the patient repeatedly** during the night, resulting in **daytime sleepiness.**

TABLE 15-2	SLEEP DISORDERS AND THEIR CHARACTERISTICS
Sleep Disorder	**Characteristics**
Sleep terror disorder	Repetitive experiences of fright in which a person (usually a child) screams in fear during sleep (see Patient Snapshot 15-3)
	The person cannot be awakened
	The person has no memory of having a dream
	Occurs during δ sleep
	Onset in adolescence may indicate temporal lobe epilepsy
Nightmare disorder	Repetitive, frightening dreams that cause nighttime awakenings
	The person usually can recall nightmare
	Occurs during REM sleep
Sleepwalking disorder	Repetitive walking around during sleep
	No memory of episode on awakening
	Begins in childhood (usually 4–8 years of age)
	Occurs during δ sleep
Circadian rhythm sleep disorder	Inability to sleep at appropriate times
	Delayed sleep phase type involves falling asleep and waking later than wanted
	Jet lag type lasts 2–7 days after a change in time zones
	Shift work type (e.g., in physician training) can result in work errors
Nocturnal myoclonus	Repetitive, abrupt muscular contractions in legs from toes to hips
	Causes nighttime awakenings
	More common in elderly
Restless leg syndrome	Uncomfortable sensation in legs, necessitating frequent motion
	Repetitive limb jerking during sleep
	Causes difficulty falling asleep and nighttime awakenings
	More common with aging, pregnancy, and kidney disease
Primary hypersomnias (Kleine-Levin syndrome and menstrual-associated syndrome [symptoms only in the premenstruum])	Recurrent periods of excessive sleepiness occurring almost daily for at least 1 month
	Sleepiness is not relieved by daytime naps
	Often accompanied by hyperphagia (overeating)
	Kleine-Levin is more common in adolescent males
Sleep drunkenness	Difficulty awakening fully after adequate sleep
	Rare, must be differentiated from substance abuse or other sleep disorder
	Associated with genetic factors
Bruxism (tooth grinding during sleep)	Can lead to tooth damage and jaw pain
	Occurs during stage 2 sleep
	Treated with dental appliance worn at night or corrective orthodontia
REM sleep behavior disorder	REM sleep without skeletal muscle paralysis
	Patients can injure themselves or their sleeping partners

REM, rapid eye movement.
Reprinted with permission from Fadem B. BRS Behavioral Science, 4th ed. Baltimore, Lippincott Williams & Wilkins, 2005:90.

a. In patients with **central sleep apnea** (more common in the elderly), little or no respiratory effort occurs, resulting in less air reaching the lungs.

b. In patients with **obstructive sleep** apnea, respiratory effort occurs and patients often **snore,** but an airway obstruction prevents air from reaching the lungs.

  i. Obstructive sleep apnea occurs most often in people 40–60 years of age.

  ii. It is more common in men (8:1 male to female ratio) and in the obese.

  iii. **Pickwickian syndrome** is a related condition in which airway obstruction caused by excessive body weight results in the patient falling asleep during daytime hours.

  iv. Sleep apnea occurs in **1–10% of the population** and is related to **depression, headaches, respiratory acidosis,** and **pulmonary hypertension.**

2. Sleep apnea may result in **sudden death** during sleep, particularly in the elderly and in infants.

D. Narcolepsy

1. Patients with narcolepsy have **sleep attacks** (i.e., fall asleep suddenly during the day) despite having a normal amount of sleep at night.

2. The percentage of **nighttime REM sleep is greatly reduced** in narcolepsy.

3. Narcolepsy is also characterized by the following:

a. **Hypnagogic or hypnopompic hallucinations,** strange perceptual experiences that occur just as the patient falls asleep or wakes up, respectively, occur in 20–40% of patients.

b. **Decreased sleep latency, short REM latency,** and **interrupted REM** (sleep fragmentation)

c. **Cataplexy and sleep paralysis:** in these states, the body is showing the characteristic motor paralysis of REM sleep while the brain is awake.

  i. **Cataplexy** is a sudden physical collapse caused by the loss of all muscle tone after a strong emotional stimulus (e.g., laughter, fear) and occurs in 30–70% of patients.

TABLE 15-3	TREATMENT OF INSOMNIA, OBSTRUCTIVE SLEEP APNEA, AND NARCOLEPSY
Disorder	**Treatment**[a]
Insomnia	Avoidance of caffeine, especially before bedtime
	Development of a series of behaviors associated with bedtime (i.e., a sleep ritual or sleep hygiene)
	Maintaining a fixed sleeping and waking schedule
	Daily exercise (but not just before sleep)
	Relaxation techniques
	Limited use of nonbenzodiazepine sleep agent (e.g., zolpidem, zaleplon, eszopiclone)
	Limited use of hypnotic benzodiazepine (e.g., temazepam)
Breathing-related sleep disorder (obstructive sleep apnea)	Weight loss (if overweight)
	Continuous positive airway pressure (a device applied to the face at night to gently move air into the lungs)
	Surgery to enlarge the airway (e.g., uvulopalatoplasty)
	Tracheostomy (as a last resort)
Narcolepsy	Scheduled daytime naps
	Stimulant agents (e.g., modafinil [Provigil]), methylphenidate [Ritalin])
	If cataplexy is present, an antidepressant may be added

[a]Treatments are listed in order of utility, from highest to lowest.

Reprinted with permission from Fadem B. BRS Behavioral Science, 4th ed. Baltimore, Lippincott Williams & Wilkins, 2005:92.

ii. **Sleep paralysis** is the inability to move the body for a brief time after waking.
4. Narcolepsy is uncommon.
   a. It occurs most frequently in **adolescents and young adults.**
   b. There may be a **genetic component.**
   c. **Daytime naps** leave the patient feeling refreshed.

E. **Treatment of sleep disorders.** The treatments of insomnia, breathing-related sleep disorder, and narcolepsy are listed in Table 15-3.

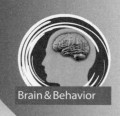

Chapter 16

The Doctor–Patient Relationship

Brain & Behavior

I. Ethical Conduct

Patient Snapshot 16-1

A competent 35-year-old woman who is 4 months pregnant tells her physician that over the past year she has been using illegal intravenous drugs and has had at least six different sexual partners. The physician explains the risks to her fetus if she is HIV positive and how prenatal treatment with zidovudine (AZT) and/or nevirapine can reduce the risks. The physician confirms that the patient understands these risks by asking her to explain them back to him. He then suggests that she be tested for the virus. The woman refuses adamantly to be tested. Acting ethically, the physician has no choice but to note the patient's refusal in her chart and continue to provide prenatal care for her. Once the child is born, however, the mother cannot refuse to have the child tested and, if necessary, treated (for more on ethical issues relating to children, see Chapter 1).

A. Informed consent

1. With the exception of life-threatening emergencies, physicians must obtain consent (verbal or nonverbal) from competent, informed adult patients before proceeding with any medical or surgical treatment.
2. Before patients can give consent to be treated by a physician, they must be informed of and understand the following:
   a. The **health implications** of their diagnosis
   b. The **health risks** and **benefits** of treatment
   c. The **alternatives** to treatment
   d. The likely **outcome if they do not consent** to the treatment
   e. That they can **withdraw consent for treatment at any time** before or during the treatment or procedure
3. Physicians also must obtain informed consent before entering a patient in a **research study.** However, if a patient's condition worsens during the study as a result of lack of treatment, placebo treatment, or exposure to experimental treatment, the patient must be taken out of the study and given the standard treatment for his or her condition.
4. Competent patients have the **right to refuse** to consent to a needed test or procedure for religious or other reasons, even if their health will suffer or death will result from such refusal. Although medical or surgical intervention may be necessary to protect the health or life of a fetus, a **competent pregnant woman has the right to refuse** such intervention (e.g., cesarean section or AZT treatment even if the fetus will die or be seriously injured without the intervention (Patient Snapshot 16-1).

B. Confidentiality

1. Physicians are expected to maintain patient confidentiality.
2. Physicians are **not required** to maintain patient confidentiality under the following conditions:
   a. The patient is suspected of **child or elder abuse**

171

      b. The patient has a significant **risk of suicide**

      c. The patient poses a serious **threat to another person** (e.g., an HIV-positive man who habitually puts his uninformed partner at risk by engaging in unprotected sex)

C. Relationships with patients

    1. **Sexual relationships** with current or former patients are inappropriate and are prohibited by the ethical standards of most specialty boards.

    2. Physicians should avoid treating family members, close friends, and employees.

    3. **Referrals** of patients to other doctors should be reserved for patients with medical and psychiatric problems outside the range of expertise or against the belief system of the treating physician (e.g., doing an abortion). It is inappropriate to refer patients to other doctors because the patients are annoying, seductive, or angry.

D. Impaired physicians

    1. Causes of impairment in physicians include **drug or alcohol abuse, physical or mental illness,** and impairment in functioning associated with **old age.**

    2. **Removing** an impaired colleague, medical student, or resident from contact with patients is an ethical requirement because patients must be protected and the impaired colleague must be helped. The legal requirement for reporting impaired colleagues depends on state regulations.

      a. An **impaired medical student** should be reported to the **dean** of the medical school or the dean of students.

      b. An **impaired resident** or **attending physician** should be reported to the person directly in charge of him or her (e.g., the residency training director or the chief of the medical staff).

      c. An impaired **physician in practice** should be reported to the state licensing board or the impaired physicians program, usually part of the state medical society.

    3. Physicians are **not required** to inform either patients or the medical establishment about another **physician's HIV-positive status** because, if the physician follows procedures for infection control, he or she does not pose a risk to patients.

II. Getting Information from Adult Patients

The Clinical Interview. The seating of the participants, the types of questions that will be asked, and techniques for interviewing are important in obtaining information from adult patients. For discussion on getting and giving information to children and adolescents, see Chapter 1.

A. Appropriate seating for the participants during clinical interactions includes avoiding having a large object such as a desk or table between the doctor and the patient and ensuring that all participants are at eye level with each other (Fig. 16-1).

B. Direct versus open-ended questions

    1. **Open-ended questions** are nonstructured, do not close off potential areas of pertinent information, and allow a variety of responses, e.g., "Tell me about the pain."

    2. **Direct questions** are those that can be answered with yes, no, or a few simple words and are used to clarify the information obtained from open-ended question, e.g., "Does the pain wake you at night?"

      a. Direct questions are also used to **elicit information quickly** in an emergency situation or when a patient has a cognitive disorder.

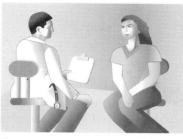 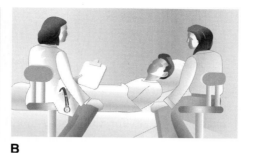

A   **B**

FIG 16-1. Seating of the participants during clinical interactions. **A.** Physician and patient interaction in an office. Note that there is no desk or other obstacle between the participants. **B.** Interaction among the physician, patient, and patient's relative in a hospital room. Note that the three participants sit in a triangular fashion with the doctor to one side of the patient's bed and the relative to the same side so that everyone is at eye level and the bed is not an obstacle between any two individuals. [Adapted with permission from Fadem B. Behavioral Science in Medicine, Baltimore, Lippincott Williams & Wilkins, 2004.]

      b. Direct questions may be preferred when a patient is **sexually provocative** toward the doctor or **overly talkative.**

C. Specific strategies and techniques, such as support, empathy, validation, facilitation, reflection, silence, confrontation, and recapitulation, used in interviewing patients are described in Patient Snapshot 16-2.

Patient Snapshot 16-2

A physician sees a 33-year-old man who sustained a severe spinal cord injury at the C5 level 3 weeks earlier in a car accident. The patient can be described as C5 quadriplegic. His fiancé, who was driving, received only minor injuries in the accident. After he recovers from his acute injuries, the patient will have no useful leg function and will require assistance with everyday function, such as bathing and getting in and out of bed. He will be totally dependent on his caretakers for both bowel and bladder function. Sexual function will also be a problem. The patient should have reasonable shoulder and proximal arm function but no finger or hand muscle function. He will require a motorized wheelchair that can be driven with modified hand controls.

As the physician begins to talk to the patient, she notes that the patient is oriented and alert but seems suspicious and agitated. He also appears to be experiencing some discomfort. When the physician asks the patient how he is feeling, he says that he is fine and then starts crying. At this time, the physician should remain attentive and concerned but should remain **silent,** allowing the patient time to gather his thoughts. After she has done this, expressions of interest and concern for the patient using **support** and **empathy** (e.g., "Finding out the extent of your injuries must have been a frightening experience for you") are appropriate.

During the interview, the doctor can maximize information gathering by encouraging the patient to elaborate on his responses using interview techniques such as **facilitation** (e.g., "Tell me more") and **reflection** (e.g., "You said that your discomfort has increased during the past week.") Information that the patient has given can be clarified by calling his attention to inconsistencies in his responses or body language using **confrontation** (e.g., "You say that you are fine, but you seem quite upset.") The interview technique of **validation** gives credence to the patient's feelings and confirms to the patient that sadness is to be expected under the circumstances (e.g., "Many people would feel down if they had been injured as you were.")

At the end of the interview, the physician should go over what the patient has told her (the interview technique of **recapitulation**) to be sure that she understands and can correctly document the information obtained during the interview.

III. Giving Information to Patients

Patient Snapshot 16-3

During his regular office visit, a 34-year-old male patient who has been taking flu-oxetine (Prozac) for the past 6 months seems uncomfortable and then says, "Could you tell me again about the side effects of this medication?" Selective serotonin reuptake inhibitors (SSRIs) such as fluoxetine have negative sexual side effects, and because of the patient's discomfort, the doctor should assume that this patient is experiencing such effects. The physician can then remind the patient that sexual side effects such as delayed orgasm are common with use of drugs such as fluoxetine. After this, the physician can elicit the patient's perspective on the problem by asking an open-ended question (e.g., "Tell me about your experience with the drug.") After determining that the patient is indeed experiencing sexual side effects, the physician can make recommendations that address the problem, for example, switching to an antidepressant medication with fewer negative sexual effects, such as bupropion (see Chapter 22).

A. Eliciting questions from patients

1. Patients are often reticent to ask questions about issues that are potentially **embarrassing** (e.g., sexual problems) or **fear provoking** (e.g., biopsy results).
2. Physicians should **anticipate** such unspoken questions, verbalize them, and then answer them truthfully and completely (see Patient Snapshot 16-3).

B. Relaying information to patients

1. Patients are usually told the **complete truth** about the diagnosis and prognosis of their illness.
2. Physicians should **avoid philosophical or religious statements,** such as, "It is not how long you live but how well you live." Information about a competent patient's illness should be **given directly to the patient** by the doctor and not relayed through relatives.
3. A physician **can delay** telling the patient the diagnosis until the patient indicates that he or she is ready to receive the news.
4. A six-step strategy for giving bad news to patients is presented in Table 16-1,

C. Making decisions for patients

1. **Physicians should not tell patients what to do** but should instead provide the information patients need to make their own decisions (e.g., what form of contraception to choose).
2. If there is disagreement among family members about the decision, the doctor's role also involves **facilitating discussion** among them so that they can all ultimately agree on the decision that has been made.

IV. Personality and Coping Styles

A. Personality

1. Personality traits and coping styles are individuals' **unique ways of responding** to the environment and interpersonal relationships.
2. These characteristics are influenced by **innate temperament** interacting with **life experiences** and are important determinants of how people react to illness.

B. Personality disorders (see also Chapter 20)

1. Personality traits that lead to **personal distress or to problems in social or occupational functioning** may be diagnosed as personality disorders.

TABLE 16-1	SPIKES: A SIX-STEP PROTOCOL FOR GIVING PATIENTS BAD NEWS
Step	**Techniques**
Setting up interview	Arrange for privacy
	Involve significant others at patient's request
	Sit down and maintain eye contact with patient
	Touch patient's arm or hand (if comfortable for patient)
	Silence your pager and do not respond to phone
Perception of patient	Find out how what patient understands about medical situation
	Determine if patient is using denial or wishful thinking
	Determine if patient has unrealistic expectations about diagnosis
Invitation	Find out how patient would like to receive diagnosis and related information
	Find out how much detail patient wishes to have
	Offer to answer questions in future
	Offer to talk to a relative or friend
Knowledge	Prepare patient for bad news
	Give positive news first
	Present bad news clearly and unambiguously
	Give information in small doses and check patient's understanding regularly
	Use nontechnical words of explanation if possible
	Avoid conveying hopelessness
Emotions/empathy	Observe patient's emotions
	Ask patient about his or her feelings
	Connect patient's emotion with reason for it (e.g., news about the illness)
	Tolerate patient's distress
	Stay near patient and wait silently for him or her to speak
	Ask patient if anyone should be called
Strategy/summary	Ask patient if he or she is ready to discuss treatment
	Evaluate patient's understanding, expectations, and hopes for future
	Share decision-making responsibility with patient
	Understand goals of patient (e.g., pain control)
	State immediate plans for care
	Schedule a follow-up visit

Reprinted with permission from Baile WF, Buckman R, Lenzi R, et al. SPIKES A six-step protocol for delivering bad news: Application to the patient with cancer. Oncologist 2000;5:302–311.

2. Personality disorders are **chronic and lifelong.**
3. The *Diagnostic and Statistical Manual of Mental Disorders,* 4th edition, text revision (DSM-IV-TR) classifies personality disorders into three clusters based on shared characteristics.
    a. **Cluster A:** paranoid, schizoid, schizotypal
    b. **Cluster B:** histrionic, narcissistic, antisocial, borderline
    c. **Cluster C:** avoidant, obsessive–compulsive, dependent
4. The way that patients interact with doctors is influenced by the patients' personality type/disorder (Table 16-2).

TABLE 16-2	**PERSONALITY TYPES AND THE DOCTOR—PATIENT RELATIONSHIP**	
Patient Snapshot	**Personality Type**	**Doctor–Patient Relationship**
A 55-year-old man who has symptoms suggesting a cardiovascular disorder refuses to have a blood test recommended by his doctor. He states that doctors often try to make money by recommending tests that people do not need.	Paranoid	Questions physician's motives and may blame physician for illness
Because he prefers to be alone, a 30-year-old man with symptoms of diabetes puts off going to the doctor. By the time he does come in, he is so ill that he must be hospitalized. The doctor finds that the patient is content with his relatively solitary lifestyle and finds no evidence of a formal thought disorder.	Schizoid	Seems detached and withdrawn and shows little or no emotional connection with doctor
An oddly dressed 42-year-old woman tells the doctor that when she became ill with scleroderma, she decided to adopt nine cats. She says that the cats bring her luck and that she can sense their thoughts.	Schizotypal	Has odd thought patterns and behaves strangely and even more inappropriately when ill
A 38-year-old woman comes to the physician's office dressed in a very low cut blouse. She reports that she is in agonizing pain but states that she feels much better when the doctor begins to examine her.	Histrionic	Reports symptoms dramatically Approaches physician in an inappropriate sexual fashion during illness
A 48-year-old man asks the doctor to refer him to a physician who graduated from a top-ranking medical school. He says he knows the doctor will not be offended because it is obvious that he is better than the doctor's other patients.	Narcissistic	Feels superior to others; is demanding; and when ill, is sensitive to a perceived lack of attention from doctor May refuse needed treatment if it threatens his or her perfect self-image
A 35-year-old man brags to his physician that he has been charged with shoplifting a number of times but has never been convicted. After he leaves, the doctor notices that a prescription pad is missing.	Antisocial	Often charming but tells lies and manipulates to get his or her way May steal from doctor's office
A 20-year old female college student asks her physician for a date and then becomes very upset when he refuses. After the interview, she tells the physician that all of the other doctors she has seen were terrible and that he is the only doctor who has ever understood her problems (use of splitting as a defense mechanism; see Table 12-1).	Borderline	Feeling of aloneness and emptiness Overidealizes and then overreacts to perceived rejection by doctor
A 45-year-old woman who works as an office assistant and lives with her elderly aunt states that family members often tell her she is too shy. She reports that she usually refuses overtures of friendship from co-workers because she is afraid that they will not like her.	Avoidant	Fears rejection by doctor and so avoids needed tests and treatment
A 33-year-old man who has diabetes reports that each night he makes up a written schedule for his behavior and for all of the food that he will eat for the next day. He spends the rest of the office visit showing the doctor extensive food lists and schedules.	Obsessive–compulsive	Fears loss of control when ill Perfectionistic and follows doctor's orders to the letter
A 42-year-old female patient recently diagnosed with hypertension asks her doctor if she can call him every morning to ask his advice about her activities, diet, and exercise program.	Dependent	Excessive need to be cared for by others results in helplessness and the desire for decision making by physician during illness

5. **Medications** can be used to treat associated symptoms such as depression and anxiety but **have no proven usefulness** in personality disorders.

C. **Coping styles**
1. Patients with **cluster A** personality types or disorders are likely to respond to their illness by becoming even more **withdrawn or suspicious.**
2. Patients with **cluster B** personality types or disorders are more likely to become **emotional and seductive** when stressed by illness.
3. Patients with **cluster C** personality types or disorders show **increased anxiety** and may be even more fearful than other patients about losing control and becoming dependent during illness.

V. Adherence

A. **Adherence** is the extent to which a patient follows the instructions of the physician. These instructions include the following:
1. Taking medications on schedule
2. Having a needed medical test or surgical procedure
3. Following directions for changes in lifestyle, such as diet or exercise

B. **Factors affecting adherence**
1. Adherence is **not related to** patient intelligence, education, sex, religion, race, socioeconomic status, or marital status.
2. Adherence **is related to** personality traits and defense mechanisms.
3. Adherence is **positively associated** with how well the patient likes the doctor and how ill the patient feels.
4. Factors associated with adherence are listed in Table 16-3.

TABLE 16-3	FACTORS ASSOCIATED WITH ADHERENCE TO MEDICAL ADVICE	
Factors That Increase Adherence		**Factors That Decrease Adherence**
Good physician–patient relationship (most important factor)		Perception of physician as cold and unapproachable
Likes physician		Anger at physician
Feels ill		Few symptoms
Limitation of usual activities		Little disruption of activities
Written instructions for taking medication		Oral instructions for taking medication
Acute illness		Chronic illness
Simple treatment schedule		Complex treatment schedule
Short time spent in waiting room		Long time spent in waiting room
Recommending one behavioral change at a time (e.g., this week, stop smoking)		Recommending multiple behavioral changes at the same time (e.g., stop smoking and start exercising and dieting)
Belief that benefits of care outweigh its financial and time costs (health belief model)		Belief that financial and time costs of care outweigh its benefits
Peer support (particularly in adolescents with chronic illnesses)		Little peer support

Adapted with permission from Fadem B. High-Yield Behavioral Science, 2nd ed. Baltimore, Lippincott Williams & Wilkins, 2001.

C. Beliefs and adherence. To be effective in helping patients, physicians need to have **respect for and work in the context of patients' beliefs** (see Chapter 12). For example:

1. Make available the **special foods** that patients believe can help them.
2. Work with patients who believe that **outside influences** (e.g., a hex or a curse imposed by the anger of an acquaintance or relative) can cause illness, for example, ask how the hex can be removed.
3. If requested by the patient, include **folk or religious healers** (e.g., *chamanes, curanderos,* and *espiritistas* among Latinos) in the treatment plan.

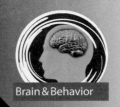
Section IV
NEUROLOGIC AND PSYCHIATRIC DISORDERS AND THEIR TREATMENT

Chapter **17**

Assessment and Classification of Patients with Behavioral Symptoms

I. Neurobiologic Assessment

Biological abnormalities and unidentified medical illnesses can cause neuropsychiatric symptoms in otherwise mentally healthy individuals and can exacerbate such symptoms in people already diagnosed with neurologic and psychiatric illnesses.

Patient Snapshot 17-1

The wife of a retired 73-year-old man tells the doctor that her husband has been acting differently over the past few months. She reports that he no longer does the crossword puzzles he formerly enjoyed and shows little interest in the television shows he had looked forward to. His wife is convinced that he is depressed or is developing Alzheimer disease. Physical and neurologic examinations are essentially normal, but ocular examination reveals bilateral central lens opacities (cataracts). After cataract surgery, the patient's interest in his environment and day-to-day activities gradually return to normal.

A. Physical examination and blood studies

1. The physical examination includes the assessment of neurologic function, particularly of **sensory systems** such as vision and hearing. Unidentified loss of sensory function can lead to withdrawal and depression, particularly in the elderly (Patient Snapshot 17-1).

2. **Skin lesions** identified in the physical examination can indicate illegal drug use or unreported domestic abuse.

3. **Blood studies** include complete blood count (CBC), erythrocyte sedimentation rate (ESR), and the **metabolic screening battery** (serum electrolyte levels, glucose level, and hepatic and renal function tests).

4. Analysis of blood B_{12} and **folate levels** and a **toxicology screen** to identify drug abuse should also be conducted for patients with neuropsychiatric symptoms.

B. Measurement of biogenic amines and psychotropic drugs

1. Altered levels of biogenic amines and their metabolites occur in some psychiatric conditions (see Chapter 11).

2. Plasma levels of some antipsychotic and antidepressant agents are measured to evaluate **patient compliance** or to determine whether **therapeutic blood levels** of the agent have been reached.

3. Laboratory tests are also used to monitor patients for complications of pharma-cotherapy.

   a. Patients taking the antimanic agent carbamazepine (Tegretol) or the antipsychotic agent clozapine (Clozaril) must be observed for blood abnormalities such as **agranulocytosis** (white blood cell count <2000), which typically presents in the emergency room as a severe throat infection.

   b. **Liver function** tests are used in patients being treated with carbamazepine and valproic acid (antimanic agents).

   c. **Thyroid function** and **kidney function** tests should be used in patients who are being treated with the antimanic agent **lithium.** Patients taking lithium can develop hypothyroidism and nephrotoxicity.

   d. Lithium levels also should be monitored regularly because of the drug's **narrow therapeutic range.**

Patient Snapshot 17-2

A 34-year-old woman visits her family physician complaining of fatigue and feeling cold all the time. Her symptoms started about 1 year earlier. The interview reveals that the patient feels that her job as a secretary is exhausting, and she wants to give it up. The patient says that these problems have made her feel sad and hopeless and that she cries frequently. Physical examination reveals that the patient has gained 8 lb in the past year. Her skin and hair appear dry, and her voice is hoarse. Laboratory studies indicate that serum concentrations of thyroid stimulating hormone (TSH) are increased and triiodothyronine (T_3) and thyroxine (T_4) are decreased. A few weeks after treatment with L-thyroxine (Synthroid) is initiated, the patient's serum thyroid hormone and TSH levels are normal. Over the next few weeks her mood and energy level gradually improve.

C. **Tests of endocrine function**

   1. **Dexamethasone suppression test (DST)**

      a. In a normal patient with a normal hypothalamic-adrenal-pituitary axis, dexamethasone, a synthetic glucocorticoid, **suppresses the secretion of cortisol.**

      b. In contrast, approximately half of patients with **major depressive disorder** have a positive DST (i.e., this suppression is limited or absent).

      c. There is some evidence that patients with a positive DST (indicating reduced suppression of cortisol) will respond well to treatment with antidepressant agents or to electroconvulsive therapy.

      d. The DST has **limited clinical usefulness.**

         i. Positive findings are not specific.

         ii. Nonsuppression is seen in conditions other than major depressive disorder, including schizophrenia, dementia, Cushing disease, pregnancy, anorexia nervosa, severe weight loss, and endocrine disorders.

         iii. Nonsuppression is also seen with use, abuse, and withdrawal of alcohol and antianxiety agents.

   2. **Thyroid function tests.** Hypothyroidism and hyperthyroidism can mimic depression and anxiety, respectively.

      a. Physical signs and symptoms of **hypothyroidism** include fatigue, weight gain, edema, hair loss, and cold intolerance (Patient Snapshot 17-2).

      b. Physical signs and symptoms of **hyperthyroidism** include rapid heartbeat (palpitations), flushing, fever, weight loss, and diarrhea.

      c. Psychiatric symptoms are associated with other endocrine disorders, such as **Addison disease** and **Cushing disease.**

D. **Neuroimaging and electroencephalogram (EEG) studies.** Structural brain abnormalities and EEG changes may be associated with specific behavioral disorders (Table 17-1).

TABLE 17-1	NEUROIMAGING AND ELECTROENCEPHALOGRAPHY IN THE BIOLOGIC EVALUATION OF THE PSYCHIATRIC PATIENT
Specific Test or Measure	**Uses and Characteristics**
Computed tomography (CT)	Identifies anatomically based brain changes (e.g., enlarged brain ventricles) in cognitive disorders such as Alzheimer disease and in schizophrenia
Nuclear magnetic resonance imaging (NMRI)	Identifies demyelinating disease (e.g., multiple sclerosis)
	Shows biochemical condition of neural tissues without exposing patient to ionizing radiation
Positron emission tomography (PET) or functional MRI (fMRI)	Localizes areas of brain that are physiologically active during specific tasks by characterizing and measuring metabolism of glucose in neural tissue
	Measures specific neurotransmitter receptors
	Requires use of a cyclotron
Single-photon emission tomography (SPECT)	Obtains similar data to PET and fMRI but is more practical for clinical use because it uses a standard γ-camera
Electroencephalogram (EEG)	Measures electrical activity in cortex
	Is useful in diagnosing epilepsy and in differentiating delirium (abnormal EEG) from dementia (often normal EEG)
	May show, in schizophrenic patients, decreased α waves, increased θ and δ waves, and epileptiform activity
Evoked EEG (evoked potentials)	Measures electrical activity in cortex in response to tactile, auditory, sound, or visual stimulation
	Used to evaluate vision and hearing loss in infants and brain responses in comatose and suspected brain-dead patients

Adapted from Fadem B. BRS Behavioral Science, 4th ed. Baltimore, Lippincott Williams and Wilkins, 2005:42.

E. Neuropsychological tests

1. Neuropsychological tests are designed to assess general intelligence, memory, reasoning, orientation, perceptuomotor performance, language function, attention, and concentration in patients with suspected neurologic problems, such as **dementia** and **brain damage** (Table 17-2).

2. In such patients, the **Folstein Mini-Mental State Examination** (Table 17-3) can follow improvement or deterioration, and the **Glasgow Coma Scale** (Table 17-4) can assess level of consciousness.

F. Other tests

1. **Drug-assisted interviewing**

   a. Administration of a sedative such as **amobarbital sodium** (the Amytal interview) before the clinical interview may be useful in determining whether organic pathology is responsible for symptomatology in patients who exhibit certain psychiatric disorders or malingering.

   b. Use of such a sedative can relax patients with conditions such as **dissociative disorder, conversion disorder** (see Chapter 21), or disorders involving high

TABLE 17-2	NEUROPSYCHOLOGICAL TESTS USED IN PSYCHIATRY
Test	**Uses**
Halstead-Reitan Battery	To detect and localize brain lesions and determine their effects
Luria-Nebraska Neuropsychological Battery	To determine left or right cerebral dominance
	To identify specific types of brain dysfunction, such as dyslexia
Bender Visual Motor Gestalt Test	To evaluate visual and motor ability through the reproduction of designs

TABLE 17-3	FOLSTEIN MINI-MENTAL STATE EXAMINATION	
Skill Evaluated	Sample Instructions to the Patient	Maximum Score[a]
Orientation	Tell me where you are and what day it is	10
Language	Name the object that I am holding	8
Attention and calculation	Subtract 7 from 100 and then continue to subtract 7s	5
Registration	Repeat the names of these three objects	3
Recall	After 5 min, recall the names of these three objects	3
Construction	Copy this design	1

[a]Maximum total score = 30; total score < 25 suggests cognitive problems; total score < 20 suggests significant impairment.

Adapted with permission from Fadem B, Simring S. High-Yield Psychiatry, 2nd ed. Baltimore, Lippincott Williams & Wilkins, 2003:8.

levels of anxiety and **mute psychotic states** (see Chapters 19 and 20), so that they can express themselves coherently during an interview.

2. **Sodium lactate administration.** Intravenous (IV) administration of sodium lactate can provoke a **panic attack** in susceptible patients and can thus help identify individuals with panic disorder (see Chapter 20). **Inhalation of carbon dioxide** can produce the same effect.

II. Psychiatric Assessment

Diagnosis of a patient with behavioral symptoms is based primarily on the history and clinical interview (see Chapter 16). Standardized testing such as IQ tests and personality tests may be done to augment the clinician's impression of the patient.

A. **Psychiatric evaluation of patients with emotional symptoms**
   1. **Psychiatric history.** The patient's psychiatric history is taken as part of the medical history. The psychiatric history includes questions about mental illness, drug and alcohol use, sexual activity, current living situation, and sources of stress.
   2. **The mental status examination (MSE) and related instruments**
      a. The MSE is a structured interview that evaluates an individual's current state of mental functioning (Table 17-5).

TABLE 17-4	GLASGOW COMA SCALE[a]		
Number of Points	Best Eye-Opening Response (E)	Best Verbal Response (V)	Best Motor Response (M)
1	No eye opening	No verbal response	No motor response
2	Opens eyes in response to painful stimulus	Makes incomprehensible sounds	Shows extension to painful stimuli
3	Opens eyes in response to verbal command	Speaks using inappropriate words	Shows flexion to painful stimuli
4	Opens eyes spontaneously	Makes confused verbal response	Withdraws from painful stimulus
5	—	Is oriented and can converse	Localizes a source of pain
6	—	—	Obeys commands

[a]Maximum total score = 15; lowest possible score = 3; total score > 12 indicates mild impairment; total score 9–12 moderate impairment; total score < 9 severe neurological impairment. The reported score is commonly broken down into components (e.g., E3, V2, M4 = GCS 9).

TABLE 17-5	THE MENTAL STATUS EXAMINATION	
Category	**Definition**	**Examples**
General presentation		
Appearance	Posture	Has a hunched over posture while standing
	Grooming	Is unshaven
Appearance for age		Appears younger than chronologic age
Clothing		Is dressed inappropriately for situation
Behavior	Mannerisms	Shows unusual facial expressions or hand movements
	Psychomotor behavior	Seems physically speeded up (agitated) or slowed down (retarded)
	Tics	Shows repetitive, nonproductive movements
Attitude toward the examiner	Cooperative	Acts helpful
	Seductive	Behaves in a sexually provocative fashion toward examiner
	Hostile	Seems angry at examiner
	Defensive	Seems to take examiner's remarks personally
Sensorium and cognition		
Level of consciousness	Alertness	Glasgow Coma Scale of 3 (is in a coma) to 15 (is completely alert)
	Lethargy	Seems mentally slowed down
	Sleepiness	Seems tired
Orientation	Person	Does not know own name or with whom he or she lives
	Place	Does not know where he or she is
	Time	Does not know the year, day, or time
Memory	Immediate	Cannot remember three words when questioned after 5 min
	Recent	Cannot remember activities in the last 12 hr (verify information to rule out confabulation)
	Remote	Cannot remember historical information about oneself that most people would know
Attention	Concentration	Cannot pay attention to the examiner without being distracted by other stimuli
		Cannot repeat a string of three to six numbers forward and backward (digit span) or spell the word *world* backward
	Cognitive ability	Cannot read a simple paragraph of text
		Cannot tell you how many states are in the United States
		Cannot multiply 8 by 6
	Spatial ability	Cannot copy a simple drawing of a triangle or a square
	Abstraction ability	Cannot describe how a pear and an apple are alike
		Cannot explain the meaning of the proverb "People who live in glass houses should not throw stones"
Speech	Timbre	Speaks too softly
	Speed	Speech is pressured (seems compelled to speak quickly)
	Articulation	Speech is not readily understandable
	Deficiencies in language	Uses words poorly or has a poor vocabulary
Mood and affect	Mood	Describes feeling depressed (low, hopeless, helpless, suicidal) or manic (high, euphoric, irritable)
	Affect	Shows decreased (blunted, restricted, or flat) external expression of mood
	Congruence and appropriateness	Described mood and visible affect are similar and are appropriate to current situation
Thought		
Form or process of thought	Associations between thoughts	Has thought patterns that make sense and follow each other logically
		Has thoughts that move rapidly from one to another (flight of ideas)

(continued)

TABLE 17-5	THE MENTAL STATUS EXAMINATION (*CONTINUED*)	
Category	**Definition**	**Examples**
		Repeats thoughts over and over (i.e., perseveration)
		Responds to rhyming sounds rather than meanings of words (i.e., echolalia)
Thought content	Compulsions	Is unable to refrain from washing one's hands
	Obsessions	Is unable to get a thought out of one's head
	Phobias	Has irrational fears (e.g., fears eating in public)
	Delusions	Believes that the CIA is after him or her
	Ideas of reference	Believes that someone in a movie is talking about him or her
Perceptual problems	Illusions	Misinterprets reality (e.g., thinks that a toy on floor in a dark room is a live pet)
	Hallucinations	Has false sensory perceptions (e.g., feels insects crawling on skin)
Judgment and insight	Judgment	Has an unusual response to a hypothetical situation (e.g., says he or she would discard a stamped, addressed letter found on sidewalk)
	Insight	Understands that he or she is ill and that he or she may have contributed to illness
Reliability	Truthfulness	Using collateral information from family or friends as well as one's clinical judgment, it becomes apparent that patient is being truthful and is contributing correct information about previous hospitalizations
Impulse control	Aggressive and sexual impulses	Using history as well as current behavior, it becomes apparent that patient cannot control his or her impulses

Reprinted with permission from Fadem B, Simring S. High-Yield Psychiatry, 2nd ed. Baltimore, Lippincott Williams & Wilkins, 2003:6–7.

    b. Commonly used objective rating scales of depression are the **Hamilton, Raskin, Zung,** and **Beck** scales.
        i. In the Hamilton and Raskin scales, an examiner rates the patient.
        ii. In the Zung and Beck scales, the patient rates him- or herself (e.g., measures include sadness, guilt, social withdrawal, and self-blame).

Patient Snapshot 17-3

An 8-year-old girl (chronological age [CA] = 8) who is having difficulty in school is given the Wechsler Intelligence Scale for Children—Revised (WISC-R). The test determines that the child is functioning mentally at the level of an average 5-year-old (mental age [MA] = 5). The child's intelligence quotient (IQ) is calculated as MA/CA × 100 or 5/8 × 100 = 63. Therefore, the category of intellectual function that best describes this child is mild mental retardation (IQ = 50–70).

B. Intelligence tests
    1. Intelligence and mental age
        a. Intelligence is defined as the ability to understand abstract concepts; reason; assimilate, recall, analyze, and organize information; and meet the special needs of new situations.
        b. Mental age (MA), as defined by Alfred Binet, reflects a person's level of intellectual functioning. **Chronological age** (CA) is the person's actual age in years.

2. **Intelligence quotient (IQ)**
   a. **IQ = MA/CA × 100.** An **IQ** of **100** means that the person's mental and chronological ages are equivalent.
   b. The highest CA used to determine IQ is **15 years.**
   c. IQ is determined to a large extent by **genetic factors;** however, environmental factors such as **poor nutrition** and **illness** during development can negatively affect **IQ.**
   d. The results of IQ tests are influenced by a person's cultural background and emotional response to testing situations.
   e. IQ is relatively **stable throughout life.** In the absence of brain pathology, an individual's IQ is essentially the same in old age as in childhood.
3. **Normal intelligence**
   a. **Normal, or average, IQ** is in the **range of 90–109.**
   b. The standard deviation in IQ scores is 15. A person with an IQ that is more than two standard deviations below the mean (IQ <70) is usually considered mentally retarded (see Chapter 2). *Diagnostic and Statistical Manual of Mental Disorders,* 4th edition, text revision (DSM-IV-TR) **classifications of mental retardation** (the overlap or gap in categories is related to differences in testing instruments) are as follows:
      i. Profound (IQ <20)
      ii. Severe (IQ 20–40)
      iii. Moderate (IQ 35–55)
      iv. Mild (IQ 50–70)
      v. A score between **71** and **84** indicates **borderline** intellectual functioning.
      vi. A person with an **IQ** more than two standard deviations above the mean (IQ >130) has superior intelligence.
4. **Wechsler intelligence tests**
   a. The Wechsler Adult Intelligence Scale—Revised (**WAIS-R**) is the most commonly used IQ test.
   b. The WAIS-R has 11 subtests: 6 verbal (general information, comprehension, arithmetic, similarities, digit span, and vocabulary) and 5 performance (picture completion, block design, picture arrangement, object assembly, and digit symbol).
   c. The Wechsler Intelligence Scale for Children—Revised (**WISC-R**) is used to test intelligence in children **6–16.5** years of age.
   d. The Wechsler Preschool and Primary Scale of Intelligence (**WPPSI**) is used to test intelligence in children **4–6.5** years of age.
5. **Related tests.** The **Vineland Social Maturity Scale** is used to evaluate skills for daily living (e.g., dressing, using the telephone) in the mentally retarded (see Chapter 3) and other challenged people, such as those with impaired vision or hearing.

C. Personality tests

1. Personality tests are used to evaluate **psychopathology** and **personality characteristics** and are categorized by whether information is gathered objectively or projectively.
2. An **objective personality test** is based on questions that are **easily scored** and statistically analyzed.
3. A **projective personality test** requires the subject to interpret the questions and the examiner to interpret the responses. It is assumed that responses are based on the subject's motivational state and defense mechanisms.
4. Commonly used objective and projective personality tests are described in Table 17-6.

TABLE 17-6		PERSONALITY TESTS	
Name of test	**Uses**	**Characteristics**	**Examples**
Minnesota Multiphasic Personality Inventory	The most commonly used objective personality test Useful for primary-care physicians because no training is required for administration and scoring	Objective test Patients answer 567 true (T) or false (F) questions about themselves Clinical scales include depression, paranoia, schizophrenia, and hypochondriasis Validity scales identify trying to look ill (faking bad) or trying to look well (faking good)	I avoid most social situations (T or F) I often feel jealous (T or F) I like being active (T or F)
Rorschach Test	The most commonly used projective personality test Used to identify thought disorders and defense mechanisms	Projective test Patients are asked to interpret 10 bilaterally symmetrical ink blot designs—for example, "Describe what you see in this figure."	
Thematic Apperception Test	Stories are used to evaluate unconscious emotions and conflicts	Projective test Patients are asked to create verbal scenarios based on 30 drawings depicting ambiguous situations—for example, "Using this picture, make up a story that has a beginning, a middle, and an end."	
Sentence Completion Test	Used to identify worries and problems using verbal associations	Projective test Patients complete sentences started by examiner	"My mother . . ." "I wish . . ." "Most people . . ."

Adapted with permission from Fadem B. BRS Behavioral Science, 4th ed. Projective test Baltimore, Lippincott Williams & Wilkins, 2005:66–67.

III. DSM-IV-TR

A. Inclusion and diagnostic criteria for mental disorders are based on a consensus of current opinions and concepts in psychiatry as described in the **DSM-IV-TR,** a classification scheme devised by the American Psychiatric Association.

B. The DSM-IV-TR is compatible with the other major psychiatric classification scheme, the **tenth revision of the International Statistical Classification of Diseases and Related Health Problems (ICD-10),** developed by the World Health Organization and used mainly in Europe and other areas outside of the United States.

C. The DSM-IV-TR includes **16 major diagnostic groupings** plus a grouping called "other conditions that may be a focus of clinical attention" (Table 17-7) and uses a **multiaxial system** that codes a patient's condition along five axes. A definitive diagnosis can be made using only the first three axes. The five axes are as follows:
1. Axis I: clinical disorders
2. Axis II: personality disorders and mental retardation
3. Axis III: general medical conditions
4. Axis IV: psychosocial and environmental problems
5. Axis V: the global assessment of functioning (GAF) scale quantifies a patient's level of function in daily life and emotional symptomology on a continuum from 1

TABLE 17-7	DSM-IV-TR CLASSIFICATIONS
Condition	**Examples**
Disorders first diagnosed in infancy, childhood, or adolescence	Mental retardation, learning disorders, communication disorder, pervasive developmental disorders, attention deficit and disruptive behavior disorders
Delirium, dementia, and amnestic and other cognitive disorders	Delirium owing to congestive heart failure, Alzheimer dementia
Mental disorders caused by a general medical condition not elsewhere classified	Personality change owing to systemic lupus erythematosus
Substance-related disorders	Alcohol-related disorders, sedative-related disorders
Schizophrenia and other psychotic disorders	Schizophrenia, schizophreniform disorder
Mood disorders	Major depressive disorder, bipolar I disorder, bipolar II disorder
Anxiety disorders	Panic disorder, specific phobia, post-traumatic stress disorder
Somatoform disorders	Conversion disorder, hypochondriasis
Factitious disorders	Factitious disorder with either predominantly psychological or predominantly physical signs and symptoms
Dissociative disorders	Dissociative amnesia, depersonalization disorder
Sexual and gender identity disorders	Paraphilias, gender-identity disorders
Eating disorders	Anorexia nervosa, bulimia nervosa
Sleep disorders	Primary sleep disorders, sleep disorders related to another mental disorder
Impulse-control disorders not elsewhere classified	Intermittent explosive disorder, kleptomania
Adjustment disorders	Adjustment disorder with depressed mood, with anxiety, with mixed anxiety and depressed mood, with disturbance of conduct
Personality disorders	Paranoid personality disorder, antisocial personality disorder
Other conditions that may be a focus of clinical attention	Medication-induced movement disorders, problems related to abuse or neglect, malingering

(inability to maintain minimal personal hygiene, danger to self) to 100 (superior social and occupational functioning, no emotional symptoms).

D. Psychiatric disorders in the DSM-IV-TR may be separated into **subtypes** or have **specifiers.**
1. The subtypes are based on the **presentation** of symptoms (e.g., schizophrenia, catatonic type).
2. The specifiers denote the **features** and **severity** of the illness and describe whether the illness is in partial or full remission (e.g., major depressive disorder with psychotic features).
3. Specifiers also disclose the patient's **history** of the disorder and can be **provisional** if the practitioner believes that the full criteria for the disorder will be met over time. The specifier can also be **not otherwise specified** (NOS) if:
   a. The illness **does not meet the full criteria** for a specific disorder because it is not listed in the DSM-IV-TR
   b. The disorder meets the criteria **for more than one condition**
   c. The disorder is the result of an **organic condition**
   d. There is **not enough information** available to allow classification of the disorder

Neurologic Disorders: Inflammatory, Traumatic/Mechanical, Neoplastic, and Vascular Disorders

Brain & Behavior

I. Inflammatory Disorders

Patient Snapshot 18-1

An 18-year-old college student with no past medical history presents to the emergency room with a chief complaint of headaches for a few weeks. She also complains of increasing malaise during the same time period. Physical examination is unremarkable. A CT scan of the head is performed, and the radiologist comments that it appears within normal limits. Subsequently, a lumbar puncture is performed with the following results: cerebrospinal fluid (CSF) color is clear; opening pressure is normal; CSF glucose is about two thirds serum glucose; CSF protein is marginally increased; and the cell count shows a few lymphocytes and no neutrophils. Given the patient's age and clinical presentation, including near-normal glucose level and mild CSF protein elevation, the emergency room physician concludes that the patient has acute aseptic viral meningitis, most likely caused by an enterovirus.

A. **Infectious disorders**
1. **Meningitis** is an inflammatory process that is localized to the covering layers of the brain, the meninges. Co-involvement of brain parenchyma and the meninges is indicated by the term **meningoencephalitis.** Infectious meningitis, the focus here, can be divided into the following categories (see also Table 11-1):
   a. **Acute pyogenic bacterial meningitis** can be caused by a number of different types of bacteria. Age and immune status of the patient determine which type is most prevalent (Table 18-1)
      i. **Signs and symptoms** of bacterial meningitis include fever, headache, photophobia, irritability, mental status changes, and neck stiffness.
      ii. Two classic indications of acute bacterial meningitis are **Kernig** and **Brudzinski signs**.
         (a) Kernig sign: inability to fully extend the knee when the hip is flexed to 90° owing to severe hamstring stiffness
         (b) Brudzinski sign: flexion of the hips and knees with passive flexion of the neck, secondary to severe neck stiffness
      iii. The CSF changes that result include cloudy or purulent appearance, increased opening pressure, neutrophilic cellular predominance, elevated protein level, and markedly decreased glucose.
   b. **Acute aseptic** or **viral meningitis** is an infectious inflammation of the meninges that is often less fulminant than its bacterial counterpart.
      i. Viral meningitis is usually self-limiting and treated symptomatically.
      ii. Up to 70% of cases are caused by an Enterovirus.
      iii. The CSF changes that result include lymphocytic proliferation (pleocytosis), mild to moderate protein elevation, and near normal glucose level.
   c. **Chronic bacterial meningitis** is most commonly caused by *Mycobacterium tuberculosis.*

TABLE 18-1	COMMON CAUSES OF MENINGITIS IN DIFFERENT GROUPS	
Age or Immune Status	**Causes**
Newborns 0–6 months	*Escherichia coli*
	Listeria
Infants and children 6 months to 6 years	*Streptococcus pneumoniae*
	Neisseria meningitidis
	Haemophilus influenzae B[a]
	Enterovirus
Children and adults 6–60 years	*N. meningitides*
	Enterovirus
	S. pneumoniae
	Herpes simplex virus (HSV)
Adults 60+ years	*S. pneumoniae*
	Gram-negative rods
	Listeria
HIV-positive patients	*Cryptococcus*
	Cytomegalovirus
	Toxoplasmosis
	Creutzfeldt-Jakob disease

[a]The incidence of meningitis owing to *H. influenzae* has declined significantly since the mid-1980s as a result of the widespread use of vaccination against this organism.

    i. Patients present with typical **signs and symptoms** such as headache, general malaise, confusion, and emesis.

    ii. CSF changes include pleocytosis of mononuclear cells or a lymphocytic/neutrophilic mixture, very high elevation in protein level, and normal to moderately reduced glucose level.

    iii. The fibrinous exudate that forms at the base of the brain can be so profound as to cause cranial nerve palsies and hydrocephalus.

2. Brain abscesses are destructive and progressive lesions caused by bacterial seeding and proliferation within the brain parenchyma.

    a. Microorganisms can be introduced to the brain by **direct extension** (e.g., mastoiditis) or **hematogenous seeding** from a distant site of infection (e.g., bacterial endocarditis).

    b. Patients often present with **focal neurologic deficits** that depend on the location of the abscess. Moreover, abscess growth causes an **increase in intracranial pressure** and can ultimately lead to uncal herniation and death.

B. Immune disorders

1. Multiple sclerosis (MS) is a progressive autoimmune demyelinating disorder of the central nervous system (CNS). It is defined clinically by the occurrence of multiple discrete episodes of neurologic dysfunction separated in time and the presence of demyelinating lesions separated in anatomic space.

    a. Epidemiology. MS is the most common demyelinating disorder. It has a peak onset between ages 20 and 40 years and is twice as common in women.

b. **Pathogenesis.** MS is believed to be the result of an **inappropriate immune response** against components of myelin sheaths. Both basic science and clinical investigation indicate that activation of CD4+ T lymphocytes by myelin antigens may be involved.

c. **Pathology.** Examination of brain and spinal cord tissue from individuals with MS demonstrates multiple irregularly shaped plaques within white matter regions, particularly in the periventricular area.
   i. On MRI scans, multiple plaques in the periventricular white matter project away from the ventricles in a finger-like fashion, known as **Dawson fingers.**
   ii. Examination of the CSF can provide supporting evidence for a diagnosis of MS in the presence of the appropriate clinical picture. The CSF typically has a mildly **elevated level of protein** and a **lymphocytic pleocytosis.**
   iii. Examination of CSF protein by electrophoresis often demonstrates the presence of **oligoclonal bands,** antibodies produced by B cells in the nervous system.

d. **Clinical presentation.** The neuropsychiatric manifestations of MS depend on the location of plaque formation. However, several findings are common:
   i. Disease involving the **optic nerve,** known as **optic neuritis,** is often the first reported manifestation of MS and commonly affects just one eye, resulting in unilateral vision loss.
   ii. MS plaques in the **brainstem** can cause cranial nerve palsies, ataxia, and nystagmus.
   iii. Involvement of **spinal cord tracts** can result in both motor and sensory symptoms.

e. **Course.** The most common pattern of disease progression is that of **relapsing-remitting MS.** In this form of MS, a patient has discrete episodes of neurologic dysfunction owing to new plaque formation. Each episode is followed by slow partial recovery. This clinical pattern can occur over months to years, after which the disease can switch to **secondary-progressive** form. In this form, the disease relentlessly progresses without the benefit of remission. Patients ultimately die of illnesses secondary to neurologic dysfunction (e.g., pneumonia secondary to aspiration).

2. **Guillain-Barré syndrome** is an immune-mediated peripheral neuropathy that can lead to death owing to respiratory muscle paralysis.
   a. **Pathogenesis.** A large proportion of cases of Guillain-Barré are preceded by a flu-like syndrome. Indeed, most cases are epidemiologically associated with prior infection by *Campylobacter jejuni,* cytomegalovirus (CMV), Epstein-Barr virus, or *Mycoplasma pneumoniae.* One theory of this disease's mechanism involves activation of a T-cell response, with subsequent peripheral demyelination as a result of macrophage activation.
   b. Examination of the CSF in a patient with suspected Guillain-Barré often demonstrates **albumin-cytologic dissociation.** In other words, there is an elevated protein level in the absence of pleocytosis.
   c. **Clinical presentation.** The clinical picture of Guillain-Barré is most commonly that of rapidly progressive **ascending paralysis.** Paralysis can last from days to weeks and is followed by gradual, full recovery.

II. Traumatic and Mechanical Disorders

A. **Concussion** is a type of brain injury often brought about by a rapid change in momentum of the head.
1. Neurologic dysfunction occurs immediately on injury and includes findings such as **loss of consciousness, temporary respiratory arrest,** and **loss of deep tendon reflexes.**

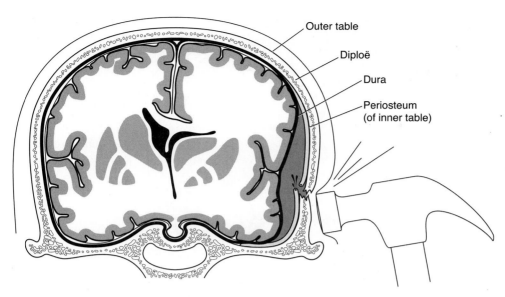

FIG 18-1. An epidural hematoma results from a laceration of the middle meningeal artery. Arterial bleeding into the epidural space forms a biconvex clot. The classic lucid interval is seen in 50% of cases. Skull fractures are usually found. Epidural hematomas rarely cross suture lines. [Fix JD. High-Yield Neuroanatomy, 3rd ed. Baltimore, Lippincott Williams & Wilkins, 2004.]

    2. Dysfunction is **temporary** and recovery is **complete,** although patients are typically amnestic to the concussive event.

B. **Diffuse axonal injury** is a more severe type of acceleration–deceleration injury to the parenchyma of the brain. A large proportion of trauma patients with this form of injury become comatose as a result.
    1. Diffuse axonal injury is caused by mechanical forces that disrupt axonal integrity and alter axoplasmic transport. It can be thought of as a shearing injury that stretches and tears axons.
    2. As indicated by the name, the deep white matter tracts of the cerebrum are most affected (e.g., corpus callosum).
    3. Microscopically, diffuse axonal injury is characterized by axonal swelling and punctate hemorrhages. On CT scan, these hemorrhages can be seen as pinpoint hyperdensities in the parenchyma.

C. **An epidural hematoma** is an accumulation of arterial blood in the potential space between the dura mater and the internal surface of the skull (Fig. 18-1). The classic epidural hematoma results from a laceration of the **middle meningeal** artery after traumatic fracture of the **temporal bone.**
    1. On CT scan an epidural hematoma appears as a **biconvex clot.** The hematoma does not traverse the suture lines of the skull because the dura is attached to the calvaria at the suture lines.
    2. Clinically, patients who have an epidural hematoma can present with a **lucid interval** after the initial trauma. This interval can last from minutes to hours and is followed by headache, obtundation, and localizing neurologic dysfunction.
    3. If not treated by prompt neurosurgical evacuation, an epidural hematoma can lead to a "blown pupil" as a result of **uncal herniation.** The profound mydriasis of the affected pupil is the result of compression of the parasympathetic fibers that travel on the outside of the oculomotor nerve.

D. **Subdural hematomas** are accumulations of venous blood that reside in the **subdural space** between the dura mater and the arachnoid (Fig. 18-2).
    1. A subdural hematoma results from tearing of the **bridging veins** that pass from the surface of the brain to drain into the dural sinuses. In elderly patients and

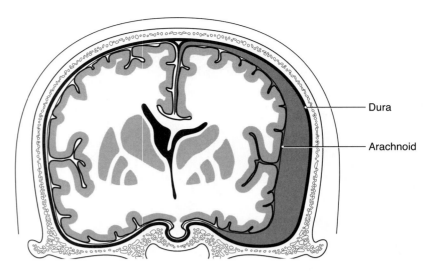

FIG 18-2. A subdural hematoma (SDH) results from lacerated bridging veins. SDHs are frequently accompanied by traumatic subarachnoid hemorrhages and cortical contusions. Sudden deceleration of the head causes tearing of the superior cerebral veins. The SDH extends over the crest of the convexity into the interhemispheric fissure but does not cross the dural attachment of the falx cerebri. The clot can be crescent shaped, biconvex, or multiloculated. SDHs are more common than epidural hematomas. SDHs always cause brain damage. [Fix JD. High-Yield Neuroanatomy, 3rd ed. Baltimore, Lippincott Williams & Wilkins, 2004.]

patients with brain atrophy owing to alcoholism, these bridging veins are stretched, making them more prone to tearing.

2. On CT scan, an acute subdural hematoma classically appears as a crescent-shaped clot that can traverse the suture lines of the skull.

3. Individuals with subdural hematomas can present with a variety of symptoms, depending on whether the bleed is **acute, subacute,** or **chronic.** Symptoms include headache, mental status changes, contralateral hemiparesis, or dementia.

III. Neoplastic Disorders

Patient Snapshot 18-2

A 62-year-old woman presents to the emergency room with a complaint of progressively worsening headaches and severe weakness on the left side of her body. These problems have been getting worse over the past 2–3 months. The emergency room physician performs a thorough physical examination, which reveals that the patient has a left-sided hemiparesis and bilateral papilledema. Because the physical examination findings and history suggest a large space-occupying lesion within the woman's skull and increased intracranial pressure, the physician sends the patient for imaging studies, including an MRI. In consultation with the hospital's neurosurgeon, who also evaluates the patient and the MRI study, the physician observes that the patient has a large frontoparietal mass that crosses the midline via the corpus callosum. There is a great deal of edema around the mass. With the woman's consent, he schedules her for surgery to treat the tumor. After the patient's surgery, the pathologist on the case reports to the surgeon that the mass is a glioblastoma multiforme, the most common and most malignant of the gliomas.

A. **Introduction.** A number of important features make neoplastic disorders of the nervous system unique.

1. Unlike neoplasia in many other organ systems, the **majority of tumors of the CNS are primary** (about two thirds); only a minority are the result of metastases (about one third). For metastatic tumors, the most common primary sites are lung (35%), breast (17%), gastrointestinal system (6%), skin/melanoma (6%), and kidney (5%).

2. A generalized anatomic distinction in the location of neoplastic lesions can be made between children and adults. About 70% of CNS tumors in children arise in the **posterior fossa.** A similar percentage of CNS tumors in adults arise in the **cerebral hemispheres.**

3. A basic histolopathologic division can be drawn in the types of primary CNS tumors. Approximately 50% are **glial** in origin, and approximately 50% are **nonglial**.

B. Figure 18-3 introduces many of the most common primary mass lesions and tumors of the CNS.

IV. Vascular Disorders

A. **Global cerebral ischemia**
1. Although the brain makes up ~**2% of body weight**, it receives ~**15% of the body's cardiac output**. Moreover, it is responsible for ~**20% of the body's oxygen consumption.**
2. Global cerebral ischemia is a varied pathologic process, the results of which depend on the severity of the insult varying from:
    a. Transient postischemic confusion to
    b. Persistent vegetative state to
    c. Brain death
3. It results from any process that causes decreased cerebral perfusion and thus oxygenation: e.g., cardiac arrest, any form of shock, and severe hypotension.
4. Different populations of cells within the nervous system are vulnerable to different intensities of ischemic insult, a phenomenon known as **selective vulnerability** (Fig. 18-4).
    a. Neurons are the most sensitive cells of the nervous system, followed by glial cells such as oligodendrocytes and astrocytes.
    b. Among neurons the following are the most vulnerable to ischemia: **pyramidal neurons of the CA1 region of the hippocampus, Purkinje neurons of the cerebellum,** and **pyramidal neurons of the neocortex.**
5. **Watershed infarcts** occur along the spectrum of global cerebral events (Fig. 18-4). They are found in wedge-shaped territories of the brain and spinal cord that lie between distal arterial fields. These areas are particularly subject to decreased perfusion. The region between the anterior cerebral artery and the middle cerebral artery is particularly vulnerable to such infarcts.

B. **Stroke**
1. **Stroke** or **cerebrovascular accident** describes the pathologic process of nervous system tissue dying secondary to prolonged ischemia.
2. **Atherosclerosis** is the major predisposing factor for stroke, and in general, results from two types of processes:
    a. **Embolization** is the release and trapping of material from a relatively distant site (e.g., atheromatous fragments, fat, air) that abruptly occludes vascular flow. Owing to the abrupt nature of this process, the blood vessels distal to the occlusion undergo necrosis and leak blood into the surrounding tissue, resulting in **secondary hemorrhage** or **hemorrhagic stroke.**

A

Germinomas
- germ cell tumors that are commonly seen in the pineal region (> 50%)
- overlie the tectum of the midbrain
- cause obstructive hydrocephalus owing to aqueductal stenosis
- the common cause of Parinaud syndrome

Brain abscesses
- may result from sinusitis, mastoiditis, hematogenous spread
- location: frontal and temporal lobes, cerebellum
- organisms: streptococci, staphylococci, and pneumococci
- result in cerebral edema and herniation

Colloid cysts of third ventricle
- make up 2% of intracranial gliomas
- are of ependymal origin
- found at the interventricular foraminia
- ventricular obstruction results in increased intracranial pressure and may cause positional headaches, "drop attacks," or sudden death

Meningiomas
- derived from arachnoid cap cells and represent the second most common primary intracranial brain tumor after astrocytomas (15%)
- are not invasive; they indent the brain; may produce hyperostosis
- pathology: concentric whorls and calcified psammoma bodies
- location: parasagittal and convexity
- gender: females > men
- associated with neurofibromatosis 2 (NF-2)

Ependymomas

Astrocytomas
- represent 20% of the gliomas
- historically benign
- diffusely infiltrate the hemispheric white matter
- most common glioma found in the posterior fossa of children

Glioblastoma multiforme
- represents 55% of gliomas
- malignant; rapidly fatal astrocytic tumor
- commonly found in the frontal and temporal lobes and basal ganglia
- frequently crosses the midline via the corpus callosum (butterfly glioma)
- most common primary brain tumor
- histology: pseudopalisades, perivascular pseudorosettes

Oligodendrogliomas
- represent 5% of all the gliomas
- grow slowly and are relatively benign
- most common in the frontal lobe
- calcification in 50% of cases
- cells look like fried eggs (perinuclear halos)

B

Choroid plexus papillomas
- historically benign
- represent 2% of the gliomas
- one of the most common brain tumors in patients < 2 years of age
- occur in decreasing frequency: fourth, lateral, and third ventricle
- CSF overproduction may cause hydrocephalus

Cerebellar astrocytomas
- benign tumors of childhood with good prognosis
- most common pediatric intracranial tumor
- contain pilocytic astrocytes and Rosenthal fibers

Medulloblastomas
- represent 7% of primary brain tumors
- represent a primitive neuroectodermal tumor (PNET)
- second most common posterior fossa tumor in children
- responsible for the posterior vermis syndrome
- can metastasize via the CSF tracts
- highly radiosensitive

Hemangioblastomas
- characterized by abundant capillary blood vessels and foamy cells; most often found in the cerebellum
- when found in the cerebellum and retina, may represent a part of the von Hippel-Lindau syndrome
- 2% of primary intracranial tumors; 10% of posterior fossa tumors

Intraspinal tumors
- Schwannomas 30%
- Meningiomas 25%
- Gliomas 20%
- Sarcomas 12%
- Ependymomas represent 60% of intramedullary gliomas

Craniopharyngiomas
- represent 3% of primary brain tumors
- derived from epithelial remnants of Rathke pouch
- location: suprasellar and inferior to the optic chiasma
- cause bitemporal hemianopia and hypopituitarism
- calcification is common

Pituitary adenomas (PAs)
- most common tumors of the pituitary gland
- prolactinoma is the most common (PA)
- derived from the stomodeum (Rathke pouch)
- represent 8% of primary brain tumors
- may cause hypopituitarism, visual field defects (bitemporal hemianopia and cranial nerve palsies CN III, IV, VI, V1, and V2 and postganglionic sympathetic fibers to the dilator muscle of the iris)

Schwannomas (acoustic neuromas)
- consist of Schwann cells and arise from the vestibular division of CN VIII
- make up 8% of intracranial neoplasms
- pathology: Antoni A and B tissue and Verocay bodies
- bilateral acoustic neuromas are diagnostic of NF-2

Brain stem glioma
- usually a benign pilocytic astrocytoma
- usually causes cranial nerve palsies
- may cause the locked-in syndrome

Ependymomas
- represent 5% of the gliomas
- histology: benign, ependymal tubules, perivascular pseudorosettes
- 40% are supratentorial; 60% are infratentorial (posterior fossa)
- most common spinal cord glioma (60%)
- third most common posterior fossa tumor in children and adolescents

FIG 18-3. Supratentorial **(A)** and infratentorial (posterior fossa) and intraspinal **(B)** tumors of the central and peripheral nervous systems. In children, 70% of tumors are infratentorial. In adults, 70% of tumors are supratentorial. *CN,* cranial nerve; *CSF,* cerebrospinal fluid. [Fix JD. High-Yield Neuroanatomy, 3rd ed. Baltimore, Lippincott Williams & Wilkins, 2004.]

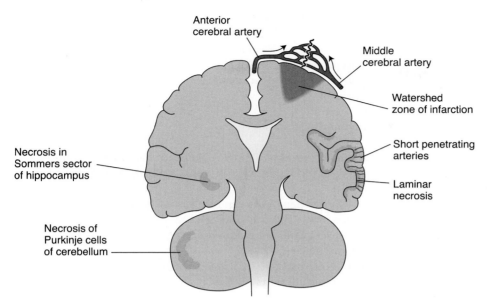

FIG 18-4. Consequences of global ischemia. A global insult induces lesions that reflect the sensitivity of individual neuronal systems (pyramidal cells of Sommer sector of the hippocampus, Purkinje cells) and the vascular architecture (watershed infarcts, laminar necrosis). [Rubin E, Gorstein F, Rubin R et al. Rubin's Pathology: Clinicopathologic Foundations of Medicine, 4th ed. Philadelphia, Lippincott Williams & Wilkins, 2005.]

    b. **Thrombosis** is clot formation within a blood vessel. This tends to occur more slowly and thus gradually deprives downstream arteries of blood. As a result, secondary hemorrhage is less likely and the tendency is toward **ischemic stroke.**

  3. The normal distribution of the brain's blood supply determines the extent and location of a stroke (Fig. 18-5). Thus the resulting neurologic deficits are as varied as the possible locations of ischemia.

  4. When local cerebral dysfunction occurs as a result of cerebral ischemia, lasts for <24 hr, and is followed by complete recovery, it is defined as a **transient ischemic attack (TIA).** Patients who have a history of TIAs are at increased risk for a stroke.

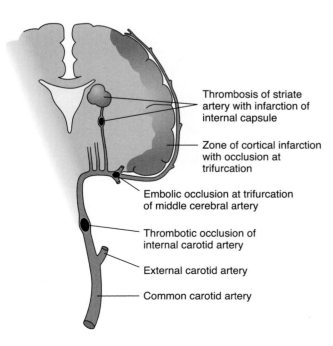

Thrombosis of striate artery with infarction of internal capsule

Zone of cortical infarction with occlusion at trifurcation

Embolic occlusion at trifurcation of middle cerebral artery

Thrombotic occlusion of internal carotid artery

External carotid artery

Common carotid artery

FIG 18-5. Distribution of cerebral infarcts. The normal distribution of the cerebral vasculature defines the pattern and size of infarcts and, consequently, their symptoms. Occlusion at the trifurcation causes cortical infarcts with motor and sensory loss and often aphasia. Occlusion of a striate branch transects the internal capsule and causes a motor deficit. [Rubin E, Gorstein F, Rubin R et al. Rubin's Pathology: Clinicopathologic Foundations of Medicine, 4th ed. Philadelphia, Lippincott Williams & Wilkins, 2005.]

C. **Spontaneous intraparenchymal hemorrhage**
1. Atraumatic intraparenchymal hemorrhage is most frequent from the **4th** to the **6th decades** of life. Around 50% of spontaneous intraparenchymal hemorrhages are the result of **hypertension**. Other important contributors are the following:
   a. **Coagulopathies** (including iatrogenic coagulopathies—think heparin, warfarin, clopidogrel)
   b. **Neoplasm**
   c. **Amyloid angiopathy**
   d. **Vasculitis**
2. **Chronic hypertension** causes pathologic changes to blood vessel walls (e.g. hyaline change, proliferative changes, necrosis) that make them weaker and prone to rupture.
   a. **Charcot-Bouchard aneurysms** can result from chronic hypertension. These are small aneurysms (<300 μm) that tend to form along the path of a vessel (not at a bifurcation) and are common to the basal ganglia. These can rupture, resulting in hemorrhage.
   b. Certain locations are particularly prone to hypertensive bleeds:
      i. **Basal ganglia–thalamus** (65%)
      ii. **Pons** (15%)
      iii. **Cerebellum** (8%)
3. The clinical features of spontaneous intraparenchymal hemorrhage depend on the location and extent of the bleed.
4. When hemorrhage extends into the ventricular system, it is known as **intraventricular hemorrhage.**
   a. This event generally portends a worse prognosis.
   b. Blood can rapidly accumulate in the ventricular system, causing compression of surrounding structures.
   c. If a patient survives more than a few days, **hydrocephalus** can result because the blood in the ventricular system clots and blocks the normal flow of CSF.

D. **Lacunar infarcts**
1. Another effect of chronic hypertension is a **lacunar infarct.** In particular, the deep penetrating arteries of the brain (e.g., to basal ganglia) undergo arteriolar sclerosis and can become occluded.
2. The results of the occlusions are **multiple small cavitary infarcts** that resemble lakes, for which these infarcts are named.
3. Again, the resulting signs and symptoms depend on location, extent, and frequency of lacunar infarcts.

E. **Subarachnoid hemorrhage and ruptured aneurysms**
1. **Cerebral aneurysms.** In general, aneurysms form as a result of changes in intravascular pressure and arterial wall integrity. Specific causes include the following:
   a. **Developmental defects** at points of arterial bifurcation that are believed to occur during embryogenesis. The results are **berry aneurysms,** or saccular aneurysms, of which >90% form at arterial branch points in the carotid system (Fig. 18-6).
   b. **Atherosclerosis** in the large cerebral vessels (e.g., carotids, basilar, vertebral arteries) causes destruction of arterial wall anatomy and aneurysm formation. Aneurysms caused by atherosclerosis tend to be elongated and **fusiform.**
   c. Aneurysms that result from infections in the walls of cerebral arteries are known as **mycotic aneurysms.** They form when septic emboli get lodged in vessels, bacteria proliferate, inflammation is triggered, and vessel walls break down.
2. Rupture of a cerebral aneurysm causes **subarachnoid hemorrhage (SAH).** More than 75% of spontaneous SAHs are the result of aneurysmal rupture.

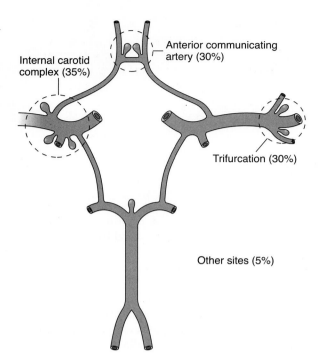

Internal carotid complex (35%)

Anterior communicating artery (30%)

Trifurcation (30%)

Other sites (5%)

FIG 18-6. Incidence of saccular aneurysms (berry aneurysms, which preferentially involve the carotid tributaries). [Rubin E, Gorstein F, Rubin R et al. Rubin's Pathology: Clinicopathologic Foundations of Medicine, 4th ed. Philadelphia, Lippincott Williams & Wilkins, 2005.]

- **a.** **Symptoms** and **signs** of SAH include sudden severe headache (e.g., "the worst headache of my life"), nausea, vomiting, meningeal signs, photophobia, and coma.
- **b.** Diagnosis of SAH is made with the aid of CT scan. Acute blood in the cisterns and fissures will appear **hyperdense** (e.g., bright). If not seen on a CT scan, a lumbar puncture can be performed. A positive lumbar puncture will demonstrate frankly bloody CSF that does not clear with collection into successive tubes or xanthochromic (e.g., pink or yellowish coloration resulting from erythrocyte breakdown) CSF. MRI is another diagnostic alternative.
- **c.** The gold standard diagnostic test for the detection of a cerebral aneurysm is **cerebral angiography.**

3. Management of SAH requires prompt neurosurgical consultation.

Chapter 19

Psychotic and Mood Disorders

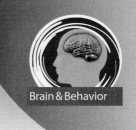

Brain & Behavior

I. Overview

The **psychotic disorders** (e.g., schizophrenia) and the **mood** disorders (e.g., major depressive disorder and bipolar disorder) are the **most serious and debilitating** psychiatric disorders.

A. Characteristics

1. **Psychotic episodes.** Patients experience periods of time in which they are out of touch with reality (psychotic episodes) in both psychotic and mood disorders. Psychotic episodes are characterized by false beliefs (i.e., delusions) such as being followed by government agents and/or false perceptions (i.e., **hallucinations**), such as hearing voices, as well as other perceptual and thought abnormalities (Table 19-1).
   a. **Schizophrenia** is characterized by repeated psychotic episodes.
   b. **Bipolar patients** commonly have psychotic symptoms in the manic phase; patients with **depression** sometimes experience such episodes (depression with psychotic features).

2. **Increased risk of suicide**
   a. **Suicide risk is high** in patients with schizophrenia. More than 50% of patients attempt suicide (often during postpsychotic depression or when having hallucinations "commanding" them to harm themselves), and 10% of those die in the attempt.
   b. Suicide attempts and suicide are also common in patients with mood disorders.
   c. These disorders and a variety of demographic, psychosocial, and physical factors are associated with increased suicide risk (Table 19-2).

3. **Level of consciousness.** Patients with mood disorders and schizophrenia have a normal level of consciousness and are oriented to person, place, and time when not experiencing psychotic symptoms.

B. Occurrence

1. Schizophrenia and bipolar disorder occur **equally in men and women** and each occurs in **1% of the population** in all cultures and ethnic groups studied.
2. Major depressive disorder is **twice as common in women** (10–20%) than in men (5–12%) and also occurs in all cultural and ethnic groups.
3. Because patients with schizophrenia tend to drift down the socioeconomic scale as a result of their social deficits (the **downward drift hypothesis**), they are often found in lower socioeconomic groups (e.g., homeless people).

C. Psychosocial etiology

1. **Biologic factors** are paramount in the etiology of **schizophrenia** and **bipolar disorder.** Psychosocial factors play much less of a role in these disorders.
2. **Both** biologic and psychosocial factors are involved in the development of **major depressive disorder.** The **psychosocial** factors include the following:
   a. **Loss of a parent** in childhood
   b. **Sexual abuse** in childhood

TABLE 19-1	SYMPTOMS OF PSYCHOSIS: DISORDERS OF PERCEPTION, THOUGHT CONTENT, THOUGHT PROCESSES, AND FORM OF THOUGHT		
Disorder of	Symptom	Definition	Example
Perception	Illusion	Misperception of real external stimuli	Interpreting appearance of a coat in a dark closet as a man
	Hallucination	False sensory perception	Seeing snakes crawling on ceiling when none exist
Thought content	Delusion	False belief not shared by others	Feeling that police are listening to one's thoughts
	Idea of reference	False belief of being referred to by others	Feeling of being discussed by someone on television
Thought processes	Impaired abstraction ability	Problems discerning essential qualities of objects or relationships	When asked what brought him or her to emergency room, patient says "an ambulance"
	Magical thinking		Knocking on wood to prevent something bad from happening
Form of thought	Loose associations	Shift of ideas from one subject to another in an unrelated way	Patient begins to answer a question about his or her health and then shifts to a statement about baseball
	Neologisms	Inventing new words	Patient refers to doctor as a "medocrat"
	Tangentiality	Getting further away from point as speaking continues	Patient begins to answer a question about his or her health and ends up talking about a sister's abortion

Reprinted with permission from Fadem B. BRS Behavioral Science, 4th ed. Baltimore, Lippincott Williams & Wilkins, 2005:99.

    c. **Loss of a spouse** or child in adulthood
    d. **Loss of health**
    e. **Low self-esteem** and negative interpretation of life events
    f. **Learned helplessness** (e.g., because attempts to escape bad situations in the past have proven futile, the person now feels helpless and essentially gives up; see Chapter 12)

D. Biologic origin
    1. **Genetic factors.** Individuals with a **close genetic relationship** to a patient with schizophrenia or mood disorders such as bipolar disorder are more likely than those with a more distant relationship to develop such disorders (Table 19-3).
    2. **Altered neurotransmitter activity** (see Chapter 11)
        a. **Dopamine**
            i. The **dopamine hypothesis of schizophrenia** states that schizophrenia results from **excessive dopaminergic activity** (e.g., excessive number of dopamine receptors, excessive concentration of dopamine, hypersensitivity of receptors to dopamine).
            ii. **Reduced dopamine activity** may be involved in symptoms of **depression.**
        b. **Serotonin and norepinephrine**
            i. The **monoamine hypothesis of mood disorders** states that **hypoactivity of serotonin and norepinephrine** are implicated in **depression** and **hyperactivity** is implicated in **mania.**
            ii. **Hyperactivity** of serotonin is also implicated in **schizophrenia.**
        c. **Glutamate.** Agents that act as antagonists of the N-methyl-D-aspartate (NMDA) subtype of glutamate receptors can
            i. Increase (e.g., phencyclidine) or decrease (e.g., memantine) psychotic symptoms
            ii. Relieve symptoms of depression

TABLE 19-2		RISK FACTORS FOR SUICIDE	
Category	Factor	Increased Risk	Decreased Risk
History	Previous suicidal behavior	Serious suicide attempt (about 30% of people who attempt suicide try again; 10% succeed)	Suicidal gesture, but not a serious attempt, was made
		Less than 3 months' time has passed since previous attempt	More than 3 months' time has passed since suicidal gesture
		Possibility of rescue was remote	Rescue was very likely
	Family history	Close family member (especially parent) committed suicide	No family history of suicide
		Having divorced parents (especially for adolescents)	Intact family
		Being <11 years old at the time of a parent's death	Parents alive through childhood
Current psychological, physical, and social factors	Psychiatric symptoms	Severe depression / Psychotic symptoms / Hopelessness / Impulsiveness	Mild depression / No psychotic symptoms / Some hopefulness / Thinks things out
	Depth of depression	Initial stages of recovery from deep depression; recovering patients may have enough energy to commit suicide	The depth of severe depression; patients rarely have clarity of thought or energy needed to plan and commit suicide
	Substance use	Alcohol and drug dependence	Little or no substance use
		Current intoxication	Not intoxicated
	Physical health	Serious medical illness (cancer, AIDS)	Good health
		Perception of serious illness (most patients have visited a physician within 6 months before suicide)	No recent visit to a physician
	Social relationships	Divorced (particularly men)	Married
		Widowed	Strong social support systems
		Single, never married	Has children
		Lives alone	Lives with others
Demographic factors	Age	Elderly (persons 65+ years of age, especially elderly men)	Children (up to age 15 years)
		Middle-aged (>55 years of age in women; >45 years in men)	Young adults (age 25–40 years)
		Adolescents (suicide is third leading cause of death in those 15–24 years of age; rates increase after neighborhood suicide of a teen or after television shows depicting teenage suicide)	
	Sex	Male sex (men successfully commit suicide three times more often than women)	Female sex (although women attempt suicide three times more often than men)
	Occupation	Professional	Nonprofessional
		Physicians (especially women and psychiatrists)	
		Dentists	
		Police officers	
		Attorneys	

TABLE 19-2		RISK FACTORS FOR SUICIDE (*CONTINUED*)	
Category	Factor	Increased Risk	Decreased Risk
		Musicians	
		Unemployed	Employed
	Race	White (66% of successful suicides are white males)	Nonwhite
	Religion	Jewish	Catholic
		Protestant	Muslim
	Economic conditions	Economic recession or depression	Strong economy
Lethality	Plan and means	A plan for suicide (e.g., decision to stockpile pills)	No plan for suicide
		A means of committing suicide (e.g., access to a gun)	No means of suicide
		Sudden appearance of peacefulness in an agitated, depressed patient (patient has reached an internal decision to kill him- or herself and is now calm)	
	Method	Shooting oneself	Taking pills
		Crashing one's vehicle	Slashing one's wrists
		Hanging oneself	
		Jumping from a high place	

Reprinted with permission from Fadem B. BRS Behavioral Science, 4th ed. Baltimore, Lippincott Williams & Wilkins, 2005:111–113.

   d. **Protein kinase C** (**PKC**) hyperactivity has been demonstrated in both schizophrenia and bipolar disorder.
 3. **Neuroanatomy**
   a. **Decreased activity of the frontal lobes** and of **limbic structures** is seen in the brains of people with psychotic and mood disorders (Fig. 19-1).
   b. **Lateral and third ventricle enlargement,** abnormal cerebral symmetry, and changes in brain density are seen in people with psychotic disorders and in those with mood disorders with psychotic features.

E. **Physical illness and related factors**
 1. **Medical conditions and nonpsychoactive medications** can cause psychotic or mood symptoms and thus mimic schizophrenia or mood disorders—*Diagnostic*

TABLE 19-3	RISK OF DEVELOPING SCHIZOPHRENIA AND BIPOLAR DISORDER IN RELATIVES OF PATIENTS	
Relationship to a Patient with the Disorder	Approximate Risk for Schizophrenia (%)	Approximate Risk for Bipolar Disorder (%)
No relationship (general population)	1	1
First-degree relative (sibling, dizygotic twin, parent)	10	20
Child of two parents	40	60
Monozygotic twin	50	70

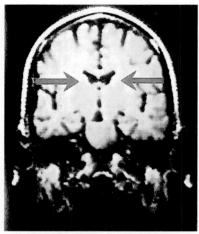

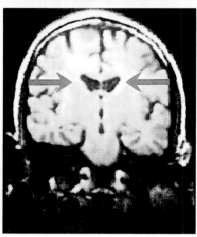

FIG 19-1. Enlarged lateral ventricles in schizophrenia. These MRI scans are from the brains of identical twins. The scan on the *top* is from the normal sibling; the one on the *bottom* is from the sibling who has been diagnosed with schizophrenia. Note the enlarged lateral ventricles in the sibling with schizophrenia, indicating loss of brain tissue. [Reprinted with permission from Bear MF, Connors BW, Paradiso MA. Neuroscience: Exploring the Brain, 3rd ed. Baltimore, Lippincott Williams & Wilkins, 2007:22–12.]

and Statistical Manual of Mental Disorders, 4th edition, text revision (DSM-IV-TR) diagnosis: psychotic disorder or mood disorder caused by a general medical condition (Table 19-4).

2. **Psychiatric illnesses** other than schizophrenia and mood disorders that may be associated with psychotic and mood symptoms include the following:

    a. **Cognitive disorders** (e.g., delirium, dementia, and amnestic disorder) (see Chapter 4)

    b. **Substance-related disorders** (see Chapter 14)

    c. **Personality disorders** (see Chapter 20)

II. Schizophrenia and Other Psychotic Disorders

Patient Snapshot 19-1

A 35-year-old man with schizophrenia states that his roommates are spying on him by listening through the electrical outlets. For this reason, he has changed roommates a number of times over the past 5 years. He dresses strangely, is dirty with unkempt hair, and seems preoccupied. He reports that he has trouble paying attention to the doctor's questions because "I am listening to my leader giving me instructions in my head." Physical examination is essentially normal. Neuroimaging reveals hypoactivity of the prefrontal cortex and limbic structures and enlarged brain ventricles.

TABLE 19-4	MEDICAL CONDITIONS AND NONPSYCHOTROPIC AGENTS ASSOCIATED WITH PSYCHOTIC AND MOOD SYMPTOMS	
Condition or Agent	**Mania and Schizophrenia**	**Depression**
Associated medical conditions	Neoplasms	Neoplasms (pancreatic and other gastrointestinal tumors)
	Rheumatologic disorders (systemic lupus erythematosus)	Viral illnesses (pneumonia, influenza, AIDS)
	Endocrine disorders (Cushing syndrome, acute intermittent porphyria)	Endocrine disorders (hypothyroidism, Addison disease)
	Neurologic disorders (Parkinson disease, Huntington disease, multiple sclerosis)	Neurologic disorders (Parkinson disease, Huntington disease, multiple sclerosis, stroke [particularly left frontal])
Nonpsychotropic agents	Analgesics (pentazocine)	Antihypertensives (reserpine, propranolol, verapamil)
	Antiarrhythmics (quinidine)	Steroid hormones (corticosteroids, progesterone)
	Anticholinergics (atropine)	Anticonvulsants
	Antibiotics (iproniazid)	Antibiotics (tetracycline)
	Antihistamines (phenylephrine)	Cardiac glycosides (digitalis)

A. **Schizophrenia,** the prototype of the psychotic disorders, is a **chronic, debilitating** mental disorder that first appears in adolescence or early adulthood.

B. **Symptoms** of schizophrenia can be classified as positive or negative.
   1. **Positive symptoms** are things **additional** to expected behavior and include delusions, hallucinations, agitation, and talkativeness.
   2. **Negative symptoms** are things **missing** from expected behavior and include lack of motivation, social withdrawal, flattened affect, cognitive disturbances, poor grooming, and poor (i.e., impoverished) speech content.
   3. These classifications can be useful in predicting the effects of antipsychotic medication (see Chapter 22).
      a. **Positive symptoms** respond well to most **traditional** and **atypical antipsychotic agents.**
      b. **Negative symptoms** respond better to **atypical** than to traditional antipsychotics.

C. **Course.** Schizophrenia has **three phases:** prodromal, psychotic, and residual.
   1. **Prodromal** signs and symptoms occur before the first psychotic episode and include avoidance of social activities; physical complaints; and new interest in religion, the occult, or philosophy.
   2. In the **psychotic phase,** the patient loses touch with reality. Positive symptoms occur during an acute psychotic episode.
   3. In the **residual phase** (time period between psychotic episodes), **the patient is in touch with reality** but does not behave normally. Rather, the patient shows negative symptoms as well as persistent disturbances of thought, behavior, appearance, speech, and affect.

D. **Prognosis.** Schizophrenia usually involves repeated psychotic episodes and a **chronic, downhill course** over years. The **prognosis is better** and the suicide risk is lower if the patient is older at the onset of the illness, is married or has other social relationships, or is female.

E. **Subtypes.** The **DSM-IV-TR** lists five subtypes of schizophrenia (Table 19-5).

TABLE 19-5	DSM-IV-TR SUBTYPES OF SCHIZOPHRENIA
Subtype	**Characteristics**
Disorganized	Poor grooming and disheveled personal appearance
	Inappropriate emotional responses (e.g., silliness)
	Facial grimacing, mirror gazing
	Onset before 25 years of age
Catatonic	Stupor or agitation, lack of coherent speech
	Bizarre posturing (waxy flexibility)
	Rare since the introduction of antipsychotic agents
Paranoid	Delusions of persecution
	Better functioning and older age at onset than other subtypes
Undifferentiated	Characteristics of more than one subtype
Residual	At least one previous psychotic episode
	Subsequent residual symptoms but no current frank psychotic symptoms

Reprinted with permission from Fadem B. BRS Behavioral Science, 4th ed. Baltimore, Lippincott Williams & Wilkins, 2005:101.

F. Other psychotic disorders. Psychotic disorders are all characterized at some point during their course by a loss of touch with reality. However, the other psychotic disorders do **not include all of the criteria** required for the diagnosis of schizophrenia (Table 19-6).

TABLE 19-6	SCHIZOPHRENIA AND OTHER PSYCHOTIC DISORDERS	
Disorder	**Characteristics**	**Prognosis**
Schizophrenia	Psychotic and residual symptoms lasting >6 months	Lifelong social and occupational impairment
Brief psychotic disorder	Psychotic symptoms lasting >1 day, but <1 month; often precipitating psychosocial factors	50–80% recover completely
Schizophreniform disorder	Psychotic and residual symptoms lasting 1–6 months	33% recover completely
Schizoaffective disorder	Symptoms of a mood disorder as well as psychotic symptoms	Lifelong social and occupational impairment (somewhat higher overall level of functioning than schizophrenia)
Delusional disorder	Fixed, persistent, nonbizarre delusional system (paranoid in persecutory type and romantic—often with a famous person—in erotomanic type); few if any other thought disorders	50% recover completely; many have relatively normal social and occupational functioning
Shared psychotic disorder (folie a deux)	Development of delusions in a person in a close relationship (e.g., spouse, child) with someone with delusional disorder (the inducer)	10–40% recover completely when separated from the inducer

Reprinted with permission from Fadem B. BRS Behavioral Science, 4th ed. Baltimore, Lippincott Williams & Wilkins, 2005:102.

Patient Snapshot 19-2

A 26-year-old medical student is brought to the emergency department by her husband. The husband tells the doctor that his wife has shown odd behavior ever since failing an exam 2 weeks earlier. In particular, she told him that her professors are trying to poison her. The woman has no prior psychiatric history and physical examination and laboratory results are unremarkable. She is given the diagnosis of brief psychotic disorder. Her paranoid delusions resolve after treatment with antipsychotic medication, and she goes home after 3 days in the hospital. About 1 month later, the patient, who is no longer taking the antipsychotic medication, shows no sign of psychotic thinking.

G. Treatment
1. **Pharmacologic treatments** for schizophrenia and other psychotic disorders include traditional antipsychotics (dopamine$_2$ receptor antagonists) and atypical antipsychotic agents (see Chapter 22). Because of their better side-effect profiles, the atypical agents are now first-line treatments.
2. **Psychological treatments,** including individual, family, and group psychotherapy, are useful for **providing long-term support** and to foster **compliance** with the drug regimen (see Chapter 23).

III. Major Depressive Disorder, Bipolar Disorder, and Other Mood Disorders

Patient Snapshot 19-3

A 65-year-old woman who was diagnosed with advanced lung cancer 3 months earlier, has lost 18 lb, wakes frequently during the night, and has very little energy. Over the past month she has been preoccupied with feelings of guilt about "people I have hurt in my life" and expresses concern that she will die alone. While weight loss, insomnia, and loss of energy are common in patients with advanced cancer, this patient's preoccupation with feelings of guilt indicate that she is experiencing a major depressive episode rather than a normal reaction to serious illness. Because antidepressants take about 3 weeks to relieve depression and this patient has a limited life span, a faster-acting treatment such as a stimulant agent or electroconvulsive therapy may be more appropriate to treat her depression.

A. Definitions
1. The mood disorders are characterized by a primary **disturbance** in **internal emotional state** causing subjective distress and problems in functioning.
2. **Given the patient's current social and occupational situation,** he or she emotionally feels the following:
   a. Somewhat worse than would be expected (**dysthymia**)
   b. Very much worse than would be expected (**depression**)
   c. Somewhat better than would be expected (**hypomania**)
   d. Very much better than would be expected (**mania**)
3. The **categories** of primary mood disorders are major depressive disorder, bipolar disorder (I and II), dysthymic disorder, and cyclothymic disorder.
4. **Symptoms** of **depression** and **mania** are given in Table 19-7

B. Epidemiology. There are **no differences** in the occurrence of mood disorders associated with ethnicity, education, marital status, or income.

TABLE 19-7	SYMPTOMS OF DEPRESSION AND MANIA	
Episode	**Symptom**	**Occurrence[a]**
Depression	Depressed mood (has feelings of sadness, hopelessness, helplessness, low self-esteem, and excessive guilt)	++++ (hallmark)
	Reduced interest or pleasure in most activities (in severe form this is called *anhedonia*, inability to respond to pleasurable stimuli)	++++
	Reduced energy and motivation	++++
	Anxiety (is apprehensive about imagined dangers)	++++
	Sleep problems (wakes frequently at night and too early in morning)	++++
	Cognitive problems (has difficulty with memory and concentration)	+++
	Psychomotor retardation (is slowed down) (seen particularly in elderly) or agitation (is speeded up)	+++
	Decreased appetite (has less interest in food and sex; in atypical depression, patients overeat)	+++
	Diurnal variation in symptoms (feels worse in morning and better in evening)	++
	Suicidal ideation (has thoughts of killing oneself)	++
	Suicide (takes own life)	+
	Psychotic symptoms (has delusions of destruction and fatal illness)	+
Mania	Elevated mood (has strong feelings of happiness and physical well-being)	++++ (hallmark)
	Grandiosity and expansiveness (has feelings of self-importance)	++++
	Irritability and impulsivity (is easily bothered and quick to anger)	++++
	Disinhibition (shows uncharacteristic lack of modesty in dress or behavior)	++++
	Assaultiveness (cannot control aggressive impulses; has problems with law)	++++
	Distractibility (cannot concentrate on relevant stimuli)	++++
	Flight of ideas (thoughts move rapidly from one to other)	++++
	Pressured speech (seems compelled to speak quickly)	++++
	Impaired judgment (provides unusual responses to hypothetical questions; e.g., says he or she would buy a blood bank if inherited money)	++++
Psychotic symptoms	Has delusions (that are often grandiose; e.g., of power and influence)	+++

[a]Approximate percentage of patients in which the sign or symptom is seen: +, <25%; ++, 50%; +++, 70%; ++++, >90%.

Reprinted with permission from Fadem B. BRS Behavioral Science, 4th ed. Baltimore, Lippincott Williams & Wilkins, 2005:109.

C. Major depressive disorder
1. **Characteristics:** recurrent episodes of depression, each continuing **for at least 2 weeks**
2. **Masked depression**
   a. As many as 50% of depressed patients seem unaware of or deny depression and thus are said to have **masked depression.**
   b. Patients with masked depression often visit primary-care doctors complaining of **vague physical symptoms.**
   c. These complaints may be **mistaken for hypochondriasis** (see Chapter 21).
   d. In contrast to patients with hypochondriasis, depressed patients show other symptoms of depression (e.g., severe weight loss, intense guilt) in addition to their physical complaints.
3. **Seasonal affective disorder (SAD)**
   a. SAD is a subtype of major depressive disorder associated with the **winter** season and short days.
   b. Many SAD patients improve in response to full-spectrum light exposure.

D. Bipolar disorder
1. In bipolar disorder, there are episodes of **both mania and depression (bipolar I** disorder) or **both hypomania and depression (bipolar II** disorder).
2. There is no simple manic disorder because depressive symptoms eventually occur. Therefore, **one episode of symptoms of mania** (Table 19-7) alone or hypomania plus one episode of major depression defines bipolar disorder.

E. Other mood disorders
1. **Dysthymic disorder** involves dysthymia continuing over a **2-year period** with no discrete episodes of illness.
2. **Cyclothymic disorder** involves periods of hypomania and dysthymia occurring over a **2-year period** with no discrete episodes of illness.
3. In contrast to major depressive disorder and bipolar disorder, dysthymic disorder and cyclothymic disorder are less severe, nonepisodic, chronic, and **never associated with psychosis.**

F. Prognosis
1. Untreated episodes of depression and mania are usually **self-limiting** and last 6–12 months and 3 months, respectively.
2. In contrast to schizophrenia in which patients are chronically impaired, in mood disorders the patient's mood and functioning typically **return to normal** between episodes.

G. Treatment
1. Treatment for **depression and dysthymia** includes **antidepressant agents**—for example, heterocyclics, selective serotonin reuptake inhibitors (SSRIs), monoamine oxidase inhibitors (MAOIs), and stimulants—as well as psychotherapy and electroconvulsive therapy (ECT) (see Chapters 22 and 23).
2. Treatment for **bipolar disorder and cyclothymic disorder** includes **mood stabilizers** (e.g., lithium and anticonvulsants), **sedative agents** (e.g., lorazepam), and **antipsychotics** (e.g., olanzapine) as well as ECT.

Chapter 20

Anxiety, Stress, Adjustment, Personality, and Eating Disorders

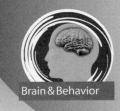

Brain & Behavior

I. Anxiety, Stress, and Adjustment Disorders

Patient Snapshot 20-1

A 40-year-old man tells his physician that he is often late for work. He attributes this problem to the fact that he gets out of bed repeatedly during the night to recheck the locks on the doors and to be sure the gas jets on the stove are turned off. His lateness is exacerbated by his need to count all of the traffic lights along the route to work. If he suspects that he missed a light, he becomes quite anxious and must then go back and recount them all. Physical examination and laboratory studies are unremarkable. The most effective long-term treatment for this patient with obsessive–compulsive disorder (OCD) is a selective serotonin reuptake inhibitor (SSRI) such as fluoxetine or fluvoxamine.

A. Fear and anxiety
1. Fear is a normal reaction to a known, external source of danger.
2. In anxiety, the individual is frightened but the source of the danger is not known, not recognized, or **inadequate to account for the symptoms.**
3. The **physiologic manifestations** of anxiety involve activation of the **autonomic nervous system** (ANS) and are similar to those of fear:
   a. Shakiness and sweating
   b. Palpitations (subjective experience of tachycardia)
   c. Tingling in the extremities and numbness around the mouth
   d. Dizziness and syncope (fainting)
   e. Gastrointestinal and urinary disturbances (e.g., diarrhea, urinary frequency
   f. Mydriasis (pupil dilation)

B. Classification of the anxiety disorders and adjustment disorder
1. The *Diagnostic and Statistical Manual of Mental Disorders,* 4th edition, text revision (**DSM-IV-TR**) **classification** of anxiety disorders includes the following:
   a. Panic disorder (with or without agoraphobia)
   b. Phobias (specific and social)
   c. Obsessive–compulsive disorder (OCD)
   d. Generalized anxiety disorder (GAD)
2. The anxiety disorders also include the **stress disorders**
   a. Post-traumatic stress disorder (PTSD)
   b. Acute stress disorder (ASD)
3. Patient snapshots and descriptions of these disorders are given in Table 20-1.

TABLE 20-1	DSM-IV-TR CLASSIFICATION OF THE ANXIETY DISORDERS AND ADJUSTMENT DISORDERS
Patient Snapshot	**Characteristics**

Panic disorder (with or without agoraphobia)

 A 23-year-old college student comes to the emergency room after experiencing a sudden onset of increased heart rate and profuse sweating during her drive to school. She states that she thinks she is having a heart attack. She notes that these episodes have occurred at least four times in the past few weeks Physical examination is essentially normal.

Episodic (about twice weekly) periods of intense anxiety (i.e., panic attacks)

Cardiac and respiratory symptoms

The conviction that one is about to die

Sudden onset of symptoms, increasing in intensity over a period of approximately 10 min and lasting about 30 min (attacks rarely follow a fixed pattern)

Attacks can be induced by administration of sodium lactate or carbon dioxide (see Chapter 17)

Strong genetic component

More common in young women in their 20s

In panic disorder with agoraphobia, characteristics and symptoms of panic disorder are associated with fear of open places or situations in which patient cannot escape or obtain help (agoraphobia)

Panic disorder with agoraphobia is associated with separation anxiety disorder in childhood (see Chapter 3)

Phobias (specific and social)

 A 28-year-old woman cannot leave her house because she is afraid that she will see a cat on the street. Because of this fear of cats, she has had to give up her job and cannot pay her bills.

In specific phobia, there is an irrational fear of certain things (e.g., elevators, snakes, or closed-in areas)

In social phobia (social anxiety disorder), there is an exaggerated fear of embarrassment in social situations (e.g., public speaking, eating in public, using public restrooms)

Because of fear, the patient avoids object or situation

Avoidance leads to social and occupational problems

Obsessive–compulsive disorder (OCD)

See Patient Snapshot 20-1

Recurring, intrusive feelings, thoughts, and images (obsessions) that cause anxiety

Anxiety is relieved in part by performing repetitive actions (compulsions)

A common obsession is avoidance of hand contamination and a compulsive need to wash hands after touching things

Repeated checking (e.g., of gas jets on stove) and counting objects are also common

Patients usually have insight (i.e., they realize that these thoughts and behaviors are irrational and want to eliminate them)

Usually starts in early adulthood but may begin in childhood

Genetic factors are involved; increased in first-degree relatives of Tourette disorder patients

Generalized anxiety disorder (GAD)

 A 42-year-old woman complains of chronic indigestion diarrhea that have been present for many years. She also reports that she has always had trouble falling asleep and asks her doctor for a prescription for sleeping pills.

Persistent anxiety symptoms, including hyperarousal and worrying, lasting 6 months or more Gastrointestinal symptoms are common

Symptoms are not related to a specific person or situation (i.e., free-loating anxiety)

Commonly starts during the 20s

(continued)

TABLE 20-1	DSM-IV-TR CLASSIFICATION OF THE ANXIETY DISORDERS AND ADJUSTMENT DISORDERS *(CONTINUED)*

Patient Snapshot	Characteristics

Post-traumatic stress disorder (PTSD) and acute stress disorder (ASD)

 A 28-year-old man who was in a house fire 2 years earlier in which some people died reports that he often has nightmares about the fire and wakes up in a cold sweat with a pounding heart. He worries about fires whenever he is at the movies and is anxious about fire even though he locates every potential exit before sitting down.

Symptoms occurring after a catastrophic (life-threatening or potentially fatal) event (e.g., war, earthquake, serious accident, rape, robbery) affecting patient or patient's close friend or relative

Symptoms can be divided into four types: reexperiencing (e.g., intrusive memories of event—flashbacks—and nightmares), hyperarousal (e.g., anxiety, increased startle response, impaired sleep, hypervigilance), emotional numbing (e.g., difficulty connecting with others) and avoidance (e.g., survivor's guilt, dissociation, social withdrawal)

In PTSD, symptoms last for >1 month (sometimes years)

In ASD, symptoms last only between 2 days and 4 weeks

Adjustment disorder[a]

 About 3 months after moving to a new city, a teenager who was formerly outgoing and a good student seems sad, loses interest in friends, and begins to do poor work in school. His appetite is normal and there is no evidence of suicidal ideation. Four months later, he has made a few friends and his schoolwork improves.

Emotional symptoms (e.g., anxiety, depression, conduct problems) causing social, school, or work impairment occurring within 3 months and lasting <6 months after a serious (but usually not life-threatening) life event (e.g., divorce, bankruptcy, changing residence)

Symptoms can persist for >6 months in presence of a chronic stressor

[a]Included here because it often must be distinguished from PTSD.

Adapted with permission from Fadem B. BRS Behavioral Science. 4th ed. Baltimore, Lippincott Williams & Wilkins, 2005:121.

C. The organic basis of anxiety

1. Neurotransmitters involved in the development of anxiety include γ-aminobutyric acid (GABA) (decreased activity), serotonin (decreased activity), and norepinephrine (increased activity) (see Chapter 11).

2. The **locus ceruleus** (site of noradrenergic neurons), **raphe nucleus** (site of serotonergic neurons), caudate nucleus (particularly in OCD), temporal cortex, and frontal cortex are likely to be involved in anxiety disorders (see Chapter 6).

3. Organic causes of symptoms of anxiety include **excessive caffeine intake,** substance abuse, hyperthyroidism, vitamin B_{12} deficiency, hypoglycemia or hyperglycemia, cardiac arrhythmia, anemia, pulmonary disease, and **pheochromocytoma** (adrenal medullary tumor).

4. If the cause is primarily organic, a diagnosis of **substance-induced anxiety disorder** or **anxiety disorder caused by a general medical condition** may be appropriate.

D. Treatment of the anxiety disorders

1. **Antianxiety agents** include benzodiazepines, buspirone, and β-blockers (see Chapter 22)

   a. **Benzodiazepines** carry a high risk of dependence and addiction and so are usually used for only a limited time to treat acute anxiety symptoms—for example, **alprazolam** (Xanax) for emergency treatment of **panic attacks.**

   b. **Buspirone** (BuSpar) is a nonbenzodiazepine antianxiety agent that, because it has **low abuse potential,** is useful as long-term maintenance therapy for patients with GAD. However, buspirone has little immediate effect on anxiety symptoms because it takes up to 2 weeks to work.

   c. **β-Blockers** such as **propranolol** (Inderal) are used to control **autonomic symptoms** (e.g., tachycardia) when performing in public or taking an examination.

2. Antidepressants (see Chapter 22)

    a. Antidepressants—**monoamine oxidase inhibitors** (MAOIs); **tricyclics;** and especially **selective serotonin reuptake inhibitors** (SSRIs) such as paroxetine (Paxil), fluoxetine (Prozac), and sertraline (Zoloft)—are the most effective long-term (maintenance) therapy for panic disorder and for OCD.

    b. The antidepressants **doxepin** (Sinequan) and **venlafaxine** (Effexor) are approved to treat GAD.

    c. Paroxetine, sertraline, and venlafaxine are also indicated in the treatment of social phobia.

3. Psychological treatment

    a. **Systematic desensitization** and **cognitive therapy** are the most effective treatments for phobias and are useful adjuncts to pharmacotherapy in other anxiety disorders. Behavioral therapies such as flooding and implosion are also useful (see Chapter 23).

    b. **Support groups** (e.g., victim survivor groups) are particularly useful for ASD and PTSD.

II. Personality Disorders

Patient Snapshot 20-2

A single 30-year-old woman who has been smoking three packs of cigarettes a day for the last 10 years asks the physician to help her stop smoking. The doctor asks the patient why she smokes so much. The patient responds, "I always feel very alone and empty inside; I smoke to fill myself up." The patient reveals that she sometimes cuts the skin on her arms with a knife to "feel something." She also notes that because she was afraid to be alone, she tried to commit suicide after a man with whom she had had two dates did not call her again. The physician notes that the patient shows characteristics of borderline personality disorders.

A. Characteristics

    1. Individuals with personality disorders show **chronic, lifelong, rigid, unsuitable patterns of relating to others** that cause social and occupational problems (e.g., loneliness, job loss) and difficulties in interactions with physicians (see Table 16-2).

    2. Those with personality disorders generally are not aware that they are the cause of their own problems (i.e., they **do not have insight**), do not have frank psychotic symptoms and **do not seek psychiatric help.**

B. Classification

    1. Personality disorders are categorized by the **DSM-IV-TR** into **clusters: A** (paranoid, schizoid, schizotypal), **B** (histrionic, narcissistic, borderline, and antisocial), and **C** (avoidant, obsessive–compulsive, and dependent).

    2. Each cluster has its own hallmark characteristics and genetic or familial associations, (e.g., relatives of people with personality disorders have a higher likelihood of having certain psychiatric disorders) (Table 20-2).

    3. For the DSM-IV-TR diagnosis, a personality disorder must be present by early adulthood. Antisocial personality disorder cannot be diagnosed until age 18; before that age, the diagnosis is conduct disorder (see Chapter 3).

C. Treatment

    1. For those who seek help, individual and group psychotherapy may be useful.

    2. Pharmacotherapy can also be used to treat symptoms such as depression and anxiety, which may be associated with the personality disorders.

TABLE 20-2	DSM-IV-TR CLASSIFICATION AND CHARACTERISTICS OF THE PERSONALITY DISORDERS
Personality Disorder	**Characteristics**
Cluster A	**Hallmark:** avoids social relationships, is "peculiar" but not psychotic
	Genetic association: psychotic illnesses
Paranoid	Distrustful, suspicious, litigious
	Attributes responsibility for own problems to others
	Interprets motives of others as malevolent
Schizoid	Long-standing pattern of voluntary social withdrawal
	No thought disorder
	Restricted emotions
Schizotypal	Peculiar appearance
	Magical thinking (i.e., believing that one's thoughts can affect course of events)
	Odd thinking and behavior without frank psychosis
Cluster B	**Hallmark:** dramatic, emotional, inconsistent
	Genetic association: mood disorders, substance abuse, and somatoform disorders
Histrionic	Theatrical, extroverted, emotional, sexually provocative, "life of party"
	In men, Don Juan in dress and behavior
	Shallow, vain, cannot maintain intimate relationships
Narcissistic	Pompous, with a sense of special entitlement
	Lacks empathy for others
Antisocial	Refuses to conform to social norms and shows no concern for others
	Associated with conduct disorder in childhood and criminal behavior in adulthood (psychopaths or sociopaths)
Borderline	Erratic, impulsive, unstable behavior and mood
	Feeling bored, alone, and empty
	Suicide attempts for relatively trivial reasons
	Self-mutilation (cutting or burning oneself)
	Often comorbid with mood and eating disorders
	Mini-psychotic episodes (i.e., brief periods of loss of contact with reality)
Cluster C	**Hallmark:** fearful, anxious
	Genetic association: anxiety disorders
Avoidant	Sensitive to rejection, socially withdrawn
	Feelings of inferiority
Obsessive–compulsive	Perfectionistic, orderly, inflexible
	Stubborn and indecisive
	Ultimately inefficient
Dependent	Allows other people to make decisions and assume responsibility for them
	Poor self-confidence, fear of being deserted and alone
	May tolerate abuse by domestic partner

Adapted with permission from Fadem B. BRS Behavioral Science. 4th ed. Baltimore, Lippincott Williams & Wilkins, 2005:134–135.

III. Obesity and Eating Disorders

Patient Snapshot 20-3

A 16-year-old ballet dancer who is 5 feet, 7 inches tall and currently weighs 95 lb tells the doctor that she needs to lose another 15 lb to pursue a career in dance. Her mood appears good. Findings on physical examination are normal except for excessive growth of downy body hair. Laboratory tests reveal evidence of hypokalemia, and X-ray examination reveals evidence of early osteoporosis. She reports that she has not menstruated in more than 1 year. The physician diagnoses anorexia nervosa.

A. Obesity
1. **Overview**
   a. Obesity is defined as being **>20% over ideal weight** based on common height and weight charts or having a **body mass index** (**BMI**; body weight [kg]/height [m^2]) of **30 or higher.**
   b. At least **25% of adults** are obese and an increasing number of children are overweight (at or above the 95th percentile of BMI for age) in the United States.
   c. Obesity is **not an eating disorder.**
   d. **Genetic factors** are most important in obesity; adult weight is closer to that of biologic rather than of adoptive parents.
   e. Obesity is more common in lower socioeconomic groups and is associated with increased risk for cardiorespiratory problems, hypertension, diabetes mellitus, sleep, and orthopedic problems.
2. **Treatment**
   a. Most weight loss achieved using commercial dieting and weight loss programs is **regained within a 5-year period.**
   b. **Bariatric surgery** (e.g., gastric bypass, gastric banding) is initially effective but has less value for maintaining long-term weight loss.
   c. Pharmacologic agents for weight loss include **orlistat** (Xenical), a pancreatic lipase inhibitor that limits the breakdown of dietary fats; **sibutramine hydrochloride** (Meridia), which blocks monoamine reuptake, thereby increasing feelings of satiety; and **phendimetrazine** (Adipost), which has amphetamine-like appetite-suppressing effects.
   d. A combination of **sensible dieting and exercise** is the most effective to way to maintain long-term weight loss.

B. Eating disorders: anorexia nervosa and bulimia nervosa
1. In anorexia nervosa and bulimia nervosa, the patient shows abnormal behavior associated with food despite a **normal appetite.**
2. The subtypes of anorexia nervosa are the **restricting type**—excessive dieting—and **binge eating–purging type**—excessive dieting plus binge eating (consuming large quantities of high-calorie food at one time) and purging (vomiting or misuse of laxatives, diuretics, and enemas).
3. The subtypes of bulimia nervosa are the **purging type** (binge eating and purging) and **nonpurging type** (binge eating and excessive dieting or exercising but no purging).
4. Eating disorders are **more common in women** and in **higher socioeconomic groups** and are more common in the United States and other developed countries because these societies value thinness.
5. Physical and psychological characteristics and treatment of anorexia nervosa and bulimia nervosa are given in Table 20-3.

TABLE 20-3	**PHYSICAL AND PSYCHOLOGICAL CHARACTERISTICS AND TREATMENT OF ANOREXIA NERVOSA AND BULIMIA NERVOSA**		
Disorder	**Physical Characteristics**	**Psychological Characteristics**	**Treatment[a]**
Anorexia nervosa	Extreme weight loss (15% or more of normal body weight) Amenorrhea (three or more consecutively missed menstrual periods) Metabolic acidosis Hypokalemia Hypercholesterolemia Mild anemia and leukopenia Lanugo (downy body hair on the trunk) Melanosis coli (blackened area of the colon if there is laxative abuse) Osteoporosis Cold intolerance Syncope	Refusal to eat despite normal appetite because of an overwhelming fear of being obese Unrealistic perception of oneself as "fat" even when one is thin Abnormal behavior dealing with food (e.g., simulating eating) Lack of interest in sex Was a "perfect" child (e.g., good student) Interfamily conflicts (e.g., patient's problem draws attention away from parental marital problem or an attempt to gain control to separate from mother) Excessive exercising (hypergymnasia)	Hospitalization directed at reinstating nutritional condition (starvation can result in death) Family therapy (aimed particularly at mother–daughter relationship) Psychoactive drugs are relatively ineffective
Bulimia and nervosa	Relatively normal body weight Esophageal varices caused by repeated vomiting Tooth enamel erosion owing to gastric acid in the mouth Swelling or infection of the parotid glands Metacarpal–phalangeal calluses (Russell sign) from the teeth because the hand is used to induce gagging Electrolyte disturbances Menstrual irregularities	Binge eating (in secret) of high-calorie foods, followed by vomiting or other purging behavior to avoid weight gain (binge eating and purging also occurs in 50% of patients with anorexia nervosa) Depression Hypergymnasia	Cognitive behavioral therapies Average to high doses of antidepressants Psychotherapy

[a]Listed in order of highest to lowest utility.

Adapted with permission from Fadem B. BRS Behavioral Science, 4th ed. Baltimore, Lippincott Williams & Wilkins, 2005:136.

Chapter 21

Psychosomatic and Neuropsychiatric Disorders

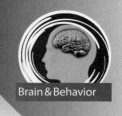
Brain & Behavior

I. Psychosomatic Illnesses and Related Disorders

A. Overview

1. At least **30%** of the **physical complaints** of medical patients are not well explained by organic illness.
2. Such patients may have underlying medical illnesses that have eluded detection—so-called **unexplained illnesses.**
3. Alternatively, such patients may have emotional conditions leading to physical symptom production: **psychosomatic or somatoform disorders** or **masked depression.**
4. Even physical complaints that can be explained by organic illness are likely to have some **psychosomatic components.**
5. Unexplained symptoms are also seen when illnesses are purposely feigned, as in **factitious disorder** and **malingering.**

B. Somatoform disorders

Patient Snapshot 21-1

A 50-year-old woman has a 25-year history of vague physical complaints including nausea, painful menses, and loss of feeling in her legs. Today she reports tenderness around the umbilicus. Physical examination and laboratory workup are unremarkable. The patient says that she has always had physical problems, particularly when she is under stress, but is puzzled that her doctors never seem to identify their cause. The physician talks with the patient about her current life stressors and sets up a follow-up appointment in 1 month's time.

1. Somatoform disorders are characterized by **physical symptoms without sufficient organic cause.**
2. The patient thinks that the symptoms have an organic cause, but the symptoms are believed to be unconscious expressions of unacceptable feelings by use of the **defense mechanism** of **somatization** (see Chapter 12).
3. The *Diagnostic and Statistical Manual of Mental Disorders,* 4th edition, text revision (**DSM-IV-TR**) **categories** of somatoform disorders include somatization disorder, hypochondriasis, conversion disorder, body dysmorphic disorder, and somatoform pain disorder (Table 21-1).
4. Most somatoform disorders are **more common in women,** although **hypochondriasis occurs equally** in men and women.
5. Useful strategies for managing patients with somatoform disorders include the following:
   a. Forming a good **physician–patient relationship** (e.g., scheduling regular appointments, providing reassurance and structured time limits)
   b. Providing a **multidisciplinary approach,** including other medical professionals (e.g., pain management, mental health services)
   c. Identifying and addressing the **psychosocial difficulties** in the patient's life that may intensify the symptoms

TABLE 21-1	DSM-IV-TR CLASSIFICATION OF THE SOMATOFORM DISORDERS
Classification	**Characteristics**
Somatization disorder (see Patient Snapshot 21-1)	History over years of at least two gastrointestinal symptoms (e.g., nausea), four pain symptoms, one sexual symptom (e.g., menstrual problems), and one pseudo-neurologic symptom (e.g., paralysis)
	Onset <30 years of age
Hypochondriasis	Exaggerated concern with health and illness lasting at least 6 months
	Concern persists despite medical evaluation and reassurance
	More common in middle and old age
	Goes to many different doctors seeking help ("doctor shopping")
Conversion disorder	Sudden, dramatic loss of sensory or motor function (e.g., blindness, paralysis, pseudo-seizures), often associated with a specific stressful life event
	More common in unsophisticated adolescents and young adults
	Patients appear relatively unworried (la belle indifference)
Body dysmorphic disorder	Excessive focus on a minor or nonexistent physical defect
	Symptoms are not accounted for by anorexia nervosa
	Onset usually in the late teens
Somatoform pain disorder	Intense acute or chronic pain not explained completely by physical disease
	Onset usually in the 30s and 40s

Patient Snapshot 21-2

A 32-year-old woman takes her 4-year-old son to a physician's office. She says that the child often experiences episodes of abdominal pain and sometimes has trouble breathing. The child's medical record shows many office visits and four abdominal surgical procedures, although no abnormalities were ever found. Physical examination and laboratory studies are unremarkable. When the doctor confronts the mother with the suspicion that she is fabricating the illness in the child, the mother angrily grabs the child and immediately leaves the office.

C. **Factitious disorder (formerly Münchhausen syndrome), factitious disorder by proxy, and malingering**
 1. While individuals with somatoform disorders truly believe that they are ill, patients with factitious disorders or who are malingering **feign mental** or **physical illness** or actually **induce physical illness** in themselves or others for psychological gain (factitious disorder) or tangible gain (malingering) (Table 21-2).
 2. Patients with factitious disorder often have worked in the medical field (e.g., nurses, technicians) and know how to persuasively simulate an illness.
 3. **Feigned symptoms** most commonly include abdominal pain, fever (by heating the thermometer), blood in the urine (by adding blood from a needlestick), induction of tachycardia (by drug administration), skin lesions (by injuring easily reached areas), and hypoglycemia (by injecting insulin).

D. **Masked depression**

Patient Snapshot 21-3

A 41-year-old man says that he has been sick to his stomach for the past 3 months. Physical examination, including a gastrointestinal workup, is unremarkable except that the patient has lost 15 lb since his last visit 1 year ago. The patient is unshaven

TABLE 21-2	FACTITIOUS DISORDER, FACTITIOUS DISORDER BY PROXY, AND MALINGERING
Condition	**Characteristics**
Factitious disorder (formerly Münchhausen syndrome)	Conscious simulation of physical or psychiatric illness to gain attention from medical personnel
	Undergoes unnecessary medical and surgical procedures
	Has a grid abdomen (multiple crossed scars from repeated surgeries)
Factitious disorder by proxy	Conscious simulation of illness in another person, typically in a child by a parent, to obtain attention for parent from medical personnel
	Is a form of child abuse because the child undergoes unnecessary medical or surgical procedures (see Chapter 13)
	Must be reported to child welfare authorities (state social service agency)
Malingering	Conscious simulation or exaggeration of physical or psychiatric illness for financial (e.g., insurance settlement) or other obvious gain (e.g., avoiding incarceration)
	Avoids treatment by medical personnel
	Health complaints cease as soon as the desired gain is obtained
	Malingering is not a psychiatric disorder

and appears slowed down. He expresses the fear that he has stomach cancer but denies depression. Despite the patient's denial, the doctor suspects that depression is related to the patient's physical complaints (masked depression) and starts him on the antidepressant fluoxetine. About 3 months later, the patient states that his gastrointestinal symptoms are gone, he has gained 7 lb, and he is feeling like his "old self."

1. Depressed patients who seem unaware of or deny depression but experience **vague unexplained physical symptoms** are said to have masked depression (see Chapter 19).
2. In contrast to patients who have somatoform disorders, treatment with **antidepressants** can relieve both the depression and the physical symptoms in patients with masked depression.

II. Dissociative Disorders

A. **Characteristics**
   1. **Memory loss** and **mental confusion** typically involve physiologic abnormalities in neural function owing to illness, injury, substance abuse, or cognitive disorder (see Chapter 4).
   2. When such loss or confusion is **solely the result of psychological factors,** the diagnosis is a dissociative disorder.
   3. The dissociative disorders are characterized by abrupt but temporary **loss of memory** (amnesia) **or identity** or by feelings of detachment.
   4. Dissociative disorders are commonly related to disturbing **emotional experiences** in the patient's **recent or remote past.**

B. **Classification and treatment**
   1. The **DSM-IV-TR** categories of dissociative disorders—dissociative amnesia, dissociative fugue, dissociative identity disorder, and depersonalization disorder—are described in Table 21-3.

TABLE 21-3	DSM-IV-TR CLASSIFICATION OF THE DISSOCIATIVE DISORDERS	
Condition	**Patient snapshot**	**Characteristics**
Dissociative amnesia	A 20-year-old marine reports that he has no memory of an encounter with the enemy in which his close friend was killed.	Inability to remember important personal information Resolves in minutes or days but may last longer
Dissociative fugue	A 35-year-old woman has been living in a town in Ohio for more than 1 year and working for the school system. She has no memory of how she got to Ohio or of her life as a secretary in Florida more than 1 year earlier.	Inability to remember important personal information Wandering away from home May involve adopting a new identity
Dissociative identity disorder (formerly multiple personality disorder)	A 30-year-old medical resident usually dresses conservatively. A friend shows her a recent video of herself at a party in a low-cut blouse. The resident does not remember going to the party or posing for the video.	At least two distinct personalities (often more) in one individual Not a psychotic disorder
Depersonalization disorder	A 40-year old man tells his physician that when he is stressed out familiar objects in the environment (e.g., his furniture) often seem strange to him. He states that he knows this is only a feeling and that the objects are really familiar.	Persistent feelings of personal detachment and unreality about one's body, social situation, or environment (derealization) Normal reality testing

2. **Treatment** of the dissociative disorders includes **hypnosis** and **amobarbital sodium interviews** and long-term **psychoanalytically oriented psychotherapy** to recover lost (repressed) memories of the disturbing emotional experiences (see Chapter 23).

III. Paroxysmal Neurobehavioral Disorders

A. Overview

1. **Paroxysmal disorders** are characterized by the **sudden onset of neurologic symptoms** (e.g., seizures, headaches, trigeminal neuralgia, syncope), occurring as a **result of neurologic, psychiatric, or medical conditions.**

2. The mainstay of **treatment and prophylaxis** for paroxysmal disorders includes the following:

   a. **Anticonvulsants** such as carbamazepine (Tegretol) or gabapentin (Neurontin)

   b. **Antidepressant agents**

Patient Snapshot 21-4

A well-groomed, mildly obese 40-year-old woman is brought to the emergency room by her husband. The husband states that his wife has been having seizures. Vital signs are normal. The patient has no history of recent head trauma, neurologic disorder, or substance use. When the physician begins to examine her, the patient starts to show facial grimacing. She then arches her back and begins to jerk her arms and legs. During this episode, which lasts several minutes, the patient's eyes are closed and she seems unresponsive, but there is no urinary incontinence or tongue biting. After the episode, neurologic examination and prolactin levels are normal. Although a similar episode is observed on the inpatient service during 24-hr electroencephalogram with audio-video monitoring, no seizure activity is demonstrated. The patient is diagnosed with pseudo-seizures and referred for cognitive–behavioral therapy.

B. Seizures

1. Seizures are a result of abnormal high-amplitude, low-frequency, synchronous brain activity caused by neurologic dysfunction. **Epilepsy** is a disorder involving repeated seizures (see Chapter 15).

2. **Pseudo-seizures** are phenomena that resemble epileptic seizures but are characterized by a **normal EEG.** They are induced by psychological factors and, like other presentations of **conversion disorder** (Table 21-1), are not consciously motivated and occur for no apparent gain.

   a. Childhood physical or sexual abuse or other **traumatic events** are often found in the history of patients with pseudo-seizures.

   b. **Cognitive–behavioral therapy** may be an effective treatment for patients with pseudo-seizures (see Chapter 23).

3. **Distinguishing** pseudo-seizures from seizures can be difficult.

   a. Patients with pseudo-seizures **do not show the elevation of prolactin** seen in many patients within 15 min of an epileptic seizure.

   b. **Closing of the eyes** is more likely to be seen during pseudo-seizures than during seizures.

   c. **Pseudo-seizures** tend not to respond to anticonvulsant medications.

C. Headaches

1. Most headaches can be **categorized** as **vascular** (e.g., migraine, cluster) or **tension** (acute or chronic) or some combination of these types (Table 21-4).

2. Many headaches have an emotional or **psychosomatic** component such as **stress** and, if chronic, may fit the classification of **somatoform pain disorder (Table 21-1).**

TABLE 21-4		HEADACHES	
Category	**Type**	**Characteristics**	**Treatment**
Vascular headaches (cause: disturbance in cranial circulation)	Migraine	Last 4 hr to 3 days	Ergotamine tartrate (Cafergot)
		Unilateral	Analgesics
		Visual disturbances (e.g., blurring)	Triptans (e.g., sumatriptan)
		Gastrointestinal disturbances (e.g., nausea)	Selective serotonin reuptake inhibitors (e.g., fluoxetine)
		Present on awakening	
		11% prevalence	
	Cluster	Up to 8 headaches per day	
		Unilateral	
		Visual and gastrointestinal disturbances	
		Pupil constriction (miosis)	
		Sagging eyelid (ptosis)	
		Intense sweating (diaphoresis)	
Tension type (cause: prolonged contraction of head and neck muscles)	Acute	Last 30 min to 7 days	Analgesics
		Bilateral	Muscle relaxants
		80% prevalence	Massage
	Chronic	Occur more than 15 days/month	Psychotherapy
		Bilateral	Biofeedback
		Present on awakening	
		3% prevalence	

D. Trigeminal neuralgia

1. **Trigeminal neuralgia** (TN) is a disorder of the **fifth and largest cranial nerve.**

2. TN is characterized by intense **lightening strike-like** unilateral facial pain occurring spontaneously or triggered by stimuli such as tooth brushing or a slight breeze on the face.

3. Anticonvulsants are the mainstay of treatment for TN but **neurosurgical procedures** may relieve pressure on or reduce sensitivity of the nerve.

E. Syncope

1. Syncope or **fainting** is defined as a temporary loss of consciousness that is followed by spontaneous recovery. It is typically the result of reduction in cerebral blood flow, as in orthostatic hypotension.

2. Syncope can also be a result of **emotional factors.**

   a. **Vasovagal syncope,** the most common type of syncope, results from a mechanoreceptor reflex and can be triggered by pain, stress, or intense emotion.

   b. **Situational syncope** is similar to vasovagal syncope but is stimulated by urination, defecation, cough, or vomiting.

IV. Impulse Control Disorders

Patient Snapshot 21-5

A well-known 25-year-old baseball player is caught taking a compact disc from a store without paying for it. He reports that although he could easily afford the compact disc, he "had the urge to just take it." This is the third time the ballplayer has been caught in an offense of this type.

TABLE 21-5	DSM-IV-TR CLASSIFICATION OF IMPULSE CONTROL DISORDERS	
Disorder	**Description**	**Treatment**
Intermittent explosive disorder	Episodic loss of self-control leading to attack on another person	Anticonvulsants (e.g., carbamazepine)
		Lithium
	More common in young men	Selective serotonin reuptake inhibitors (SSRIs)
		Antiandrogens
Kleptomania (see Patient Snapshot 21-5)	Need to take things without paying for them even when one can afford items	Behavior therapy (aversive conditioning, systematic desensitization, see Chapter 12)
	Taking rather than having object is intent	SSRIs
Pyromania	Repetitive fire setting	Behavioral therapy
	Overwhelming interest in and attraction to fires	Family therapy for children
Trichotillomania	Need to pull out one's hair	SSRIs
	Obvious hair loss	Behavioral therapy
	Eating hair may lead to bezoars (hair ball that obstructs gastrointestinal tract)	
Pathologic gambling	Need to gamble that negatively affects family and work relationships	Gamblers Anonymous
		SSRIs
Impulse control disorder not otherwise specified	For example, compulsive buying, internet compulsion, mobile phone compulsion, compulsive sex behavior	SSRIs
		Behavioral therapy

A. **Characteristics**
   1. Patients with impulse control disorders are characterized by the **inability to resist** engaging in behavior that is **ultimately of harm** to themselves or to other people.
   2. Usually, there is **increased tension** before the behavior **followed by relief** or pleasure after the behavior is completed.

B. **Cause, differential diagnosis, and treatment**
   1. Inability to control one's impulses is related to neurotransmitter abnormalities, particularly **low levels of serotonin** (see Chapter 11), and social factors such as family dysfunction in childhood.
   2. The **differential diagnosis** of impulse control disorders includes faking (malingering) to avoid prosecution or societal censure for engaging in illegal or unacceptable behavior.
   3. Like the paroxysmal disorders, the **pharmacologic treatment** of the impulse control disorders primarily involves **anticonvulsants** and **antidepressants**.

C. **Description and treatment** of the impulse control disorders—**kleptomania, pyromania, intermittent explosive disorder, pathologic gambling, trichotillomania,** and impulse control disorders not otherwise specified (NOS)—are listed in Table 21-5.

Chapter 22

Neuropsychopharmacology

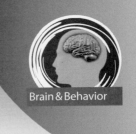

Brain & Behavior

I. Overview

A. Pharmacologic agents are used to treat the **neurotransmitter abnormalities,** which are believed to be involved in the symptoms of a variety of psychiatric and neurologic disorders (Table 22-1). Somatic therapies and psychotherapies are also used to treat patients with these illnesses (see Chapter 23).

B. Although normalization of neurotransmitter levels by pharmacologic agents can ameliorate many of the symptoms, these agents **do not cure** neurological or psychiatric disorders.

II. Antipsychotic Agents

Patient Snapshot 22-1

The physician treating the 32-year-old patient with schizophrenia in Patient Snapshot 11–2 decided to halt haloperidol and start the patient on clozapine, an atypical agent. Over a period of 10 days, the clozapine dose was increased to 250 mg/day and the patient's psychotic symptoms resolved. He also showed improvement in his negative symptom (e.g., he became more animated and motivated). A few weeks later, however, a persistent fever (101.5°F) associated with a severe sore throat, malaise, and mouth ulcers appeared. Laboratory testing revealed a granulocyte count of <1000 and the patient was diagnosed with agranulocytosis. Clozapine therapy was stopped and the patient was started on a broad-spectrum antibiotic as well as another atypical antipsychotic, aripiprazole.

A. Overview
1. Antipsychotic agents (formerly called neuroleptics or major tranquilizers) are used in the treatment of **schizophrenia** and in the treatment of psychotic symptoms associated with other psychiatric disorders.
2. Antipsychotics are also used to treat nausea, hiccups, intense agitation, and Tourette disorder.
3. Although antipsychotics are commonly taken daily by mouth, noncompliant patients can be treated with long-acting **depot** forms, such as **haloperidol decanoate** administered intramuscularly every 4 weeks.
4. Antipsychotic agents can be classified as **traditional or atypical,** depending on their mode of action and side effect profile.

B. Traditional antipsychotic agents
1. Traditional antipsychotic agents act primarily by **blocking central D₂** receptors.
2. Although negative symptoms of schizophrenia, such as withdrawal, may improve with continued treatment, traditional antipsychotic agents are **most effective against positive symptoms** such as hallucinations and delusions (see Chapter 19).

TABLE 22-1	USES OF NEUROPSYCHOPHARMACOLOGIC AGENTS		
Type of Agent (example)	**Neurologic Conditions**	**Psychiatric Conditions**	**Other Conditions**
Acetylcholinesterase inhibitor (rivastigmine)	Alzheimer disease	Psychotic symptoms	Glaucoma
	Myasthenia gravis	ADHD	Smooth muscle dysfunction
Antianxiety (diazepam)	Epilepsy	Anxiety disorders	Insomnia
	Huntington disease	Psychotic disorders	Muscle tension
	Dystonias	Substance withdrawal	
Anticholinergic (benztropine)	Parkinson disease	Extrapyramidal symptoms from use of antipsychotics	Gastrointestinal conditions (e.g., gastric ulcer)
Antidepressant (fluoxetine)	Chronic pain	Mood disorders	Enuresis
		Anxiety disorders	Premenstrual disorder
Anesthetic (opioid)	Chronic pain	Substance withdrawal	Anesthesia induction
Antihypertensive (β-blocker)	Stroke	Anxiety disorders	Hypertension
	Intention tremor	Substance withdrawal	
Antipsychotic (haloperidol)	Tourette disorder	Psychotic disorders	Nausea
	Huntington disease	Agitation	Hiccups
	Sydenham chorea		
Dopamine agonist (levodopa)	Parkinson disease	Extrapyramidal symptoms from use of antipsychotics	Prolactinoma
	Primary dystonias		
Mood stabilizer (lithium, valproic acid)	Seizures	Bipolar disorder	Extra aggressiveness
	Dystonias	Impulse control disorders	Migraine prophylaxis
N-methyl-D-aspartate receptor antagonist (memantine)	Alzheimer disease	Schizophrenia	
	Stroke		
	Huntington disease		
Stimulant (methylphenidate)	Narcolepsy	Depression	Appetite suppression in obesity
	ADHD		

ADHD: attention deficit hyperactivity disorder

3. Traditional antipsychotics are classified according to their potency.
   a. Low-potency agents, such as chlorpromazine (Thorazine) and thioridazine (Mellaril), are associated primarily with **nonneurologic** adverse effects (e.g., sedation, anticholinergic effects) (Table 22-2).
   b. High-potency agents, such as haloperidol (Haldol), trifluoperazine (Stelazine), fluphenazine (Prolixin), and perphenazine (Trilafon), are associated primarily with **neurologic** adverse effects (Table 22-2).
      i. Neurologic adverse effects that are caused primarily by decreased dopamine (e.g., extrapyramidal effects) are treated by decreasing the drug dosage or by adding an anticholinergic agent (e.g., benztropine).
      ii. Neurologic adverse effects caused by supersensitivity of dopamine receptors (e.g., tardive dyskinesia) are treated primarily by switching the patient to an atypical or low-potency agent.

C. Atypical antipsychotic agents: clozapine (Clozaril), risperidone (Risperdal), olanzapine (Zyprexa), quetiapine (Seroquel), ziprasidone (Geodon), and aripiprazole (Abilify)
   1. In contrast to traditional antipsychotic agents, atypical antipsychotics affect not only dopaminergic but also **serotonergic** systems.

TABLE 22-2	ADVERSE EFFECTS OF ANTIPSYCHOTIC AGENTS
System	**Adverse Effects**
Nonneurologic adverse effects; more common with traditional, low-potency agents	
Circulatory	Orthostatic (postural) hypotension
	Electrocardiogram abnormalities (e.g., prolongation of QT and PR intervals)
	Thioridazine is most cardiotoxic in overdose
Endocrine	Increase in prolactin level results in gynecomastia (breast enlargement), galactorrhea, erectile dysfunction, amenorrhea, and decreased libido
Hematologic	Leukopenia; agranulocytosis
	Usually occur in the first 3 months of treatment
Hepatic	Jaundice; elevated liver enzyme levels
	Usually occur in the first month of treatment
	More common with chlorpromazine
Dermatologic	Skin eruptions, photosensitivity, and blue-gray skin discoloration
	More common with chlorpromazine
Ophthalmologic	Irreversible retinal pigmentation with thioridazine
	Deposits in lens and cornea with chlorpromazine
Anticholinergic	Peripheral effects: dry mouth, constipation, urinary retention, and blurred vision
	Central effects: agitation and disorientation
Antihistaminergic	Weight gain and sedation
	Chlorpromazine is most sedating
Neurologic adverse effects; more common with traditional high-potency agents	
Extrapyramidal	Pseudoparkinsonism (muscle rigidity, shuffling gait, resting tremor, mask-like facial expression)
	Akathisia (subjective feeling of motor restlessness)
	Acute dystonia (prolonged muscular spasms; more common in men <40 years of age)
	Treat with anticholinergic (e.g., benztropine) or antihistaminergic (e.g., diphenhydramine) agent
Other	Tardive dyskinesia (abnormal writhing movements of the tongue, face, and body; more common in women and after at least 6 months of treatment); to treat, substitute low-potency or atypical antipsychotic agent
	Neuroleptic malignant syndrome (high fever, sweating, increased pulse and blood pressure, dystonia, apathy; more common in men and early in treatment; mortality rate ~20%); to treat, stop agent, give a skeletal muscle relaxant (e.g., dantrolene), and provide medical support
	Decreased seizure threshold

2. Because of their better side effect profiles, atypical agents, particularly risperidone and olanzapine, are now **first-line** agents for treating psychotic symptoms.
3. **Advantages** of atypical agents over traditional agents
    a. Atypical agents may be **more effective** when used to treat the **negative,** chronic, and refractory symptoms of schizophrenia (see Chapter 19).
    b. They are less likely to cause neurologic adverse effects.
4. **Disadvantages** of atypical agents

 a. Atypical agents may increase the likelihood of hematologic problems, such as **agranulocytosis,** with clozapine as the most problematic agent (Patient Snapshot 22-1).

 b. They may also increase the likelihood of **seizures,** anticholinergic side effects, and pancreatitis as well as **weight gain** and **type 2 diabetes** (particularly clozapine and olanzapine).

III. Antidepressant Agents

Patient Snapshot 22-2

A 35-year-old woman is brought to the emergency department by her husband after a neighbor reported that she was running down the street singing loudly. The woman, who is speaking very quickly, tells the doctor that she was trying to get enough money to cure AIDS by entertaining people in the street. The patient is a secretary and has two school-aged children. Her history reveals that over the previous 5 years, she has had two episodes of major depression for which she did not seek treatment but otherwise showed no behavioral abnormalities. Her husband notes that a few weeks earlier the patient's family doctor gave her "nerve" pills because she was becoming depressed again. Because antidepressants can precipitate a manic episode in potentially bipolar patients, this episode may have been triggered by the medication (probably an antidepressant) prescribed by the family physician.

A. Overview

 1. Heterocyclic antidepressants (HCAs), selective serotonin reuptake inhibitors (SSRIs), selective serotonin and norepinephrine reuptake inhibitors (SSNRIs), monoamine oxidase inhibitors (MAOIs), and atypical antidepressants are used to treat depression. These agents also have other clinical uses (Table 22-3).

 2. All antidepressants are believed to increase the availability of serotonin and/or norepinephrine in the synapse via **inhibition of reuptake mechanisms** (HCAs, SSRIs, SSNRIs) or blockade of the enzyme monoamine oxidase that breaks down the monoamines (MAOIs). Both of these mechanisms ultimately lead to **downregulation of postsynaptic receptors** and improvement in mood (see Chapter 11).

 3. Because of their more positive side effect profile, **SSRIs,** such as fluoxetine (Prozac), are now used as **first-line agents.**

 4. All antidepressants take **3–6 weeks** to work, and all have **equal efficacy.**

 5. Antidepressant agents do not elevate mood in nondepressed people and have **no abuse potential.** They can, however, **precipitate a manic episode** in a potentially bipolar patient (Patient Snapshot 22-2).

B. Heterocyclic agents

 1. **Heterocyclic antidepressants block reuptake of norepinephrine and serotonin** at the synapse. Some also block reuptake of dopamine, for example, amoxapine (Asendin).

 a. These agents also block muscarinic acetylcholine receptors, resulting in **anticholinergic effects** (e.g., dry mouth, blurred vision, urine retention, constipation). As such, they are contraindicated in patients with **glaucoma.**

 b. Histamine receptors are also blocked by heterocyclic agents, resulting in antihistaminergic effects (e.g., **weight gain** and **sedation**).

 2. Other adverse effects include **cardiovascular effects** such as orthostatic hypotension, neurologic effects such as tremor, and general effects such as weight gain and sexual dysfunction.

 3. Heterocyclics are dangerous in overdose.

TABLE 22-3	ANTIDEPRESSANT AGENTS	
Agent (current or former brand name)	Effects	Clinical Uses in Addition to Depression
Heterocyclic agents (HCAs)		
Amitriptyline (Elavil)	Sedating Anticholinergic	Depression with insomnia Chronic pain
Clomipramine (Anafranil)	Most serotonin-specific of the HCAs	Obsessive-compulsive disorder (OCD) Panic disorder
Desipramine (Norpramin)	Least sedating of the HCAs Least anticholinergic of the HCAs Stimulates appetite	Depression in the elderly Eating disorders
Doxepin (Adapin, Sinequan)	Sedating, antihistaminergic Anticholinergic	Generalized anxiety disorder Peptic ulcer disease
Imipramine (Tofranil)	Likely to cause orthostatic hypotension	Panic disorder with agoraphobia Enuresis Eating disorders
Maprotiline (Ludiomil)	Low cardiotoxicity May cause seizures	Anxiety with depressive features
Nortriptyline (Aventyl, Pamelor)	Least likely of the HCAs to cause orthostatic hypotension	Depression in the elderly Pruritus (itching) Patients with cardiac disease
Selective serotonin reuptake inhibitors (SSRIs)		
Fluoxetine (Prozac, Sarafem)	May cause agitation and insomnia initially Sexual dysfunction May uniquely cause some weight loss	OCD Premature ejaculation Panic disorder Premenstrual dysphoria (fluoxetine) Social phobia (paroxetine)
Paroxetine (Paxil)	Most sedating SSRI Most anticholinergic SSRI Sexual dysfunction	Hypochondriasis Chronic pain Post-traumatic stress disorder
Sertraline (Zoloft)	Most likely of the SSRIs to cause gastrointestinal disturbances (diarrhea) Sexual dysfunction	Paraphilias
Fluvoxamine (Luvox)	Currently indicated only for OCD	
Citalopram (Celexa)	More cardiotoxic that other SSRIs Low cytochrome P450 effects	
Escitalopram (Lexapro)	Most serotonin-specific of the SSRIs Low cytochrome P450 effects Fewer side effects than citalopram	
Selective serotonin and norepinephrine reuptake inhibitors (SSNRIs)		
Duloxetine (Cymbalta)	Rapid symptom relief Few sexual side effects	Refractory depression Urinary stress incontinence
Venlafaxine (Effexor)	Rapid symptom relief Few sexual side effects Low cytochrome P450 effects Increased diastolic blood pressure at higher doses	Refractory depression Generalized anxiety disorder

TABLE 22-3	ANTIDEPRESSANT AGENTS (*CONTINUED*)	
Agent (current or former brand name)	**Effects**	**Clinical Uses in Addition to Depression**
Monoamine oxidase inhibitors (MAOIs)		
Phenelzine (Nardil) Tranylcypromine (Parnate)	Hyperadrenergic crisis precipitated by ingestion of pressor amines in tyramine-containing foods or sympathomimetic drugs	Atypical depression Eating disorders Panic disorder Social phobia Pain disorders
Other antidepressants		
Amoxapine (Asendin)	Antidopaminergic effects (parkinsonian symptoms, galactorrhea, sexual dysfunction) Most dangerous in overdose	Depression with psychotic features
Bupropion (Wellbutrin, Zyban)	Insomnia Seizures Sweating Fewer adverse sexual effects Norepinephrine and dopamine reuptake inhibition (no effect on serotonin) Decreased appetite	Refractory depression (inadequate clinical response to other antidepressants) Smoking cessation (Zyban) Seasonal affective disorder Adult attention deficit hyperactivity disorder SSRI induced sexual dysfunction
Mirtazapine (Remeron)	Targets specific serotonin receptors and causes fewer adverse effects	Refractory depression Insomnia
Trazodone (Desyrel)	Sedation Rarely, causes priapism Hypotension	Insomnia

C. SSRIs and SSNRIs
1. SSRIs and SSNRIs selectively block the reuptake, respectively, of serotonin only and of both norepinephrine and serotonin.
2. SSRIs and SSNRIs have little effect on dopamine, acetylcholine, or histamine systems.
3. Because of this selectivity, SSRIs and SSNRIs cause **fewer side effects** and are safer in overdose, in the elderly, and in pregnancy than heterocyclics and MAOIs.
4. SSNRIs may work more quickly (2–3 weeks) and cause fewer sexual side effects than SSRIs.

D. MAOIs
1. MAOIs inhibit the breakdown of neurotransmitters by monoamine oxidase type A (**MAO-A**) in the brain in an irreversible reaction.
2. These agents may be particularly useful in the treatment of **atypical depression** (see Chapter 19) and treatment resistance to other agents.
3. A major drawback of use of MAOIs is **a potentially fatal reaction** when they are taken in conjunction with **tyramine-rich foods** or **sympathomimetic drugs**. This reaction occurs because of the following:
   a. **MAO metabolizes tyramine, a pressor,** in the gastrointestinal tract.
   b. If MAO is inhibited, ingestion of **tyramine-rich foods**—for example, aged cheese, beer, wine, broad beans, beef or chicken liver, and smoked or pickled meats or fish—or **sympathomimetic drugs**—such as ephedrine, methylphenidate (Ritalin), phenylephrine (Neo-Synephrine), and pseudoephedrine (Sudafed)—can increase tyramine levels.

       c. Increase in tyramine can cause elevated blood pressure, sweating, headache, and vomiting (a **hypertensive crisis**), which in turn can lead to **stroke and death.**

   4. MAOIs and SSRIs used together can cause a potentially life-threatening drug–drug interaction, **the serotonin syndrome,** marked by autonomic instability, hyperthermia, seizures, and coma.

   5. Other adverse effects of MAOIs are similar to those of the heterocyclics, including danger in overdose.

IV. Mood Stabilizers

A. Lithium (carbonate and citrate)

   1. Lithium is used **to prevent** both the manic and depressive phases of bipolar disorder.

   2. It may be used also to increase the effectiveness of antidepressant agents in depressive illness and to control aggressive behavior (see Chapter 13).

   3. **Adverse effects** of chronic use of lithium include the following:

       a. Congenital abnormalities (particularly of the cardiovascular system—for example, Ebstein anomaly of the tricuspid valve)

       b. Hypothyroidism

       c. Tremor

       d. Renal dysfunction, nephrogenic diabetes insipidus

       e. Cardiac conduction problems

       f. Gastric distress

       g. Mild cognitive impairment

   4. Lithium **takes 2–3 weeks to work.** Antipsychotics are, therefore, the initial treatment for psychotic symptoms in an acute manic episode.

   5. Because of **potential toxicity,** blood levels of lithium must be maintained at 0.8–1.2 mEq/L.

B. Anticonvulsants such as carbamazepine (Tegretol), oxcarbamazepine (Trileptal), and valproic acid (Depakene, Depakote)

   1. **In neurology,** anticonvulsants are used to treat seizure disorders and dystonias. They decrease seizure activity by modifying **neuronal excitability** through alteration in **ion channels.**

   2. **In psychiatry,** anticonvulsants are used to treat bipolar disorder, particularly the **rapid cycling** type (i.e., more than four episodes annually) and **mixed episodes** (mania and depression occurring concurrently).

       a. The mechanism of action of anticonvulsants in bipolar disorder is not clear.

       b. They are believed to decrease excessive neural activity by increasing γ-aminobutyric acid (**GABA**) release.

   3. Carbamazepine may be associated with severe adverse effects such as **aplastic anemia and agranulocytosis.**

   4. **Valproic acid** may be particularly useful for treating bipolar symptoms resulting from cognitive disorders (see Chapter 14) and for prophylaxis of migraine headaches.

   5. **Adverse effects** of valproic acid include gastrointestinal and liver problems, congenital neural tube defects, and alopecia (hair loss).

   6. Other anticonvulsant agents that appear to have mood-stabilizing effects include lamotrigine (Lamictal), gabapentin (Neurontin), topiramate (Topamax), and tiagabine (Gabitril).

V. Antianxiety, Antihypertensive, and Anesthetic Agents

In **neurology,** antianxiety agents, anesthetics, and some antihypertensive agents are useful in controlling seizures, muscle spasticity, and pain. In **psychiatry,** these agents are used to treat patients with acute anxiety as well as sleep disorders and substance withdrawal (Table 22-1).

A. Benzodiazepines (BZs)

1. BZs activate binding sites on the **GABA$_A$ receptor,** thereby increasing chloride conductance and decreasing neuronal and muscle-cell firing.
2. These agents have a short, intermediate, or long onset and duration of action and may be used to treat disorders other than anxiety disorders (Table 22-4).
3. Their characteristics of action are related to their clinical indications and their potential for abuse—for example, short-acting agents are good hypnotics (sleep inducers) but have a higher potential for abuse than longer-acting agents.
4. BZs commonly cause **sedation** but have few other adverse effects. One important side effect occurs after chronic use followed by withdrawal. This can lead to **increased seizure potential.**
5. **Tolerance and dependence** may occur with chronic use of these agents (see Chapter 14).
6. **Flumazenil** (Mazicon, Romazicon) is a BZ receptor antagonist that can reverse the effects of BZs in cases of overdose or when BZs such as midazolam (Versed) are used for sedation during a surgical procedure.

TABLE 22-4	ANTIANXIETY AGENTS (GROUPED ALPHABETICALLY BY DURATION OF ACTION AND CATEGORY)	
Agent (brand name)	**Duration of Action**	**Clinical Uses in Addition to Anxiety**
Benzodiazepines		
Clorazepate (Tranxene)	Short	Adjunct in management of partial seizures
Oxazepam (Serax)	Short	Alcohol withdrawal
Triazolam (Halcion)	Short	Insomnia
Alprazolam (Xanax)	Intermediate	Depression; panic disorder; social phobia
Lorazepam (Ativan)	Intermediate	Psychotic agitation, alcohol withdrawal, acute control of seizures
Temazepam (Restoril)	Intermediate	Insomnia
Chlordiazepoxide (Librium)	Long	Alcohol withdrawal (particularly for agitation)
Clonazepam (Klonopin)	Long	Seizures, mania, social phobia, panic disorder, obsessive–compulsive disorder
Diazepam (Valium)	Long	Muscle relaxation, analgesia, anticonvulsant, alcohol withdrawal (particularly for seizures)
Flurazepam (Dalmane)	Long	Insomnia
Nonbenzodiazepines		
Zolpidem (Ambien)	Short	Indicated only for insomnia
Zaleplon (Sonata)	Short	Indicated only for insomnia
Eszopiclone (Lunesta)	Short	Indicated only for insomnia
Ramelteon (Rozerem)	Short	Indicated only for insomnia
Buspirone (BuSpar)	Very long	Anxiety in the elderly, generalized anxiety disorder

B. Nonbenzodiazepine antianxiety agents
1. **Buspirone** (BuSpar), an azaspirodecanedione, is not related to the BZs.
   a. In contrast to BZs, buspirone is **nonsedating** and is **not associated with dependence, abuse,** or **withdrawal.**
   b. It is used primarily to treat conditions causing chronic anxiety in which BZ dependence can become a problem [e.g., **generalized anxiety disorder** (see Chapter 20)].
   c. Buspirone **takes up to 2 weeks to work** and may not be acceptable to patients who are accustomed to taking the fast-acting BZs for their symptoms.
2. **Zolpidem, zaleplon, eszopiclone,** and **ramelteon** are short-acting sedating agents unrelated to the BZs and used to treat **insomnia.**

C. Antihypertensive agents
1. The **β-antagonists** (β-blockers) such as propranolol (Inderal) and **α-adrenergic receptor antagonists** such as clonidine (Catapres) **decrease the autonomic hyperarousal** associated with some psychiatric conditions.
2. These agents are particularly useful for treating symptoms associated with **anxiety disorders** and **withdrawal** from opioids and sedatives.

D. Analgesics and anesthetics
1. Analgesics such as **opioids** and nonsteroidal anti-inflammatory drugs (**NSAIDs**) such as ibuprofen are used to treat severe and mild pain, respectively.
2. **Antidepressants** and **antipsychotics** also have a role in pain control, particularly in treating **neuropathic pain** (pain caused by neuronal damage).

VI. Stimulants

A. Amphetamines (e.g., methylphenidate, dextroamphetamine)
1. These agents are useful in the rapid treatment of **depression** in terminally ill or elderly patients.
2. They are also useful in patients with **depression refractory to other treatments** and in those at risk for the development of adverse effects of other agents for depression.
3. They are approved by the U.S. Food and Drug Administration (FDA) for treating **narcolepsy** and **ADHD.**
4. Disadvantages include their **addiction potential** (see Chapter 14) and tendency to decrease appetite.

B. Modafinil (Provigil)
1. Modafinil is a highly selective **noradrenergic receptor blocker** with stimulant properties
2. It is used in combination with antidepressants for patients with treatment-resistant depression and alone to treat **narcolepsy.**
3. In contrast to the amphetamines, modafinil is not believed have abuse potential.

VII. Agents for Specific Neuropsychiatric Conditions

A. Agents used in the treatment of dementia (see Chapter 4)
1. **Acetylcholinesterase inhibitors** (**AChEIs**), such as tacrine (Cognex), donepezil (Aricept), rivastigmine (Exelon), and galantamine (Reminyl), block the enzyme that breaks down **acetylcholine,** thereby improving cholinergic transmission.

2. **Memantine** (Namenda), an *N*-methyl-D-aspartate (NMDA) receptor antagonist, may decrease stimulation of the NMDA receptor by **glutamate,** thereby preventing further neuronal damage.

3. In some patients with Alzheimer disease, these agents may slow the progression of memory loss and may even result in **transient improvement in memory** and other cognitive function. However, data indicate that the effectiveness of these medications, particularly memantine, is largely limited to patients with more advanced disease.

B. Agents used in the treatment of addictions (see Chapter 14)
   1. **Agents used to treat alcoholism include** disulfiram (Antabuse), naloxone (Narcan), naltrexone (ReVia), and acamprosate (Campral)
   2. **Agents used to treat opioid addiction**
      a. Methadone, L-α-acetylmethadol acetate (LAMM), and buprenorphine (Temgesic) are used to decrease the severity of **withdrawal symptoms** or to **maintain** patients physically addicted to opioids.
      b. Naloxone and naltrexone are used **prophylactically** to block the positive effects of abused opioids.

C. Agents used in the treatment of stroke
   1. **NSAIDs** such as aspirin and ibuprofen and **anticoagulants** such as heparin have a role in preventing blood clotting and thus have a role in ischemic stroke prevention and treatment.
   2. **Thrombolytic agents** (e.g., streptokinase) have an important role when used in the first few hours after a thrombohemolytic stroke.
   3. Because they counteract excessive stimulation by the neurotoxic neurotransmitter glutamate, **NMDA receptor antagonists** such as memantine may also prove useful in the treatment of stroke.

D. Agents used in the treatment of multiple sclerosis (MS)
   1. MS is believed to be an **autoimmune** demyelinating disorder (see Chapter 18).
   2. Treatment for MS can be divided into agents that are disease specific or symptomatic.
      a. **Disease-specific** agents act to suppress or modulate the immune system and include **corticosteroids** (e.g. methylprednisolone or prednisone), **β-interferons** (Avonex or Rebif), **glatiramer acetate** (a mixture of amino acid tetramers), **mitoxantrone** (a synthetic antineoplastic agent), and **natalizumab** (a monoclonal antibody to an adhesion molecule important for lymphocyte motility). Other agents include general immunosuppressants such as cyclophosphamide, methotrexate, and cyclosporine.
      b. **Symptomatic agents** include **baclofen** for contractures and **cholinergic agents** to improve bladder emptying. Other agents are β-blockers for intention tremor, antipsychotics or typical antidepressants for neuropathic pain, and stool softeners for constipation.

E. Agents used in the treatment of movement disorders
   1. **Movement disorders** that occur in neurologic conditions such as Parkinson disease and as a result of treatment with antipsychotic agents result from a combination of factors, including decreased availability of **dopamine** in the substantia nigra (see Chapter 4).
   2. Treatment of movement disorders includes **dopamine agonists** and **anticholinergic agents.** A number of specific agents are used to treat Parkinson disease.
      a. **Amantadine** is an indirect dopaminergic agonist with some anticholinergic effects. It is most useful in the early stages of the illness.
      b. **Trihexyphenidyl** is a widely used anticholinergic and is most useful in the treatment of the tremor of parkinsonism.

c. **Bromocriptine, pergolide, lisuride,** and **cabergoline** are dopamine agonists that are often used in conjunction with dopamine-replacement therapy to potentiate its effects.

d. **Levodopa** (L-dopa) is the most potent anti-Parkinson treatment. It is a precursor to dopamine that can traverse the blood–brain barrier, unlike dopamine itself. However, it is metabolized in the periphery by dopa decarboxylase, which can reduce its effectiveness and trigger side effects. Therefore, levodopa is most often prescribed with a peripheral dopa decarboxylase inhibitor such as **carbidopa.**

Chapter 23

Other Neuropsychiatric Therapies

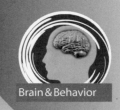

Brain & Behavior

I. Somatic Therapies

Patient Snapshot 23-1

The patient was born in 1918 in Boston and was known as Rosie to friends and family. Her mild mental retardation may have stemmed from brain damage at birth. As she got older, she developed changeable moods. She also began to demand the freedom to come and go at will. Her father worried that his daughter's condition would lead her into situations, such as pregnancy, that could damage the family's reputation. Lobotomy, a surgical procedure in which the frontal lobes are severed from the rest of the brain, was just beginning to be used. The procedure was indicated in patients with severe mental disorders or uncontrollable behavior. At the age of 23, Rosie had a prefrontal lobotomy. Unfortunately, as a result of the surgery she was left with psychomotor retardation and the inability to speak more than a few words. She had to be institutionalized for the rest of her life. Rosie—Rosemarie Kennedy—the older sister of President John F. Kennedy, died in 2004 at the age of 86.

A. Surgery for psychiatric disorders

1. Neurosurgery for behavioral abnormalities or **psychosurgery** was used in the past to treat patients with psychiatric disorders. Negative outcomes (Patient Snapshot 23-1), physician abuse of the procedures, and improvements in psychopharmacology have made most forms of psychosurgery **obsolete.**

2. However, advances in neuroanatomic understanding and stereotactic techniques have made psychosurgery a relevant treatment option for certain patients with psychiatric disorders.

   a. Bilateral **stereotactic ablation** of the anterior cingulum may be useful for medically refractory cases of obsessive–compulsive disorder (**OCD**) (see Chapter 20).

   b. **Vagus nerve stimulation** is a procedure in which a pacemaker-like device is placed under the skin of the chest wall with a wire running to the vagus nerve in the neck. Mild pulses of electrical energy are the sent to the brain via the vagus nerve. This procedure has been shown to increase serotonergic and noradrenergic transmission in the brain and may be useful in relieving **depression** (see Chapter 19).

   c. Subthalamic placement of electrodes for **deep brain stimulation** may relieve symptoms of **depression** and **OCD** in patients co-afflicted with Parkinson disease (see Chapter 4).

3. In the future, neurosurgical interventions for psychiatric disease are more likely to involve the stereotactic application of constructive therapies (e.g., gene therapies, stem cell implants), rather than ablative therapies.

B. Surgery for neurological disorders. Recent advances in neurosurgery have provided surgical options for treatment of neurologic disorders such as Parkinson disease and epilepsy.

1. **Thalamotomy and pallidotomy** are used to treat Parkinson disease (see Chapter 4).
2. **Vagus nerve stimulation** is also used to treat epilepsy (see Chapter 15).

C. **Electroconvulsive therapy (ECT) and related therapy**
   1. **Uses of ECT**
      a. ECT provides **rapid, effective, safe** treatment for some psychiatric disturbances.
      b. It is most commonly used to treat **major depressive disorder** that is **refractory to antidepressants.**
      c. ECT may also be indicated for serious depressive symptoms of any type (e.g., **psychotic depression**), particularly when rapid symptom resolution is imperative because of **suicide risk** (see Chapter 19).
      d. ECT is particularly useful for treating **depression in the elderly** because it may be safer than long-term use of antidepressant agents.
   2. The **mechanism of action** of ECT is **unknown;** it may alter neurotransmitter function in a manner similar to that of treatment with psychoactive agents.
   3. **Administration**
      a. ECT involves inducing a **generalized seizure** lasting 25–60 sec by **passing an electric current across the brain.**
      b. Before seizure induction, the patient is **premedicated** (e.g., with atropine) followed by administration of a short-acting general anesthesia (e.g., methohexital) and a muscle relaxant (e.g., succinylcholine) to prevent injury during the seizure.
      c. Improvement in mood typically **begins after a few ECT treatments.** A maximum response to ECT is usually seen after 5–10 treatments given over a 2- to 3-week period.
   4. **Problems associated with ECT**
      a. The major adverse effects of ECT are **memory problems.** These problems include **acute confusional state** (lasts for about 30 min after treatment and then remits), **anterograde amnesia** (inability to put down new memories, which resolves within a few weeks), and **retrograde amnesia** (inability to remember events occurring up to 2 months before the ECT course; these memories rarely return).
      b. **Increased intracranial pressure** or recent (within 2 weeks) myocardial infarction are the **major contraindications** for ECT.
      c. The mortality rate associated with ECT is very low and is comparable to that associated with the induction of general anesthesia.

D. **Rapid transcranial magnetic stimulation (rTMS)**
   1. In rTMS, an **electric current** is applied to the scalp to generate a **magnetic field** about 2 cm deep to stimulate cortical interneurons lying parallel to the surface of the brain.
   2. In contrast to ECT, in rTMS the **patient is awake,** neither premedication nor anesthetic is needed, and a seizure is not induced.
   3. While rTMS currently has **no approved psychiatric indication,** research suggests that it improves symptoms in some patients with refractory major depressive disorder, psychotic depression, obsessive–compulsive disorder, and post-traumatic stress disorder.

II. Psychotherapies

A. **Psychoanalysis and related therapies**
   1. Psychoanalysis and related therapies (e.g., psychoanalytically oriented psychotherapy, brief dynamic psychotherapy) are **psychotherapeutic treatments** based on Freud's concepts of the mind (see Chapter 12).

2. The central strategy of these therapies is to **uncover experiences** that are **repressed in the unconscious mind** and integrate them into the person's conscious mind and personality, using techniques such as free association, dream interpretation, and analysis of **transference reactions** (see Chapter 12).

3. In **psychoanalysis,** people receive treatment **4–5 times a week for 3–4 years;** related therapies are briefer and more direct (e.g., brief dynamic psychotherapy is limited to 12–40 weekly sessions).

B. Behavioral therapy and cognitive–behavioral therapy (CBT)
1. Behavioral therapy and CBT are based on **learning theory** (see Chapter 12)—that is, symptoms are relieved by unlearning maladaptive behavior patterns and altering negative thinking patterns.
2. In contrast to psychoanalysis and related therapies, the person's history and **unconscious conflicts are irrelevant** and thus are not examined in behavioral and cognitive therapies.
3. Characteristics of specific behavioral and cognitive therapies (e.g., systematic desensitization, aversive conditioning, flooding and implosion, token economy, and biofeedback) are listed in Table 23-1.

TABLE 23-1	BEHAVIORAL AND COGNITIVE THERAPIES: USES AND STRATEGIES
Type of Therapy: Most Common Use(s)	**Strategy**
Systematic desensitization: treatment of phobias (irrational fears; see Chapter 20)	In past, through process of classical conditioning (see Chapter 12), person associates an innocuous stimulus with a frightening stimulus. In present, increasing doses of fear-provoking stimulus are paired with a relaxing stimulus to induce a relaxation response. Because one cannot simultaneously be fearful and relaxed (reciprocal inhibition), person shows less anxiety when exposed to fear-provoking stimulus in future
Aversive conditioning: treatment of paraphilias or addictions (pedophilia, smoking)	Classical conditioning is used to pair a maladaptive but pleasurable stimulus with an aversive or painful stimulus (a shock) so that the two become associated. Person ultimately stops engaging in maladaptive behavior because it automatically provokes an unpleasant response
Flooding and implosion: treatment of phobias	Person is exposed to an actual (flooding) or imagined (implosion) overwhelming dose of feared stimulus. Through process of habituation person becomes accustomed to stimulus and is no longer afraid
Token economy: to increase positive behavior in a person who is severely disorganized (psychotic), autistic, or mentally retarded	Through process of operant conditioning (see Chapter 12), desirable behavior (hair combing) is differentially reinforced by a reward or positive reinforcement (token). Person increases desirable behavior to gain reward
Biofeedback: to treat hypertension, Raynaud disease, migraine and tension headaches, chronic pain, fecal incontinence, and temporomandibular joint pain	Through process of operant conditioning, person is given ongoing physiologic information (e.g., blood pressure measurement), which acts as reinforcement (when blood pressure drops). Person uses this information along with relaxation techniques to control visceral changes (heart rate, blood pressure, smooth muscle tone)
Cognitive therapy: to treat mild to moderate depression, somatoform disorders, eating disorders	Weekly, for 15–25 weeks, person is helped to identify distorted, negative thoughts about himself or herself. Person replaces these negative thoughts with positive, self-assuring thoughts, and symptoms improve

Adapted with permission from Fadem B. Behavioral Science, 4th ed. Baltimore, Lippincott Williams & Wilkins, 2004:164.

TABLE 23-2	TARGETED POPULATIONS FOR GROUP, FAMILY, MARITAL/COUPLES, SUPPORTIVE, INTERPERSONAL, AND STRESS MANAGEMENT THERAPIES
Type of Therapy	**Targeted Population**
Group therapy	People with a common problem (e.g., rape victims, alcohol abusers)
	People with personality disorders or other interpersonal problems
	People who have trouble interacting with therapists as authority figures in individual therapy
Family therapy	Children with behavioral problems
	Families in conflict
	People with eating disorders or substance abuse
Marital, couples, sex therapy	Heterosexual or homosexual couples with communication or psychosexual problems
Supportive therapy	People who are experiencing a life crisis
	Chronically mentally ill people dealing with ordinary life situations (e.g., finding a job)
Interpersonal therapy	People with emotional difficulties owing to problems with interpersonal skills
Stress management	People with anxiety disorders or stress-related illnesses (e.g., headaches, hypertension)

Adapted with permission from Fadem B. Behavioral Science, 4th ed. Baltimore, Lippincott Williams & Wilkins, 2004:165.

C. **Other psychotherapies**
1. Other psychotherapies include **group, family, marital/couples, sex, supportive,** and **interpersonal therapy** as well as **stress management techniques.**
2. Targeted populations for these therapies are given in Table 23-2.

Index

Page numbers in *italics* denote figures; those followed by a t denote tables.

Hemorrhage
  spontaneous intraparenchymal, 196
  subarachnoid, 196–197
Heparin, for stroke, 231
Heroin
  dopamine response, 155
  effects of use and withdrawal, 158t
  laboratory findings, 160t
  patient snapshot, 160–161
  substance abuse, 159
  treatment for abuse, 161t
Heterocyclic agents, 225, 226t
Hippocampal formation, 86
Histamine
  functions and location, 134t
  side effects, 136
HIV infection, dementia with, 39
Homeostasis, brain
  blood–brain barrier, 131, 131–132
  brain metabolism, 130–131
  choroid plexus, 132
  CSF biology, 132, 132–133, 133t
  patient snapshot, 130
Homeostatic functions of the hypothalamus, 84
Homosexuality
  development, 11–12
  occurrence, 12
Homunculus, 108
Hormones, effect on aggression, 148
Horner syndrome, 96, 122
Humor (defense mechanism), 142t
Hunger center, 84
Huntingtin, 43, 44
Huntington disease
  behavioral manifestations, 27t
  diagnosis, 43
  genetic associations, 43
  gross anatomic changes, 44, 44
  microscopic anatomic changes, 44
  neurophysiologic factors, 43–44, 44
  patient snapshot, 42–43
  psychiatric associations, 43
  therapy, 44–45
Hydrocephalus, 1, 23, 25, 77
Hydroxyindoleacetic acid, 148
Hyperkinesis, in Huntington disease, 43
Hyperpolarization, 125, 126
Hypersomnias, 168t
Hypertensive crisis, 228
Hyperthyroidism, 180
Hypnosis, for dissociative disorders, 218
Hypochondriasis, 215, 216t
Hypoglossal nerve
  anatomy, 63, 64
  functional components, 63t
  nuclei, path, and function, 67t
Hypokinesia, in Parkinson disease, 40
Hypothalamohypophysial tract, 82, 83, 84
Hypothalamus
  afferent and efferent connections, 82, 82t
  anatomy, 82
  autonomic nervous system regulation, 122
  behavioral functions, 84–85
  circadian rhythm, role in, 162
  homeostatic functions, 84
  hypothalamohypophysial tract, 82, 83, 84
Hypothyroidism, 180

I

Ibuprofen, for stroke, 231
ICD-10 (International Statistical Classification of
    Diseases and Related Health Problems,
    tenth revision), 186
Identification (with the aggressor), 142t
Identity, 10–11, 141, 141t
Identity disorder, dissociative, 218t
Imaginary friends, 9
Imipramine, 226t
Immune disorders
  Guillain-Barré syndrome, 190
  multiple sclerosis, 189–190
Implicit/nondeclarative memory, 80, 81t

Implosion, 235t
Impulse control disorders, 220–221, 220t
Infarct
  cerebral, distribution of, 195
  lacunar, 196
  watershed, 193, 195
Infectious disorders
  brain abscesses, 189
  meningitis, 188–189, 189t
Inferior cerebellar peduncle, 60t
Inferior colliculi, 61t, 99
Inflammatory disorders
  immune, 189–190
  infectious, 188–189, 189t
Informed consent, 171
Inhibitory postsynaptic potential (IPSP), 125
Insomnia, 167, 169t
Intellectual stimulation, effect on brain growth, 5
Intellectualization (defense mechanism), 142t
Intelligence
  genetic factors, 140
  tests, 184–185
Intelligence quotient (IQ), 185
Intercostal nerves, 52
Intermittent explosive disorder, 220t
Internal capsule, 72, 72, 88, 89, 92, 93, 99
Internal vertebral venous plexus, 54
International Statistical Classification of Diseases
    and Related Health Problems, tenth
    revision (ICD-10), 186
Interpersonal therapy, 236, 236t
Interventricular foramina, 71, 71, 77
Intervertebral disk herniation, 53
Interviewing
  adolescents, 12–13
  children, 12
  clinical interview, 172–173, 173
Intimacy versus isolation, stage of (Erikson), 15
Intrafusal muscle fibers, 87, 88
Ion channels, 125
IPSP (inhibitory postsynaptic potential), 125
IQ (intelligence quotient), 185
Ischemia
  global cerebral, 193, 195
  stroke, ischemic, 195
  transient ischemic attack (TIA), 195
Isolation of affect (defense mechanism), 142t

K

K+ ions, 124, 124–126
Kallmann syndrome, 27t
Kernicterus, 130
Kernig sign, 188
Ketamine
  effects of use and withdrawal, 158t
  substance abuse, 160
Kinesin, 123
Kinesthesia, 87
Kinetic labyrinth, 100–101
Kinocilium, 100
Kleptomania, 220t
Klüver-Bucy syndrome, 86
Knee-jerk reflex, 55

L

L-α-acetylmethadol acetate (LAMM), 159, 231
Labyrinthine artery, 75
Lacrimal pathway, 64
Lactate
  astrocytic production of, 130
  as energy source for brain, 130
Lacunar infarcts, 196
Lamination, law of, 89
Language
  neuroanatomy of, 79–80, 80, 80t
  skills, development in children, 6t–7t, 9
Lateral corticospinal tract, 51
Lateral funiculus, 92
Lateral geniculate body, 94, 95
Lateral lemniscus, 99

Lateral spinothalamic tract, 51, 51t, 60t
Learned helplessness, 144, 199
Learned stimulus, 143
Learning
  classical conditioning, 143–144
  habituation, 143
  methods, 143
  operant conditioning, 144, 145t, 146
  sensitization, 143
Lentiform nucleus, 111
Lesbian sexual orientation, 34
Lesch-Nyhan syndrome, 27t
Levodopa (L-dopa), 40, 42, 232
Lewy body
  dementia, 39, 39
  in Parkinson disease, 42
Libido, age influence on, 16
Life expectancy, 20–21, 21t
Life support, requests for cessation of artificial, 22,
    47
Light-near dissociation, 96
Lisuride, 232
Lithium, 180, 228
Locus ceruleus, 41, 210
Logical thought, development in children, 10
Longevity, 21
Lorazepam, 229t
Lower motor neuron (LMN) signs, 56, 111t
Lumbar cistern, 53
Lumbar tap, 53
Lumbosacral plexus, 52
Luria-Nebraska Neuropsychological Battery, 181t
Lysergic acid diethylamine (LSD)
  effects of use and withdrawal, 158t
  serotonin response to, 155
  substance abuse, 160

M

Macula utriculi, 101
Magnetic stimulation, rapid transcranial, 234
Major depressive disorder
  characteristics, 207
  dexamethasone suppression test, 180
  electroconvulsive therapy (ECT) for, 234
  insomnia from, 167
  masked depression, 207
  occurrence, 198
  patient snapshot, 205
  psychosocial factors, 198–199
  seasonal affective disorder (SAD), 207
  symptoms, 198, 199t
Malingering, 216, 217t
Mania
  neurotransmitter activity association, 138t
  symptoms, 206t
MAOIs (monoamine oxidase inhibitors), 42, 211,
    227–228, 227t
Maprotiline, 226t
Marijuana substance abuse, 160
Marital/couples therapy, 236, 236t
Marriage, and behavior influences, 146
Masked depression, 207, 217
Masturbation, 11
Medial geniculate body, 99
Medial lemniscus, 60t, 87–88, 89
Medial longitudinal fasciculus, 102–103, 103
Medulla, 58, 59, 60t
Meissner corpuscles, 90, 91
Melanin deposits in Parkinson disease, 42
Memantine, 37, 231
Memory
  loss in cognitive disorders, 35, 36t, 37t
  loss with dissociative disorders, 217
  types, 80–82, 81t
Ménière disease, 99
Meninges, spinal, 53–54
Meningitis, CSF profile in, 78t, 133, 133t
Meningocele, 24t
Meningoencephalitis, 188
Meningomyelocele, 1
Menopause, 16–17
Mental age, 184